The Relationship Between Coagulation, Inflammation and Endothelium—A Pyramid Towards Outcome

Edited by

Bruce D. Spiess, M.D.

Professor and Chief of Cardiothoracic Anesthesia
Director of Research
Department of Anesthesiology
Medical College of Virginia
Richmond, Virginia

With 9 contributors

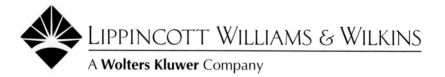

LIPPINCOTT WILLIAMS & WILKINS
A **Wolters Kluwer** Company

The Relationship Between Coagulation, Inflammation and Endothelium—A Pyramid Towards Outcome

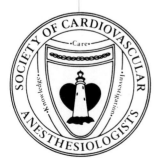

A Society of
Cardiovascular Anesthesiologists
Monograph

Accurate indications, adverse reactions, and dosage schedules for drugs are provided in this
book, but it is possible that they may change. The reader is urged to review the package information data of the manufacturers of the medications mentioned.

Printed in the United States of America
(ISBN 0-781-72758-8)

00 01 02 03 04
1 2 3 4 5 6 7 8

Publication Committee of the
Society of Cardiovascular Anesthesiologists

Current Members of SCA Publication Committee

Jeffrey R. Balser, M.D., Ph.D.
Nashville, Tennessee

Elliott Bennett-Guerrero, M.D.
New York, New York

Mark Chaney, M.D.
Chicago, Illinois

David J. Cook, M.D.
Rochester, Minnesota

Patricia M. Gramling-Babb, M.D.
Chicago, Illinois

Tim Grayson
Baltimore, Maryland

Joseph P. Mathew, M.D.
Durham, North Carolina

Johanna C. Schwarzenberger, M.D.
New York, New York

Michael K. Urban, M.D., Ph.D.
New York, New York

Preface

Cardiopulmonary bypass (CPB) creates profound changes throughout every organ system in the body. Many of us who are specialists in cardiothoracic anesthesia have devoted much of our adult life to studying and understanding those changes so that we can deliver optimum patient care. The evolution of extracorporeal support has been tremendous yet we are still confronted with a number of problems that have, as of yet, no ultimate solutions. Performing "minimally" invasive cardiac surgery without cardiopulmonary mechanical support might be one way of sidestepping some of the problems. However, as those new techniques are perfected and more procedures can be completed there still remain a vast majority of cardiovascular surgical cases that will require mechanical support. There is no doubt that the bypass machine, in one form or another will be with us for quite some time to come.

We believe, in our hearts, that outcomes must and can be improved. Last year the monograph session and the published manuscript were on that very subject—outcome research in cardiac surgery. Today we can measure a great number of adverse events that potentially occur during and after CPB. Myocardial infarctions occur in 3–10% of patients undergoing coronary artery bypass grafting. We know that strokes occur in 1–9% of patients undergoing CPB. Neuropsychiatric defects are very common (30–60%) immediately after surgery and persist in a significant number of patients (15–30%). Infection is less often studied but is a significant negative outcome with wound dehiscence, pneumonia and urinary tract infections. Pulmonary dysfunction, as defined by prolonged mechanical ventilation, is well studied but plagues us in a small segment of the population. Extensively investigated is the risk of perioperative bleeding and the need (use) of blood transfusions. The research involved in measuring and studying these adverse outcomes has been great, as evidenced by last year's monograph. The cataloguing of events and risks in certain sub-groups is very important for us practitioners to understand the scope of what we do. But, this outcomes research confirms why we must continue to find ways to minimize the frequency of these adverse events.

The adverse outcomes that do occur signal that our understanding and predictive capacity for events is very imperfect. Therefore the scientific study of cardiothoracic bypass is an intellectual endeavor very much needed. To affect those negative outcomes we must continue to seek answers about deviations of homeostasis caused by CPB.

CPB is an unnatural phenomenon that has its effects on every organ system but its contact point is with the blood of the patient. Historical teaching has held that the CPB machine causes "contact" activation and therefore sets off a wild cascade of reaction in the patient's blood because of the unnatural surface characteristics of the CPB machine. The charge characteristics of the tubing and membrane oxygenators may not be as activating as historical teaching would have us believe. More recent research has shown that patient's who lack factor XII (Hageman Factor) or contact activation factor still display all of the "usual" coagulopathic responses to the CPB machine. Therefore, historical teaching may be just that: history. Perhaps other more complex mechanisms are the basis of the coagulopathy of CPB.

Contemporary biologic research has moved far ahead of the days of the late 1950's and early 1960's so that those early ideas of CPB's inciting events must be discarded. We still believe that somehow through blood's interaction with the CPB system pathologic changes do occur. Great strides have occurred in the study of vascular biology. Indeed, 1998's monograph focused upon the many new advances in vascular biology. The inflammatory system has also seen unparalleled advances as mankind strives to understand the AIDS crisis and a number of other immunologic diseases. Blood transfusion has been critically studied in a response to the AIDS crisis as well; and in CPB, a number of advances with regards to coagulation and blood transfusion have made that a very exciting topic.

These three facets of the circulatory system, though widely studied today with great biologic advances, need to be approached with some new and modern thinking for us to move forward. The three, vascular endothelium, inflammation, and coagulation, are all highly interactive.

Systems do not truly exist in nature but are man-made categorizations created for the convenience of our study and understanding. Each "system" is directly linked to another series of biochemical or cellular events. The coagulation "system" is a prime example of a man-made categorization. One might say that in the final analysis, the function of coagulation is to prevent catastrophic blood loss in the event of injury. As medical students we can easily understand that and as biologists or evolutionists that makes sense as well. When coagulation was originally studied it was examined in that context and a number of clinical tests were devised for the laboratory that could ferret out congenital or acquired protein deficiencies. These tests allowed the early workers in coagulation to create a model (system) of protein coagulation. That model has since shaped our thinking ever since. It has created great advances but it (the model) has limited thinking as well. The coagulation monitors developed to help define the system have never been effective in predicting abnormal bleeding in surgery and they have proven woefully inadequate in guiding replacement therapy in CPB surgery. But the thinking and teaching has provided a way for medical students to grasp the biochemical steps involved in making the final protein fibrin. What has been neglected, until recently appreciated, is that those biochemical steps all occur on the surface of cell membranes. Which cell membranes? Platelets, endothelial cells and, to a great extent, white cells. The understanding of binding sites, ligands and cellular signaling has shown us that coagulation does not occur de novo in the plasma. Rather, it is a very carefully regulated process.

Coagulation does not occur alone. It is an event that is part of a larger homeostatic series of events, what should be termed vascular homeostasis. Coagulation is as much a part of stopping the loss of vascular circulating volume as it is a part of a greater inflammatory event (creating a sight and method for white cell attack) and of atherosclerosis as well as other processes (e.g., vascular regeneration).

Vascular homeostasis is therefore dependent on a complex series of interactions between endothelial cells, coagulation proteins and cells and inflammatory signals and cell lines. This monograph will examine not so much the events within each area but the interactions between what had previously been conceived of as distinct "systems." It is in the interactions that we may find some solutions to problems that lead to the adverse outcomes of CPB.

Much of the research that has been done in CPB, particularly in relationship to coagulation and bleeding for example, has focused upon describing the pathophysiology of an average (mean event) of a population undergoing CPB. Most recently we have begun to appreciate that although some "usual changes" occur with CPB, the variability of response is what drives outcome in a particular individual. In coagulation we now know that responses can be 250-500 fold different from one patient to the next in fibrinolytic events. Is it any wonder that some patients bleed more than others and some get a good or usual response to antifibrinolytic agents whereas others have very unique events? The variability in response is what creates unique outcomes. We cannot find ways of preventing single or isolated events by simply studying or looking for the "mean" response. We must actively pursue ways of predicting, treating and avoiding the unique events.

Vascular homeostatic interactions must be somehow involved with many of the adverse events that we are striving to avoid. Conceptually one might consider the three "systems" to be the base of a large pyramid of vascular homeostasis (figure 1). The peak of that pyramid would lie directly over the center of the base if all three sides of the pyramid were of equal shape and area. If however one side was displaced or mis-shapen then the peak of the resulting pyramid would be off center. The equal sided pyramid might be conceptually what happens with normal vascular homeostasis. With CPB in any given patient there will be pulls and adjustments to the side wall triangles of the pyramid. If coagulation, inflammation or endothelium function is greatly deranged then the end resultant peak will be off center. Perhaps the direction it points and the degree of deviation from center will be a result of the amount of abnormality in any of the components. The vascular homeostatic normality is maintained by a very high degree of buffering. Coagulation events, for example, are met with controlling proteins (examples: antithrombin III, aprotinin, protein C, S and others). These buffering agents keep individual stimuli from overcoming the entire organism. So it is also with endothelial function and inflammatory events. The complex interplay is what creates layers or redundant buffering that keeps any single stimulus from overcoming the organism.

CPB however is a massive stimulus. It has a tendency to overwhelm the buffering capacity of vascular homeostasis. Perhaps an individual patient has a great propensity for inflammatory cellular reactivity or fibrinolytic responsiveness. Then those events might escape from control by other processes and so overwhelm the homeostasis as to drive the triad to be dysfunctional. The peak of the pyramid would shift. An end result might well be one of the adverse outcomes first discussed. Bleeding, pulmonary dysfunction (ARDS) and thrombotic complications (MI, stroke) may all be manifestations of perturbations of vascular homeostasis. This monograph will focus on the complex interactions of vascular homeostasis and how individual reactivity might well drive outcomes.

Chapter One is unique and provides a wonderful opening into this subject. It looks at some bits of information that we know about the evolution of certain molecules and cell types. Not all living creatures on Earth have the same cells in their blood. Furthermore, when one looks at the phylogeneitic appearance of some proteins and cell lines one might be able to understand more of the function of those proteins or cells. As organisms became more complex in evolution, their "need" for circulatory systems and specialized cells grew. Hence, the development of more redundant and interactive proteins, signals and cells. CPB was certainly never "planned for" in evolution and understanding some evolutionary background provides a unique and "out of the box" perspective.

Chapter Two is of key importance. The blood constantly interacts with the endothelial cells. The endothelium is the largest surface area organ in the body and is very active in maintaining homeostasis. If damaged it looses its anticoagulant function and becomes prothrombotic. It also creates a focus for white cell adhesion and up regulation of a wide range of inflammatory reactions. This chapter is not meant to be a complete update on the status of vascular biology but it will focus on how "normal" endothelium functions. For a more complete vascular biology summary the reader is referred to the monograph of 1998. Rather this chapter is meant to focus upon how endothelium maintains homeostasis in the microenvironment of a few cells or at the blood endothelial interface when function is at rest or normal.

Chapter Three goes beyond normal endothelial function and talks about what might happen if the endothelium is damaged. Abnormal reactions may occur within a few cells or over a much wider region. Unfortunately we have a rather primitive way of studying such endothelial events in the whole organism. We can only look for markers of prior events in blood taken from either an artery or a vein. From such venipuncture data we must draw conclusions about distinct events somewhere in the vascular tree. In vitro studies can look at hypothetical events and endothelial responses but I would remind the reader that such research, although very useful, is outside of a number of the homeostatic controls that would occur in a complete human. Abnormalities in the endothelium must assuredly be responsible for a number of the adverse events attributed to CPB. We are in a very early age of study of the microenvironment.

Chapter Four looks at the inflammatory events that can affect not only the endothelium but also the coagulation proteins and platelets. One is impressed by how many different proteins, cell surface binding sites and messengers are common to both platelets and white cells. Fibrin, for example, has sites on both cell surfaces. Nitric oxide produced from normal endothelial cells repels and deactivates white cells and platelets, what a beautiful homeostatic mechanism. CPB has been termed a perfect place to study profound inflammation. At times the responses seem to be akin to those seen in sepsis. This chapter will again focus upon the complexity of interaction and homeostasis.

Chapter Five takes some of the concepts seen in chapter four and also in the endothelial chapters and discusses them in relationship to platelets functioning. Platelets are damaged and/or suppressed by CPB. In some patients the amount of dysfunction is greatly out of proportion to the length of bypass or the types of events that have occurred. We cannot at this time predict who will have those deviant responses nor can we totally prevent them. A great deal of research has been done on bleeding and platelet dysfunction with CPB, but what of platelets interactions with white cells in creating inflammatory events or upregulating other tissue damage? Are there potentials for being pro-thrombotic?

Chapter Six gives us a contemporary view of coagulation. All of us were brought up in the protein centered coagulation teaching of medical schools. That is acceptable for passing courses in medical school and rote memorization allowed passage of those exams . But, that is not how human biology controls clot function in vivo. This contemporary view will express a great deal to do with the platelet and its surface as well as the membrane/protein interactions of other cell lines. The last 5–7 years have seen the understanding of glycoprotein binding sites and the ability to pharmacologically manipulate these sites. Those manipulations as well as understanding the genetic polymorphism of these sites may well lead us in the future to be better able to predict adverse outcomes.

Chapter Seven examines the fibrinolytic events that occur with CPB. Debate has long raged about whether platelet dysfunction or fibrinolysis was the most common event of CPB leading to abnormal blood loss. It probably matters only to the academics, which are more common, but the two are intimately related. Fibrinolysis is of key importance to all of cardiovascular disease and is a risk for atherosclerosis, MI, stroke and also post CPB bleeding. We now know that extreme variability is the rule rather than the exception in terms of fibrinolysis and CPB. Some genetic differences do exist within expression of proteins and structure of proteins within the fibrinolytic system. Therefore it may be common in the future to know what risk factors there are surrounding CPB and fibrinolysis.

Chapter Eight is different from the other chapters in that it examines only one drug—heparin—and asks the question, is it a cause of some derangement in CPB. Heparin is the anticoagulant almost universally utilized for CPB. It has a wide range of biologic effects that reach far beyond binding to ATIII and creating anticoagulation. Much of the research stating that CPB causes certain events may be biased in their conclusions because of the use of heparin. Until this date, conducting CPB without heparin has rarely been possible. Therefore, every conclusion about CPB is dependent upon the use of heparin. Does heparin predispose the vascular homeostatic system to have certain adverse events? This chapter is meant to provoke thinking in the clinician and researcher and to hopefully stimulate the correct future questions to be asked of research.

Chapter Nine is the concluding chapter and perhaps the most difficult to research and write. It discusses the clinical implications for which all the other chapters provide scientific and biological background. Today some data does exist showing that perturbations of this vascular homeostatic pyramid lead to patient outcomes. One example is the mounting evidence that hematocrit after CABG effects outcome. Higher hematocrit is associated with more MIs and perhaps other adverse events. Blood transfusions have long been associated with adverse events. Might they play a role in the complex vascular homeostasis interaction? The chapter will also make some predictions into the future regarding where we might be going to test individuals prior to surgery and to prevent adverse outcomes.

Vascular homeostasis is what we have in normal health. It is shifted in CPB in one way or another. How severely the homeostatic control is shaken will greatly affect how a patient does during surgery. It is important to change our focus and thinking in cardiovascular anesthesia and surgery. If we are to be able to affect outcome in individuals then we must look at research that embraces and understands the variability of response. We must understand the complex interplay of vascular endothelium, coagulation and inflammation if we are to understand the reactive pyramid that is vascular homeostasis. Future researchers and clinicians would be well served to think beyond the limits of their initial teaching and to ask probing questions regarding the effects of CPB on the individual. No one drug (Aprotinin, lysine antifibrinolytics, DDAVP) can be expected to work the same in each individual or to prevent bleeding. So many other medications and strategies have been proposed as ways to treat or prevent complications but answers should never by sought as panaceas for all patients. Perhaps the future will hold ways for us to predict how the individual might react to the homeostatic insult that is CPB.

Contributors

Gilbert Blaise, M.D.
Professeor
Department of Anesthesiology
University of Montreal
Notre Dame Hospital
Montreal (Quebec) Canada

Simon C. Body, M.D.
Assistant Professor
Harvard Medical School;
Department of Anesthesia
Perioperative and Pain Medicine
Brigham and Women's Hospital
Boston, Massachusetts

Edward M. Boyle, Jr., M.D.
Cardiothoracic Surgery Resident
Department of Surgery
University of Washington
Seattle, Washington

Wayne L. Chandler, M.D.
Associate Professor of Laboratory
  Medicine
University of Washington
Seattle, Washington

Mark H. Ereth, M.D.
Assistant Professor of
  Anesthesiology
Mayo Clinic
Rochester, Minnesota

Jerrold H. Levy, M.D.
Professor of Anesthesiology
Emory University School
  of Medicine
Director of Cardiothoracic
  Anesthesiology
Emory Healthcare
Atlanta, Georgia

Elizabeth N. Morgan, M.D.
Senior Cardiothoracic Surgery
  Research Fellow
Department of Surgery
University of Washington
Seattle, Washington

Christine Stowe Rinder, M.D.
Associate Professor
Departments of Anesthesiology &
  Laboratory Medicine
Yale University School of Medicine
New Haven, Connecticut

David Royston, M.D.
Consultant in Cardiothoracic
  Anesthesia
Royal Brompton & Harefield
  Hospital
Harefield, Middlesex
United Kingdom

Bruce D. Spiess, M.D.
Professor and Chief of
  Cardiothoracic Anesthesia
Director of Research
Department of Anesthesiology
Medical College of Virginia
Richmond, Virginia

Edward D. Verrier, M.D.
Professor and Vice Chairman of
  Surgery
Chief of the Division of
  Cardiothoracic Surgery
University of Washington
Seattle, Washington

Contents

Preface   vii

Contributors   ix

1   1
The Evolution of Coagulation and
Inflammation
David Royston, M.D.

2   31
The Endothelium at Rest
Gilbert Blaise, M.D.

3   79
The Endothelium Disturbed: The
Procoagulant Response
Edward M. Boyle, Jr., M.D.,
Elizabeth N. Morgan, M.D.,
Edward D. Verrier, M.D.

4   91
The Relationships Between Coagulation,
Inflammation and Endothelium:
Inflammation Responds
Jerrold H. Levy, M.D.

5   107
Platelets and Their Interactions
Christine Stowe Rinder, M.D.

6   129
A Contemporary View of Coagulation
Mark H. Ereth, M.D.

7   147
The Fibrinolytic Response during
Cardiopulmonary Bypass—Pro or Anticoagulant?
Wayne L. Chandler, M.D.

8   169
Heparin: Beyond an Angicoagulant
Bruce D. Spiess, M.D.

9   191
Coagulation and Inflammation Polymorphism:
Impact on Cardiovascular Outcomes
Simon C. Body, M.B., Ch. B., F.A.N.C.Z.A.

Index   225

David Royston, M.D.

The Evolution of Coagulation and Inflammation

1

Our survival depends on an effective defense against a foreign invader. This is true over the full spectrum of life forms—from single cell animals to whole nations of people. Cellular host defense mechanisms have been evolving ever since the first organisms hundreds of millions of years ago encountered their environment and had to decide if they were touching versions of themselves or "non-self." Non-self could be good or bad for the organism because it was either to be consumed as food or be the consumer of, or intruder into, the other organism! With time, specialized cells and mechanisms evolved that separated the recognition, gathering, and degradation of food from primary host defense functions. The mechanisms involved, on a primitive biochemical level, are so similar as to be regarded as identical. As evolution has advanced, these systems have become more complex and interactive with higher vertebrates using many different tactics and mechanisms for expanding their host defense systems. However, the basic principles still apply.

In the simplest of terms, the essential goal of any organism is to preserve the integrity of "self" by recognizing injury and non-self. Once recognized, systems integrate to conduct a process whereby the insult is walled off from the rest of the body and the injury or invasion is repaired or degraded and destroyed. These immune and hemostatic processes have much in common with each other, and also seem to have a continuing development from the basic digestive process.

The series of articles in this monograph are directed toward improving our understanding of the body's response to the stimulus of

The Relationship Between Coagulation, Inflammation, and Endothelium, edited by
Bruce Spiess, Lippincott Williams & Wilkins, Baltimore © 2000.

surgery with cardiopulmonary bypass. This understanding relies on (1) defining those aspects of the response considered normal and necessary for the organism to counteract the stimulus and those that are inappropriate, unwanted, and potentially harmful; (2) deciding which aspects of the abnormal response merit interruption or interference; and (3) finding physical or pharmacologic approaches to achieve this.

The current trend for investigating ever more basic scientific mechanisms leaves the impression that the big picture of events has moved out of focus under the intensity of mechanistic scrutiny. This introduction to the monograph pursues the concept that parts of this complex jigsaw puzzle can be put in place by considering the evolutionary aspects of the immune and hemostatic processes. Using this approach we may be able to define those aspects of the system that are "fundamental" in triggering and enhancing an abnormal response, and those that may be "epiphenomena." Two main approaches or models will be used as pointers toward the potentially important pieces of the host defense puzzle.

The first approach is to consider the most primitive of creatures still existing today and to dissect out the various factors in their self-preservation systems that have been preserved in the human process. Conservation of a system or mechanism throughout the evolutionary process implies that nature has bestowed a fundamental requirement and importance on this process. The example I will use of a relevant but primitive immune/hemostatic system is the horseshoe crab (*Limulus polyphemus*) (Figure 1–1). This animal has a single cellular element,

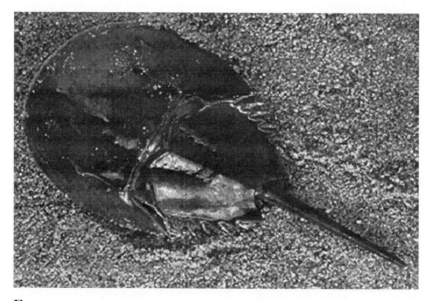

FIGURE 1–1. The horseshoe crab (*Limulus polyphemus*).

which is used for oxygen carriage, hemostasis, and host defense and a primitive coagulation system. Once activated, the animal has a method of controlling this process. The potential relevance of these components to humans is discussed below.

The second approach is the ability to sequence polypeptides and the genes that control their manufacture, which is producing a considerable amount of data that tells us about the likely origins of the defense system. If one knows gene and protein sequences, then a library of similar or like polypeptides from a wide variety of species can be derived. When scientists analyze sequence homology and use statistical probabilities, they can predict when these polypeptides first appeared in nature, how they changed with time, and when these changes occurred. The use of sequence homology in this way is of particular interest with regard to the coagulant process.

Throughout the text, reference will also be made to natural genetic "experiments." There are an increasing number of identified genetic defects that affect the hemostatic and immune systems. Some deficiencies are not seen in nature or cannot be bred into laboratory animals. These defects probably reflect the presence of a "lethal gene." The absence of a gene or its product being incompatible with life suggests that this aspect of the process is absolute and fundamental. Examples of this are the in utero lethality associated with absence of the gene for tissue factor (TF) production and also for the specific antagonist of TF. This antagonist, TF pathway inhibitor (TFPI), has three serine protease inhibitor domains. Absence of the first domain produces a lethal defect.

The final aspect of this article will be to point out, where appropriate, the relationship between the immune and hemostatic systems. One such example is the role of clotting proteins in the inflammatory response. In higher orders of animals, such as mammals, fibrinogen is regarded as the final common protein in the coagulant part of the hemostatic system. However, fibrinogen is also crucial to the response of the immune system. This interplay parallels the role of the horseshoe crab's primary coagulant protein. Studies in fibrinogen-depleted animals have shown how fibrinogen association with leukocytes is an absolute requirement to mount a competent inflammatory response in vivo. For example, defibrinogenated animals fail to accumulate neutrophil infiltrates after intraperitoneal injection of bacteria.[1] Fibrinogen is also important in the monocyte-mediated response to biomaterials[2] and in the platelet cooperative pathway. In this system, fibrinogen binding stimulates the platelet to initiate the neutrophil oxidative burst, which may lead to a destructive injury to normal tissues.[3] These aspects suggest that studies of the fundamental interplay between hemostatic and immune systems may be useful in understanding the genesis of organ and tissue dysfunction we categorize as postoperative systemic inflammatory response syndrome (SIRS).

The approach used in this article to better understand the inflammatory/hemostatic process contains an obvious weakness. Although the pivotal mechanisms of initiation and activation can be deduced from primitive systems, the degree and balance of the human response is less certain. An example from the hemostatic process is the conversion of fibrinogen to fibrin. The biochemical process in humans is very similar to that in early invertebrates and relies on the activity of a protease, derived originally from a digestive enzyme, on the inactive molecule. However, the effectiveness in the human of that process and whether it is associated with a hypocoagulable, normal, or hypercoagulable state within a vessel and tissue seems to be critically dependent on the endothelium of that particular vascular bed.[4] This apparently diverse response of the endothelium is due principally to altered expression and balance between protease and antiprotease molecules because the fundamental biochemistry of each of the molecules in these reactions, as demonstrated in the "test tube," has not been altered.

The relevance of a specific mechanism of injury to a specific tissue or organ is also becoming apparent. An increasing body of evidence points to a difference in the likelihood of a potential injury being produced by a specific inflammatory process depending on the organ being investigated. This potential is graphically illustrated by the leukocyte adhesion molecule deficiency syndrome. Neutrophils in these patients display impaired adherence in vitro and an increased intravascular half-life in vivo, which suggests that they do not adhere to injured endothelium in an appropriate manner. This has been demonstrated by intravital microscopy of gut, but similar techniques have shown that these neutrophils are released normally during vigorous exercise from the "marginated pool" and will sequester normally within the pulmonary vasculature. This has its correlate in the clinical picture of disease in these patients, with mortality usually caused by overwhelming mucous membrane and skin infection, and rarely caused by pneumonia.

Therefore, these biological variables question the relevance of a specific mechanism involved in the response in a particular organ or tissue after a noxious challenge that has the same effect in a separate tissue. This aspect cannot be directly addressed by the analytical tools and examples used in this article. Of more importance is the interpretation of negative data. The lack of evidence to implicate a specific mechanism in injury of one tissue does not preclude the pivotal involvement of that mechanism in injury to a separate tissue or organ. This aspect of altered inflammatory responses to the same challenge by vascular bed or organ will be addressed more specifically in relation to the complement system and complement-dependent inflammatory processes.

PRIMITIVE HOST DEFENSE SYSTEMS: LESSONS FROM A LIVING FOSSIL

Approximately 400 to 600 million years ago, a number of animals developed, including the jawless fish, annelids, molluscs, and the horseshoe crab.[5] These primitive creatures lack an adaptive immune system but have a highly integrated innate immunity. The innate systems found in these creatures have been preserved into mammalian and primate lines.[6] Because the horseshoe crab is still alive today, it has been the focus of studies with respect to its primitive host defense and hemostatic systems.[6] The components of these systems and their interactivity provide a unique basis for insight into the evolution of hemostasis and inflammation. In turn, studies of these fundamental systems may be useful in planning therapeutic strategies in patients with SIRS.

In simple terms, a primitive animal form can be regarded as having two sides, an outside and an inside. The basic process of any defense system is to prevent the outside from entering into the creature, a process we will call immunity or inflammation. In addition, the animal does not want to have its intraluminal or intravascular components leaking out, and therefore can prevent this by a process we will call hemostasis.

In the crab, this defense is undertaken by the same mechanism.[6] The mechanism relies on three elements. The first is a cellular element, which can move to the site of injury or invasion and recognize nonself. This single-cell element has been termed an amoebocyte, hemocyte, or coelomocyte. The hemocyte is particularly sensitive to the presence of substances such as sugars and lectins on the surface of Gram-negative bacteria and especially the endotoxin released by bacteria. In the presence of endotoxin, the amoebocyte will clump together and form an amorphous gel as discussed below. The ability to aggregate when in contact with endotoxin forms the basis of the limulus lysate amoebocytic assay that is used to detect endotoxin in humans. In the presence of bacterial endotoxin, the hemocyte also rapidly degranulates, by exocytosis, to release the contents of small (S) and large (L) granules. L-granules contain at least 24 proteins, the majority of which are clotting factors, serine protease inhibitors (serpins), and various lectins. These compounds start the process of opsonization in preparation for the contents of the S-granules, which have greater antimicrobial actions. The most important granule coagulation protein is coagulogen. This protein is the basic element of the horseshoe crab's clotting system and has a functional similarity with vertebrate fibrinogen with its ability to form a relative insoluble gel. The cleavage of coagulogen is obtained at two specific amino acid sequences (Arg-Gly and Arg-Thr); these sites in the fibrinogen molecule of higher animals are cleaved by thrombin. Indeed, the octapeptide sequence released from the cleavage of coagulogen exhibits a high sequence homology with primate fibrinopeptide B.[7] The cleavage in the horseshoe crab is undertaken by a number of factors, including factors C, B, and G, which are serine proteases. Factors C and G can be autocatalytically activated by lipopolysaccharide and (1,3)-b-D-glucan, the latter being a major cell wall component of fungi. The activation of these two zymogens to produce enzymatically active serine protease molecules results in the conversion of coagulogen to an insoluble coagulin gel. This clot is softer than a mammalian fibrin clot.

In parallel with the process of coagulin gel formation, various agglutinins/lectins that induce cell aggregation are released from L-granules. Thus, the invaders in the hemolymph are engulfed and immobilized by the clot and are subsequently killed by antimicrobial substances released from the granules. In addition to an antimicrobial peptide, tachyplesin and its analogues, the S-granule also contains at least six small proteins that show antimicrobial activities against Gram-negative and Gram-positive bacteria and fungi.

It is obvious that if the crab is being invaded by foreign organisms and the inflammatory/hemostatic process is activated, this defense system must be localized. Otherwise, autocatalytic activation of factors C and G will lead to a catastrophic consumptive coagulopathy. The horseshoe crab achieves control by inhibition of the serine proteases involved in gel formation and cell immobilization using serine protease inhibitors or serpins. Whereas mammalian plasma contains many proteins, horseshoe crab hemolymph contains just three major proteins: hemocyanin, C-reactive protein, and α_2-macroglobulin. The potential importance of α_2-macroglobulin will be discussed later. The large granules contain three different forms of serine protease coagulation inhibitor categorized as LICI-1, LICI-2, and LICI-3; other serine protease inhibitors not associated with coagulation; α_2-macroglobulin; and the cysteine protease inhibitor cystatin.

This sequence of (1) a cellular element that can clump and stick to an injury or invasion, (2) a zymogen protein that can be activated to bind and hold together the cellular element to prolong its residence time at the site of injury or invasion, and (3) an activator of this process based on one or more serine proteases is repeated throughout the evolutionary process. In addition, it is apparent that serine protease inhibitors are fundamentally required in the control and localization of the initial response of the innate hemostatic and inflammatory process.

It may be surprising that many of the aspects of the immune system that currently have an extremely high profile in terms of research endeavor and basic science understanding are not found in this specific animal species. The most interesting of these from an evolutionary and interventional standpoint are the immunoglobulin superfamily, the complement system, and the nitric oxide pathway. These will be discussed in more detail.

At this point, it is convenient to discuss the evolution of the coagulation system and its control, with particular emphasis on structural relationships and evolutionary development.

HISTORICAL DEVELOPMENT IN COAGULATION

Most coagulation factors are identified by roman numerals, with the active form denoted by the lower case *a*. They generally circulate in an inactive zymogen form and become active after proteolytic cleavage; most are serine proteases related to the digestive enzyme trypsin. The exceptions to this are factor VII (FVII), which circulates as an active protease (as does tissue-type plasminogen activator [tPA]), and factor XIII, which has transglutaminase activity to cross-link proteins. The horseshoe crab also has transglutaminase enzymatic activity. Other factors in the coagulation process, such as TF, factor V, factor VIII, and high-molecular-weight kininogen, act as cofactors. High-molecular-weight kininogen is also important because it is the source of bradykinin and is enzymatically active in the generation of kallikrein, thus again reflecting the close links between hemostasis and inflammation.

Historically the human blood coagulation system is conveniently divided into two pathways: the TF (extrinsic) pathway and the contact factor (intrinsic) pathway, with each producing activated factor X (FXa). These pathways were identified and categorized during experiments on the effects of sufficiency and deficiency of the various factors on assays of plasma coagulation. The intrinsic and extrinsic pathways meet at a final common pathway whereby factor Xa converts prothrombin to thrombin, which then acts on fibrinogen. This is an over simplification of the system because proteins from each pathway can influence one another. However, it is often used as a basis for investigation of hemostatic disorders because the laboratory-based tests of coagulation focus on each of these separate pathways. The prothrombin time is a test tube variant of the extrinsic pathway and activated clotting time (ACT) or activated partial thromboplastin time (aPTT) of the intrinsic system.

Although the pathways and proteins involved in fibrin formation and lysis are well established in the minds of all students of hematology, a look back into history reveals a different interpretation for the role of these proteins in the initiation and amplification of clot formation, degradation, and repair.

COAGULATION FROM AN EVOLUTIONARY VIEWPOINT: LESSONS FROM PROTEIN AND SEQUENCE HOMOLOGY

Figure 1–2 diagrams the evolutionary diversification of various proteins involved in the coagulation process.[6] The time when diversification occurs is derived from a number of statistical and biological end points and is also based on an anticipated rate of mutation of 0.66 gene substitutions per million years during pre-primate evolution.[8] The time scale on the figure is not linear, with the partitioning of chymotrypsin occurring about 500 million years ago and that of human and vampire bat tPA about 25 million years ago.

Observation of the pattern of divergence of these proteases and zymogens from their common ancestors brings a new bias on the interpretation of the organization of the coagulation system. Use of this evolutionary viewpoint suggests that some of these proteins may serve a closely interrelated function. These groupings are not obvious using the conventional wisdom of hemostatic control with its basis in laboratory

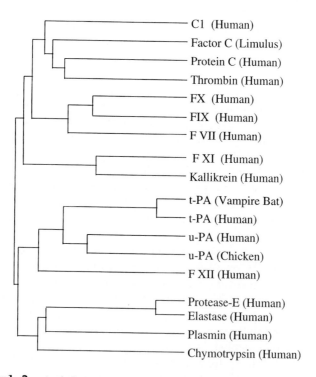

FIGURE 1–2. A phylogenetic tree of various serine proteases from vertebrate and invertebrate animals. Modified from Iwanaga and Kawabata.[6]

tests of coagulation. The interplay between compounds in this new model raise some intriguing questions with regard to their precise role in mammalian host defense systems.

All of the factors listed in Figure 1–2, in their active state, are serine proteases. This evolutionary map suggests that the active center of all these proteases should be related to the digestive enzymes trypsin and chymotrypsin. This is indeed true, as is the fact that a polyvalent inhibitor of trypsin such as aprotinin will inhibit all of these proteins in test tube experiments.

Figure 1–2 highlights the pattern and time of diversification between groups of proteins. The reader will appreciate that other attributes can also be explored using this type of analysis. An example of this would be to explain the evolutionary reason for the separation between vitamin K–dependent (protein C, prothrombin, and factors IX, X, and VII) and vitamin K–nondependent proteins. However, for the present article, each of the groups of proteins drawn in Figure 1–2 will be discussed as if they were separate entities.

Conventional wisdom would have placed plasmin with the various compounds that make up the response to activation or repair processes. However, plasmin and elastase are nonspecific digestive enzymes related to chymotrypsin. It is obvious that having gastric juice coursing through the vascular tree is not compatible with survival. This implies that these enzymes have maintained their prominence in this arm of the protease tree by some novel mechanism to protect their function. This may be related to the evolution of a specific control process, such as a specific protease inhibitor, that confines their activity to the site of their intended action. This is true for plasmin. Free plasmin binds to its serine protease inhibitor, α_2-plasmin inhibitor, within about one hundredth of a second. However, this process takes many minutes if the plasmin is bound to fibrin, which is its intended substrate.

Factor XII is contained in the group of proteins normally considered to be involved in fibrinolysis and repair rather than the induction of clot formation. This position supports evidence from clinical practice that patients with factor XII deficiency have a defect related to impaired clot lysis rather than initiation of coagulation and bleeding.[9] Factor XII–deficient patients have a higher risk of venous thromboembolism than Factor XII–sufficient humans.[10] This is despite prolonged activated coagulation times (such as aPTT or ACT), which suggest that the factor XII–deficient patients are anticoagulated. Thrombin generation during a period of extracorporeal circulation is also increased in patients who are deficient in factor XII, which implies that activation of thrombin by foreign surface interaction is not essential in this process.[11] Whether activation of factor XII is essential for activation of the inflammatory contact process during bypass in humans is unknown. However, the inflammatory response to bypass is reduced in patients who are given aprotinin therapy. Whether this a specific action associated with factor XIIa inhibition is unknown.

The use of polypeptide sequence homology raises other interesting questions regarding the role in nature of factor XII and the plasminogen system. These techniques have shown that factor XII has significant homology with growth factors such as hepatic growth factor.[12] The urinary-type plasminogen activator system is also involved in growth, especially in relation to cancer tissues and angiogenesis.[13] Other growth factors associated with plasminogen are also implicated in these processes, which suggests an important place for these factors in tissue repair after injury.[14] This suggestion is in total variance to the conventional wisdom that factor XIIa is mainly an initiator of the response to injury.

The proximity on the evolutionary scale of kallikrein to factor XI is also supported by their molecular structure. Factor XI circulates in the plasma while bound to high-molecular-weight kininogen.[15] The amino acid sequence of factor XI shows 58% identity with human plasma prekallikrein.[16] In addition, these factors have a similarity in tertiary structure with a serine protease catalytic component attached to four-repeated amino acid sequences held together by disulfide bonds and described as apple domains. Both factor XI and prekallikrein can be activated by factor XIIa; thrombin and factor IXa can also achieve this function. This may be a mechanism to produce retrograde activation of factor XII to stimulate the lytic pathway and reparative growth factors.

The proximity between factors VII, IX, and X suggests that they also serve a closely interrelated function as borne out by current concepts of the coagulation system. They are all dependent on vitamin K as a cofactor for activity. There is overwhelming evidence that expression of TF is the primary initiator of the coagulation cascade.[17] No significant homology exists between TF and any other published protein sequence in current databases. This suggests that the evolutionary divergence of TF has not occurred with a viable alternative; absence of TF is a lethal defect. Early models of coagulation tended to assign TF to a subordinate role,[18] but it is now widely accepted that the extrinsic pathway is critical as TF:FVIIa activates both factor X and factor IX. Circulating factor VII is an unusual coagulation protein for two reasons: (1) the nonactivated (zymogen) form has some proteolytic activity, and (2) about 1% of the circulating form exists as the active enzyme, factor VIIa. The inherent catalytic activity of zymogen factor VII indicates that the simple complexing of factor VII and TF is sufficient to initiate coagulation without a cascade of proteolytic events. The zymogen or active form can bind readily to TF and the complex has enough activity to cleave factor X to factor Xa. Factor Xa will then rapidly convert the FVII:TF complex to FVIIa:TF, and this positive feed-back can thus potentiate the reaction. This autocatalytic, positive feedback is also observed in other parts of the immune or inflammatory system.

This TF-dependent process is conducted close to or within a membrane surface. TF requires phospholipid and has a large transmembrane domain, which helps to retain the TF:FVIIa:FX activating complex at the cell surface. This process ensures that coagulation is localized to the site of injury. The newly created factor Xa remains phospholipid-bound and forms a complex with factor V and prothrombin (the prothrombinase complex). Factor Xa then cleaves prothrombin to form thrombin that is free from the phospholipid surface. Thrombin has a positive feedback on the coagulation cascade.

In addition to activating factor X, the FVIIa:TF complex can also cleave factor IX to form factor IXa, which can then, itself, activate factor X (Figure 1–3). This illustrates the lack of division of the contact factor and TF pathways in vivo.

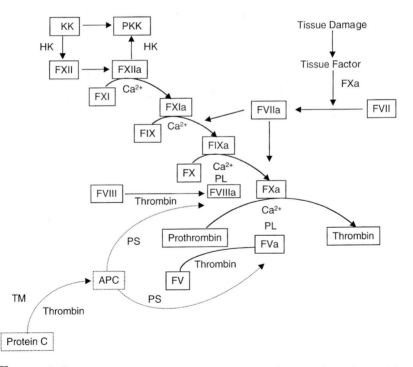

FIGURE 1–3. The coagulation cascade. The contact factor pathway (intrinsic) and the tissue factor pathway (extrinsic) interact in the generation of thrombin.

Many cell types synthesize TF, but, significantly, endothelial cells do not normally express TF on their surfaces, which is consistent with a quiescent hemostatic system. Induction of de novo synthesis of TF by endothelial cells, monocytes, and macrophages is initiated by a number of agonists.[19] However, this synthesis requires signal processing and intracellular synthetic functions to increase TF expression some hours after the provoking challenge. TF thus operates at two levels: (1) immediate exposure of the injured subendothelium to blood causes the binding of factor VII to preformed TF and, consequently, to fibrin formation; and (2) induction of TF synthesis causes the development of a procoagulant state that may be important in the amplification of SIRS during the hours or days after surgery but cannot be involved in the initiation process.

The most intriguing part of the diversification pathway in Figure 1–2 is where complement factor C1, Limulus factor C, human thrombin, and protein C are shown. The early and continued diversification of the human proteins implies strongly that both thrombin and protein C, which are also both vitamin K dependent, serve a similar function. This is difficult to relate to our current concept of these compounds if we consider that thrombin is only a procoagulant and protein C is an anticoagulant. The primary role of thrombin seems to be the catalytic conversion of fibrinogen to fibrin. This is also the role of factor C on coagulogen in Limulus polyphemus. However, thrombin can become an anticoagulant by two distinct mechanisms.

First, thrombin acts as a anticoagulant through the protein C system. Protein C is activated by the action of thrombin with surface bound thrombomodulin as the receptor. Activated protein C acts as an antagonist of the coagulation system by cleaving factor V, thus preventing its activity in the prothrombinase complex. The second mechanism by which thrombin can become an anticoagulant is more fascinating and intriguing. Recent observations have shown that thrombin in close proximity to a surface can become a powerful anticoagulant and that this process relies on nothing more complex than subtle changes in sodium concentrations within specific sites in the molecule.[20,21]

These observations support an increasing trend of the concept that molecules free in plasmatic systems behave in an entirely different and sometimes divergent manner than the way they behave when associated with a cell surface. This may help explain why we have had difficulty unraveling the inflammatory response. It may well be that many of the experiments performed in test tubes or in peripheral blood samples have little, if any, relevance to the reactions that are occurring on our vascular endothelial surfaces.

Thrombin also has a number of other actions on such apparently diverse targets as inflammatory cells, myocytes, and neuronal tissues that may be important in the systemic inflammatory response.

The close evolutionary relationship between thrombin, protein C, factor C of the horseshoe crab, and C1 is discussed in more detail below.

A similar type of analysis related to evolutionary development of serine protease inhibitors is outside the scope of this article because of space constraints. However, one interesting observation is that the molecular structure of the polyvalent inhibitor aprotinin is conserved in many systems. Particularly, the first domain of TFPI has striking sequence homology with aprotinin.[22] Absence of this first domain is a lethal defect in mammals, which suggests that the inhibitory structure of the aprotinin molecule is of fundamental importance in certain pivotally important processes.

EVOLUTIONARY DEVELOPMENT OF THE REPAIR PROCESS: INTERLEUKINS

In addition to the various processes involved with the development of a hemostatic/immune plug, there is also the need to dismantle the process of repair. The repair process is accomplished over a more prolonged time period and likely requires different cellular and humoral elements than those involved in initiating the immune response. A prerequisite of this process is a signaling system that instructs the cell element to convert from an injury/invasion limitation response to a repair process. The substance released from one cell element telling another cell element to change its functional status is now termed a cytokine. Mammalian cytokines include the interferons, the interleukins, tumor necrosis factor (TNF) and lymphotoxin, granulocyte colony-stimulating factor, macrophage colony-stimulating factor, and granulocyte-macrophage colony-stimulating factor, and transforming growth factor β. The fact that, at present, individual genetic deficiency of any cytokine has not been identified in humans suggests a critical need for these molecules in regulating mammalian host defense responses. Cytokines are also found in many invertebrates. In particular, interleukin-1 (IL-1) -like molecules have been identified and categorized.[5]

Interleukins in Early Animals

Crab IL-1 shares many biological activities with vertebrate IL-1 when assayed in several vertebrate systems. Besides the ability of crab IL-1 to stimulate lymphocytes, the molecule also activates fibroblast proliferation, protein synthesis, and prostaglandin release. In the invertebrate, IL-1 stimulates phagocytosis and proliferation of the amoebocyte. This primordial cell is the equivalent of the mononuclear phagocyte or macrophage. Crab IL-1 is also involved in encapsulation, a universal host defense mechanism of the crab, which has the generation of granuloma in higher mammals as its correlate.

At a more acute level, the crab, along with other invertebrates, has been shown to generate TNF-like activity. The compound from the crab has been shown to have similar cytotoxic activity to that found in mammals.

There are several other molecules found within the crab that have cytokine-like properties. The majority of these factors are able to stimulate production of the coelomocyte or encourage encapsulation. These proteins and cytokines are also found in many species of insects and their larvae.[23]

The evidence from the crab of both IL-1–like and TNF-like activities suggests an important role for cytokines in augmenting the host defense system. At present, no other members of the vertebrate cytokine family with potential functional homologues in the crab or other invertebrates have been identified. However, it is unlikely that those compounds associated with advanced immune responses such as IL-4, IL-5, or IL-7 or in cellular defenses against viral infection such as interferon will be found in invertebrates.

Interleukin Receptors in Early Animals

Two major goals have created much interest in the identification of interleukin receptors in invertebrates. First, scientists are searching for interleukins that primarily have roles in nonspecific host defenses that have not been identified in the basic innate immune process such as IL-6. Second, and especially important, is the fact that interleukin receptors in vertebrates are members of the immunoglobulin supergene family. Included in this family are the immunoglobulins, T-cell receptors, and histocompatibility antigens, which make up the adaptive immune system. However, as yet, no immunoglobulin-like molecules have been discovered or recognized in lower orders of animals, which is in keeping with the dominance of the innate immune system in nature. Based on evolutionary concerns, the significance of the components of the immunoglobulin supergene family in the initial acute response is, at best, not clear and, at worst, highly questionable.

This specific aspect of the evolution of the inflammatory response is of considerable relevance to other articles in this monograph. One aspect is related to the role of intercellular adhesion molecules (ICAM-1 and ICAM-2) and platelet endothelial-cell adhesion molecule in the initiation of SIRS and other mechanisms involved with SIRS after cardiac surgery. Currently, there is considerable interest in these molecules because they are required for the process of rolling and sticking of neutrophils to endothelium. The endothelial cell surface ligands for neutrophil-expressed CD11a/CD18 and CD11b/CD18 are ICAM-1 and ICAM-2, respectively. These endothelial cell ligands for neutrophil integrins are also single-chain glycoproteins of the immunoglobulin supergene family. The inability to identify these systems and molecules in lower orders of animals suggests that the early innate inflammatory cell responses do not require adhesion molecules of the immunoglobulin class. An admittedly controversial position could thus be taken to suggest that, from these evolutionary data, these factors are not causally related to the genesis of the inflammatory processes of cardiopulmonary bypass-related tissue injury.

The role of effector molecules and their binding sites leads to discussion of the complement system, which is thought to be of major importance in the early response to a foreign surface such as the cardiopulmonary bypass circuit.

EVOLUTIONARY DEVELOPMENT OF THE COMPLEMENT SYSTEM

The complement system is an effector of both the acquired and the innate immune systems of higher animals such as humans. The origins of the system have been traced back at least to starfish and snails[24] and, as with interleukin receptors, predates the appearance of antibodies, T-cell receptors, and the major histocompatible molecules of the adaptive immune system. The complement system of vertebrates involves more than 30 different proteins including the components labeled C1 through C9 and factors B, I, and H. These proteins interact by means of two enzyme cascades described as the classical and alternative pathways that share a common terminal pathway. At present we believe that the system accomplishes three major functions in man: (1) the production of C3a and C5a, which are associated with chemotaxis, smooth muscle contraction, and an increase in vascular permeability; (2) the coating of pathogenic organisms with molecules (opsonins) that are recognized by the phagocytic cells of the host; and (3) the formation of a terminal membrane attack complex (MAC) that is able to lyse microorganisms.

We now recognize that genes belonging to several families encode the complement components. The three principle components of the early or initiating parts of this system (C3, C4, and C5) belong to a single family, which also includes α_2-macroglobulin—the same protein that is found in the horseshoe crab and that is synthesized in human liver in response to inflammation and infection. The intriguing part about the macroglobulin and complement interaction at this level is related to the biologically unique mechanism of their binding to a foreign material. Understanding this leads to a reappraisal of the relevance of each of the components of the complement pathway in human tissue injury.

Weak and Strong Protein Binding

Binding of protein to foreign materials is a requirement of a humoral recognition event. In mammals, different parts of the immune system achieve this in different ways. However, the vast majority of the systems require molecules that are polymeric because an interaction between a monomer and the structure it recognizes is by low-affinity binding through hydrogen bonding or van der Waals forces. It is therefore only when these structures are displayed in a repeated array on the surface of a pathogen or in an immune complex that high avidity binding occurs.

In contrast, tight binding without the need for multiple recognition sites can be achieved through covalent bonding. This is where the molecules of macroglobulin and the principle complement components (C3 and C4) differ from all other polypeptides found in humans. These three agents bind to form ester and amide bonds on the surface of their target because of a unique internal thioester bridge.[25]

All of these proteins are synthesized as a single chain of an approximate size of 180kDa with the thioester bond situated approximately halfway along the molecule. Upon cleavage of the molecule, a conformational change takes place, and this thioester area becomes highly reactive. The protein becomes covalently bound to any nearby large molecule via an ester or amide bond. In the case of the complement components, this leads to the covalent deposition of C3 and C4 on the target cell and immune aggregates on which they are activated.

Macroglobulin has been described in arthropods and mollusc species that lack C3, as well as in starfish and vertebrates.[26] Macroglobulin shows overall sequence similarity to the complement components C3, C4, and C5.[25] The close relationship between the three principle members of the complement system and macroglobin has led to considerable debate about which of the various components came first and, therefore, is most important and basic in the initiation of foreign surface recognition and activation.[27] Three possible concepts for divergence between the various components of this system have been proposed (Figure 1–4). The evidence suggesting that scheme A is the most likely comes from further investigation of the evolutionary chemistry of these compounds. As evolution has progressed, the gene for C5 seems to have diverged from macroglobulin prior to the common ancestor of C3 and C4, which diverged later.[27]

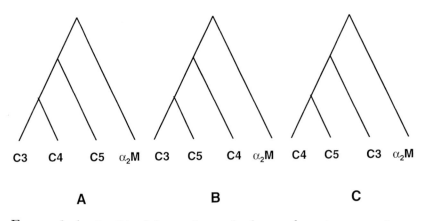

C3   C4   C5   α₂M   C3   C5   C4   α₂M   C4   C5   C3   α₂M

A   B   C

FIGURE 1–4.   Possible phylogenetic trees for the complement components, C3, C4, and C5 with α₂-macroglobulin (α₂M) as an outgroup.[27]

This relationship suggests that the generation of a lytic MAC is the principle mechanism of attack of the complement system and that C3 dependent processes are relatively new, in evolutionary terms. Based on protein evolution, other lines of evidence supporting this argument include the following: (1) Lytic activity is demonstrated in lower orders of animals such as the horseshoe crab, which implies a significant need for this process. In the crab, C-reactive protein seems to be associated with the complement-like lytic system.[28] This system provides activation of C1, without the need for an antibody as in the classical pathway, by C-reactive protein bound to the polysaccharide of the bacteria. As shown in Figure 1–2, C1 is associated with coagulation factors, which provides further evidence of a close and fundamental link between the immune and hemostatic process. Over recent years, evidence has begun to emerge showing that the macroglobulin of the crab is also involved in a lytic mechanism. This lytic activity is only partially depleted by inactivation of the thioester bond of the macroglobulin. However, macroglobulin function in this process is unclear but it is probably acting as some kind of opsonin. (2) The terminal pathway involves a set of molecules that are not homologous to any in the classical or alternative pathway. The most important of these molecules are the MAC constituents, which show evidence of evolutionary relationships both to each other and to the cytolytic proteins perforin and cytolysin.[29–31] Perforin and cytolysin are found in human phagocytic cells and have been implicated in a wide variety of nonspecific destructive and inflammatory processes including graft-versus-host disease, apoptosis, and rheumatoid arthritis. The only role played by the classical or alternative pathways in the generation of MAC is the activation of C5. Thus, the key step that allowed the evolution of the complement MAC was the gene duplication that gave rise to C5. This duplicate was then free to lose its thioester bond and acquire a C6 binding site, thereby linking the complement system with a presumably preexisting cytolytic system.

In addition to these arguments about the relative importance of the various aspects of the complement system from an evolutionary standpoint, there is also evidence from clinical correlates.

Significant activation of the complement system, as judged by a rise in plasma concentration of C3a, occurs in a number of clinical situations. In particular, the contact of blood with a foreign surface in cardiopulmonary bypass and dialysis systems is well recognized as a significant complement activator. We also know that complement is activated in patients who have sepsis and sepsis syndrome.

Is this overactivity fundamentally and causally implicated in any initial or continuing deleterious effect on organ function? At present the main body of evidence suggests this is not the case. First, we recognize that complement activation can be significantly inhibited during open-heart surgery by either modifications to the surface of the oxygenator, typically by surface coating with heparin,[32,33] or by pharmacologic intervention with corticosteroids.[34] However, with both of these treatments there has been difficulty in demonstrating a significant benefit to the patient in terms of reduced tissue or organ injury after bypass.[35] Second, we recognize that the degree of complement activation in patients with sepsis syndrome, which is shown as raised plasma C3a concentration, is unrelated to the development or degree of pulmonary injury and impaired lung function.[36] Indeed, there is some evidence to suggest that the use of high doses of corticosteroids in the presence of sepsis[37] and cardiopulmonary bypass[38] may do more harm than good, although it seems unlikely that this is as a result of inhibition of complement activation alone.

Because we cannot easily justify a role for excess complement activation in augmenting injury, we should question what happens if we have no or limited complement available for activation. A number of humans are deficient in certain complement components. A deficiency in the third component renders patients more sensitive to infection by certain groups of encapsulated bacteria such as meningococcus, pneumococcus, and neisseria. Deficiency of C3 is, as far as is known, not associated with any significant life-threatening illness. In the same way, animals bred to be genetically deficient in this complement component develop abnormal lung function after extracorporeal circulation of the same type and magnitude as animals sufficient in complement.[39] Initially, therefore, it seems that modifications to complement and its activation would not be a prime focus for a therapeutic intervention based on evolutionary and clinical grounds.

This line of thinking, concerning modifications to C3, does not seem to be as robust when discussing the MAC (C5b-9) complex. In the presence of complement activation, inhibition of the C5b-9 complex by the use of either a serine protease inhibitor[40] or an antibody against the terminal complex[41]confers significant improvements in myocardial performance. Inhibition of complement activation to prevent the formation or action of the membrane attack complex may confer significant patient benefit not observed with the inhibition of activation of C3a alone.

There is a caveat to this interpretation of the complement activation story in relation to cardiopulmonary bypass and SIRS. The prior arguments suggest that the most primitive cell defense mechanism, in evolutionary terms, is through the membrane attack complex. These are associated with cell and tissue injury, whereas activation of C3 alone may be of less relevance. However, the effects of complement activation as measured by C3a concentration has almost entirely been investigated against altered pulmonary function. This is despite studies in animals and humans showing this to be an inappropriate target organ because the evidence suggests it is unlikely to be effected by C3a-mediated inflammatory processes. However, exuberant complement activation related to the membrane attack complex, possibly in conjunction with a period of ischemia-reperfusion, may play a significant part in myocardial injury.

BIOCHEMICAL EVOLUTION: ARE THERE LESSONS FROM THE NITRIC OXIDE STORY?

We now recognize that nitric oxide is a pivotal player in a variety of physiological and pathophysiological processes. Many of these actions are considered positive attributes for the molecule, including tumoricidal, bactericidal, antiproliferative, and vasodilating effects.[42] However, there is also evidence for the association of nitric oxide with adverse outcome (eg, its actions on vascular smooth muscle). Vascular endothelial-derived nitric oxide acts on the abluminal myocyte to produce relaxation and vasodilatation, thereby increasing blood flow. This effect may be of significant benefit in patients with critical myocardial perfusion. In particular, nitric oxide–dependent vasodilatation is thought to be important in the response to ischemia-reperfusion injury of the myocardium.

In contrast, abnormal nitric oxide activity or production may lead to a deleterious effect on the patient. We recognize that nitric oxide has a direct depressant action on the cardiac myocyte and is thought to be the principle mechanism for the myocardial depression produced by IL-6.[43] Moreover, excess nitric oxide production is implicated in the profound vasodilation associated with septic shock.[44]

As astonishing as it may seem to the reader, the innate defense system of the horseshoe crab does not use nitric oxide. The question therefore is where does nitric oxide fit into the puzzle in humans: (1) Is it a fundamentally important part of the initiation of inflammation? (2) Is it a secondary system which may be more protective than harmful? (3) Will uncontrolled secondary activity lead to worsening outcome?

The answer to these questions may come from consideration of the evolutionary aspects of the enzymatic system used to generate nitric oxide, nitric oxide synthase (NOS). The nitric oxide synthases constitute a family with three distinct isoforms that have certain characteristics outlined in Table 1–1. They were originally derived from neurones, cytokine-induced macrophages, and endothelial cells, hence their names of neuronal (nNOS), inducible (iNOS), and endothelial constitutive (ecNOS). The three isoforms are now understood to be distributed across a wide variety of cell types, and cells may express more than one isoform of NOS, which can complicate interpretation of data.[45,46] The pattern of expression in humans is not as well established as in laboratory animals. Certain confounding factors are also recognized. The most important, in relation to the inflammatory process, is that nitric oxide is not expressed by stimulated human neutrophils.[47]

The question is whether study of evolutionary developments of NOS can help us to define the following: (1) What were these enzyme systems derived from? (2) How are they controlled? (3) What can they produce and what is the functional effect of this? In turn can we use this information to address the question of whether inhibition of production or activity will do good or harm to the patient?

TABLE 1–1. Characteristics of Nitric Oxide Synthase Isoforms

Isoform	nNOS	iNOS	eNOS
Chromosome location	12	17	7
Cell prototype	Neurons	Hepatocyte Macrophage	Endothelial cells
Gene size	>200 kb	~37 kb	~21 kb
Amino acids in protein	1434	1153	1203
Localization	Cytosol/ membrane	Cytosol	Membrane
Calcium dependent	+++	−	++
Calmodulin dependent	+	+	+

NOS, nitric oxide synthase; nNOS, neuronal NOS; iNOS, inducible NOS; eNOS, endothelial NOS.

WHAT IS NITRIC OXIDE SYNTHASE? WHAT ARE ITS EVOLUTIONARY ROOTS?

Nitric oxide synthases are a family of complex hemeproteins that catalyze the five-electron oxidation of L-arginine to form nitric oxide and citrulline. NOS activity has an absolute dependence on molecular oxygen and NADPH together with flavine mononucleotide and flavin dinucleotide as cofactors. In this regard it has great similarity to cytochrome P-450.[45,46] This biochemical and structural similarity to cytochrome P-450 helps us understand why NOS, and thus nitric oxide, is not pivotal in host defense in primitive creatures. Cytochrome P-450 was simply not a major player during this period of evolution. The reason for this is, itself, relatively simple.

As anesthesiologists, we recognize that P-450 enzymes catalyze the oxidation of a number of chemicals, including the majority of drugs and xenobiotics. These enzymes are also important in oxidation of endobiotics such as steroids, fatty acids, eicosanoids, and prostaglandins. During evolution of the horseshoe crab, these functions were largely unnecessary or poorly developed. The reason for this is probably related to the atmosphere of the planet.

An oxidizing atmosphere probably started to develop about 570 million years ago with a rise to about 50% of our present atmospheric level of oxygen around the start of the Devonian Period approximately 400 million years ago, a time that animals were thought to colonize the land.[48] The dramatic rise in atmospheric oxygen probably directed the functions of a primitive microsomal P-450 toward using dioxygen for the metabolism of, first, endogenous compounds and, subsequently, xenobiotics. The modifications of P-450 to oxidize endogenous compounds is first noted for steroidogenesis, which produced differences in gender and, thus, sexual reproduction.[48] The need for animals to detoxify xenobiotics developed as plant life also evolved. Plant toxins were being increasingly produced by the flora of the time to protect themselves from attack by insects and, more importantly, insect larvae. It is interesting to speculate that the current exponential growth in the family of cytochrome P-450 enzymes, presently numbering approximately 500 isoforms, may reflect the increasing development of a toxic oxidizing environment.

Based on the close relationship between cytochrome P-450 and NOS, it is not surprising that many NOS-dependent processes can be modified by inhibitors and activators of cytochrome P-450. Examples include imidazole antifungals such as ketoconazole[49,50] and thiopentone.[51,52] Similarly, nitric oxide is released from precursors such as nitrates by the action of P-450 enzymes.

NOS IN HUMANS

The genes for the production of the three human NOS isoforms identified to date (endothelial constitutive, neuronal, and macrophage cytokine-inducible) are found on human chromosomes 7, 12, and 17, respectively. These enzymes are unique in two ways. First, they each contain a cysteine thiolate heme prosthetic group (protoporphyrin IX), which makes them the only mammalian proteins that catalyze a hydroxylation reaction (P-450–based reaction) and NADPH reduction (a cytochrome P-450 reductase function) within the same protein—an attribute shared only by the bacterial flavoprotein from *Bacillus megaterium*, cytochrome P-450BM-3.[53] Second, nNOS and macrophage iNOS are the only known soluble cytochrome P-450–type enzymes.[46] The remainder, together with ecNOS, are surface bound. The membrane association of ecNOS is related to a N-terminal myristoylation site not found in nNOS or iNOS.[46] This site acts to bind the NOS to the endothelial cell membrane. The specific function of this site is unclear, but it may provide the ability for the endothelium to respond, by increasing surface NO production, to signals from agonists or from shear stress changes produced in response to alterations in blood flow.

HOW ARE THESE ENZYMES CONTROLLED?

Regulation of NOS Genes

Characterization of the organization of the human nitric oxide synthase genes reveals that, although they are structurally related, the mechanisms by which they are regulated are distinct. Expression of the mRNA for ecNOS and iNOS is regulated at the level of transcription and mRNA stability. The mRNA transcripts derived from the nNOS gene are characterized by a remarkable degree of structural diversity. The full-length reading frame of the nNOS gene is 4302 bp and encodes a protein of 1434 amino acids. However, deletion and frame-shift during reading may produce a number of related proteins derived from the gene, which includes a putative N-terminal protein of 561 amino acids. This diverse protein production by the nNOS gene is of interest in two areas. First, we understand that NOS functions as a dimer in the enzymatic synthesis of NO.[54] The production of various truncated proteins by the nNOS gene suggests evolutionarily preserved functions, probably unrelated to nitric oxide production, in neural systems. Second, this ability of nNOS to produce truncated polypeptides may explain certain preliminary reports of NOS-like activity in the hemocyte of a mollusc, the freshwater snail *Viviparus ater*.[55] The intriguing aspect is that this enzyme binds to an antibody against a rat nNOS leading to the following speculations: (1) There is a NOS-like enzyme in early animals that does not yet produce nitric oxide but is involved in host defense. In the absence of L-arginine, nNOS can generate reactive oxygen intermediates, namely superoxide anion and hydrogen peroxide.[56,57] In addition, NOS can donate electrons directly to various acceptor molecules and reduce compounds such as cytochrome c[58] with deleterious effects on the cell. (2) We may be missing a fundamental role of nNOS in neural tissues that is unrelated to its ability to produce nitric oxide.

Regulation of Synthetic Activity

Cofactors, in addition to oxygen and NADPH, required for NOS activity are tetrahydrobiopterin (a purine derived from cGMP metabolism) together with calcium and calmodulin.

Current data on the calcium-calmodulin control process shows differences between the various isoforms. nNOS and eNOS are critically dependent on elevated intracellular calcium concentration. This promotes the binding of calmodulin to the enzyme, which, in turn, allows NADPH-derived electrons to be passed to the heme group. However, there is still controversy over whether calcium and/or calmodulin are cofactors for the cytokine-inducible form of NOS. Purified rat liver NOS (induced by lipopolysaccharide treatment in vivo) is calmodulin-dependent and is only partially responsive to changes in calcium.[59] An elevated concentration of intracellular calcium is not necessary to initiate enzyme activity in macrophage iNOS, whereas calmodulin binding is obligatory.[60] Interestingly, calmodulin is a tightly bound subunit of macrophage iNOS even though this enzyme is clearly not regulated by exogenous calcium.[61] This property may mean that iNOS is tonically active in the presence of substrate (NADPH, dioxygen, and L-arginine).[62]

Because of the complexities of calcium/calmodulin activation of NOS, caution should be used when characterizing NOS isoforms based exclusively on being calcium-dependent or calcium-independent. Nonetheless this may be of great interest for anesthesiologists because many agents and adjuncts used in anesthetic practice inhibit calmodulin and calmodulin-sensitive processes. This suggests that if nitric oxide is important in postcardiopulmonary bypass SIRS, then modifications to the anesthetic technique alone may alter the pattern of the response.

A second aspect of the control process is related to the observation that each of the three NOS isoforms has a consensus sequence for phosphorylation by protein kinase. Protein kinase C and cAMP-dependent protein kinase can phosphorylate nNOS.[63] Similarly, the phosphorylation of serine residues in response to treatment with bradykinin has been shown for eNOS.[64] It is interesting to speculate if this is the mechanism involved in the bradykinin/nitric oxide–mediated response to ischemia-reperfusion.

NOS AND INFLAMMATORY RESPONSES

The combination of similarities and differences makes the role of NOS and nitric oxide in the initiation of the uncontrolled inflammatory response of SIRS difficult to define. The evolutionary development and varied expression of NOS suggest a protective rather than destructive role for these enzymes.

The diversity of the development of NOS may also explain why the current therapeutic approach to inhibition or enhancement of all isoforms may not be successful. Indiscriminate inhibition of all forms of NOS with, for example, false substrate may increase our knowledge of the mechanism of action of these systems in a variety of disease processes. However, they may also remove the positive attributes (ie, antiproliferative, bactericidal, and cytostatic properties) of nitric oxide during tissue injury or inflammation. This may explain the adverse global effects of false substrates, despite appropriate and desired cardiovascular effects, in patients with septic shock.[65] Based on our current knowledge, selective targeting of individual NOS with enzyme inhibitors will be difficult unless there are tissue-specific, posttranslation modifications that afford unique properties to each of the separate enzymes.

COMMENT AND CONCLUSIONS

A number of points emerge from the above discussions. They are based on evolutionary evidence and are thought provoking. However, many are also controversial because they do not follow current dogma.

The most basic, fundamental and innate response to injury follows a simple pattern: (1) a cellular element, which can clump and stick to an injury or invasion; (2) a zymogen protein that can be activated to bind and hold together the cellular element; and (3) an activator of this process based on one or more serine proteases. This suggests that, with our currently available pharmacologic and interventional armamentarium, augmenting the natural serine protease inhibitor-related control of the process will be most globally effective.

Based on conventional laboratory tests, the role of proteins in the coagulation system is inconsistent with the view from an evolutionary standpoint. This later view suggests the following: (1) Activation of factor XII and the plasminogen system are more fundamental in repair than in initiation of a response to injury. (2) Factor XI may be more important than factor XII in recognition of a foreign surface. (3) The coagulation system has a surface-related integrated core component that has a poor relationship with conventional concepts of separate intrinsic and extrinsic systems. (4) The proximity and evolutionary conservation of mammalian thrombin and invertebrate factor C suggest a pivotal need for their enzymatic function. The incorporation of protein C in the same group, coupled with the ability of thrombin to change function, suggests a potentially important role for thrombin in the repair process.

Interleukins are conserved in evolution, and genetic deficiency in humans is presumably a lethal gene. Both of these facts suggest a crucial role for these compounds in the process of inflammation and immunity. However, the primary function of interleukins seems to be protective and reparative rather than destructive. Mortality in patients with meningococcal septicemia is highest in families with the lowest TNF and highest IL-10 response,[66] implying that not all TNF is bad nor is all IL-10 good.

The importance of complement-dependent lytic pathways in tissue injury may have been underestimated. This may, in part, be because investigations of injury in inappropriate tissues used unconvincing biochemical end points despite their ease of measurement. It is axiomatic that making an observation does not, in itself, define the indisputable importance or unequivocal relevance of that observation.

The ability of the primary effector cell to move to and adhere to the site of injury is pivotal in the early inflammatory process. The mechanism of this activity has, at least in research terms, been made more complex by the development and appearance of the immunoglobulin gene superfamily of molecules and receptors. Interpretation of current data is made more complex because of the diversity in a response by both tissue and challenge. As with the cytokines, there is a suggestion that the ability of a neutrophil to roll, stick, and transmigrate may not be important in the initial injury but may influence repair and recovery. ICAM-1–deficient animals, although more susceptible to infection with *Haemophilus influenzae*, die less often from this infection than their ICAM-sufficient brethren.[67] If human genetic deletion is used as a model, then inhibition of neutrophil adhesion molecules may lead to more wound but no greater lung problems.

Evolution has progressed, with expansion and development of animal species, without the expression of nitric oxide implying we can live without it as part of the inflammatory process. Presently, there is considerable debate about the relevance of nitric oxide in central neuronal transmission and cardiovascular control. However, there is little, if any, evidence that NOS-deficient animals are susceptible to infections or have an abnormal inflammatory response. However, similar to interleukins, TF, and TFPI, there are no reports of patients with any NOS deletion, which suggests that this may be a lethal deletion.

References

1. McRitchie DI, Girotti MJ, Glynn MF, Goldberg JM, Rotstein OD: Effect of systemic fibrinogen depletion on intraabdominal abscess formation. J Lab Clin Med 118:48–55, 1991
2. Tang L, Eaton JW: Fibrin(ogen) mediates acute inflammatory responses to biomaterials. J Exp Med 178:2147–2156, 1993
3. Wu X, Helfrich MH, Horton MA, Feigen LP, Lefkowith JB: Fibrinogen mediates platelet-polymorphonuclear leukocyte cooperation during immune-complex glomerulonephritis in rats. J Clin Invest 94:928–936, 1994
4. Rosenberg RD, Aird WC: Vascular-bed–specific hemostasis and hypercoagulable states. N Engl J Med 340:1555–1564, 1999
5. Beck G, Habicht GS: Primitive cytokines: Harbingers of vertebrate defense. Immunol Today 12:180–183, 1991
6. Iwanaga S, Kawabata S: Evolution and phylogeny of defense molecules associated with innate immunity in horseshoe crab. Front Biosci 3:D973-D984, 1998
7. Nakamura S, Takagi T, Iwanaga S, Niwa M, Takahashi K: Amino acid sequence studies on the fragments produced from horseshoe crab coagulogen during gel formation: Homologies with primate fibrinopeptide B. Biochem Biophys Res Commun 72:902–908, 1976
8. Britten RJ: Rates of DNA sequence evolution differ between taxonomic groups. Science 231:1393–1398, 1986
9. Lammle B, Wuillemin WA, Huber I, Krauskopf M, Zurcher C, Pflugshaupt R, Furlan M: Thromboembolism and bleeding tendency in congenital factor XII deficiency: A study on 74 subjects from 14 Swiss families. Thromb Haemost 65:117–121, 1991
10. Halbmayer WM, Mannhalter C, Feichtinger C, Rubi K, Fischer M: Factor XII (Hageman factor) deficiency: A risk factor for development of thromboembolism: Incidence of factor XII deficiency in patients after recurrent venous or arterial thromboembolism and myocardial infarction. Wien Med Wochenschr 143:43–50, 1993
11. Burman JF, Chung HI, Lane DA, Philippou H, Adami A, Lincoln JC: Role of factor XII in thrombin generation and fibrinolysis during cardiopulmonary bypass. Lancet 344:1192–1193, 1994
12. Miyazawa K, Wang Y, Minoshima S, Shimizu N, Kitamura N: Structural organization and chromosomal localization of the human hepatocyte growth factor activator gene: Phylogenetic and functional

relationship with blood coagulation factor XII, urokinase, and tissue-type plasminogen activator. Eur J Biochem 258: 355–361, 1998

13. Duffy MJ, Maguire TM, McDermott EW, O'Higgins N: Urokinase plasminogen activator: A prognostic marker in multiple types of cancer. J Surg Oncol 71:130–135, 1999

14. Donate LE, Gherardi E, Srinivasan N, Sowdhamini R, Aparicio S, Blundell TL: Molecular evolution and domain structure of plasminogen-related growth factors (HGF/SF and HGF1/MSP). Protein Sci 3:2378–2394, 1994

15. Thompson RE, Mandle R Jr, Kaplan AP: Association of factor XI and high molecular weight kininogen in human plasma. J Clin Invest 60:1376–1380, 1977

16. Meijers JC, McMullen BA, Bouma BN: The contact activation proteins: A structure/function overview. Agents Actions Suppl 38: 219–230, 1992

17. Camerer E, Kolsto AB, Prydz H: Cell biology of tissue factor, the principal initiator of blood coagulation. Thromb Res 81:1–41, 1996

18. Davie EW, Fujikawa K, Kisiel W: The coagulation cascade: Initiation, maintenance, and regulation. Biochemistry 30:10363–10370, 1991

19. Prydz H, Pettersen KS: Synthesis of thromboplastin (tissue factor) by endothelial cells. Haemostasis 18:215–223, 1988

20. Hall SW, Gibbs CS, Leung LL: Strategies for development of novel antithrombotics: Modulating thrombin's procoagulant and anticoagulant properties. Cell Mol Life Sci 53:731–736, 1997

21. Leung LL, Gibbs CS: Modulation of thrombin's procoagulant and anticoagulant properties. Thromb Haemost 78:577–580, 1997

22. Royston D: Preventing the inflammatory response to open-heart surgery: The role of aprotinin and other protease inhibitors. Int J Cardiol 53(Suppl):S11–S37, 1996

23. Beck G, O'Brien RF, Habicht GS: Invertebrate cytokines: The phylogenetic emergence of interleukin-1. Bioessays 11:62–67, 1989

24. Nonaka M, Azumi K, Ji X, Namikawa-Yamada C, Sasaki M, Saiga H, Dodds AW, Sekine H, Homma MK, Matsushita M, Endo Y, Fujita T: Opsonic complement component C3 in the solitary ascidian, *Halocynthia roretzi*. J Immunol 162:387–391, 1999

25. Dodds AW, Law SK: The phylogeny and evolution of the thioester bond-containing proteins C3, C4 and α_2-macroglobulin. Immunol Rev 166:15–26, 1998

26. Bender RC, Bayne CJ: Purification and characterization of a tetrameric α-macroglobulin proteinase inhibitor from the gastropod mollusc *Biomphalaria glabrata*. Biochem J 316:893–900, 1996

27. Hughes AL: Phylogeny of the C3/C4/C5 complement-component gene family indicates that C5 diverged first. Mol Biol Evol 11:417–425, 1994

28. Armstrong PB, Armstrong MT, Quigley JP: Involvement of α_2-macroglobulin and C-reactive protein in a complement-like hemolytic system in the arthropod, *Limulus polyphemus*. Mol Immunol 30:929–934, 1993

29. Campbell RD, Law SK, Reid KB, Sim RB: Structure, organization, and regulation of the complement genes. Annu Rev Immunol 6:161–195, 1988

30. Ishikawa H, Shinkai Y, Yagita H, Yue CC, Henkart PA, Sawada S, Young HA, Reynolds CW, Okumura K: Molecular cloning of rat cytolysin. J Immunol 143:3069–3073, 1989

31. Lichtenheld MG, Olsen KJ, Lu P, Lowrey DM, Hameed A, Hengartner H, Podack ER: Structure and function of human perforin. Nature 335:448–451, 1988

32. Jansen PG, te Velthuis H, Huybregts RA, Paulus R, Bulder ER, van der Spoel HI, Bezemer PD, Slaats EH, Eijsman L, Wildevuur CR: Reduced complement activation and improved postoperative performance after cardiopulmonary bypass with heparin-coated circuits. J Thorac Cardiovasc Surg 110:829–834, 1995

33. Ovrum E, Mollnes TE, Fosse E, Holen EA, Tangen G, Abdelnoor M, Ringdal MA, Oystese R, Venge P: Complement and granulocyte activation in two different types of heparinized extracorporeal circuits. J Thorac Cardiovasc Surg 110:1623–1632, 1995

34. Engelman RM, Rousou JA, Flack JE III, Deaton DW, Kalfin R, Das DK: Influence of steroids on complement and cytokine generation after cardiopulmonary bypass. Ann Thorac Surg 60:801–804, 1995

35. Ovrum E, Am Holen E, Tangen G, Ringdal MA: Heparinized cardiopulmonary bypass and full heparin dose marginally improve clinical performance. Ann Thorac Surg 62:1128–1133, 1996

36. Weinberg PF, Matthay MA, Weslen O, Roskos KV, Godstein TM, Murray JF: Biologically active products of complement and acute lung injury in patients with the sepsis syndrome. Am Rev Respir Dis 130:791–796, 1984

37. Bernard GR, Luce JM, Sprung CL, Rinaldo JE, Tate RM, Sibbald WJ, Kariman K, Higgins S, Bradley R, Metz CA, et al: High-dose corticosteroids in patients with the adult respiratory distress syndrome. N Engl J Med 317:1565–1570, 1987

38. Chaney MA, Nikolov MP, Blakeman B, Bakhos M, Slogoff S: Pulmonary effects of methylprednisolone in patients undergoing coronary artery bypass grafting and early tracheal extubation. Anestri Analg 87:27–33, 1998

39. Gillinov AM, Redmond JM, Winkelstein JA, Zehr KJ, Herskowitz A, Baumgartner WA, Cameron DE: Complement and neutrophil activation during cardiopulmonary bypass: A study in the complement-deficient dog. Ann Thorac Surg 57:345–352, 1994

40. Homeister JW, Satoh P, Lucchesi BR: Effects of complement activation in the isolated heart: Role of the terminal complement components. Circ Res 71:303–319, 1992

41. Fitch J, Rinder C, Smith B, Smith M, Rollins S: Terminal complement components produce platelet and leukocyte activation during simulated extracorporeal circulation. Anesth Analg 80:SCA15, 1995

42. Moncada S, Palmer RM, Higgs EA: Nitric oxide: Physiology, pathophysiology, and pharmacology. Pharmacol Rev 43:109–142, 1991

43. Panas D, Khadour FH, Szabo C, Schulz R: Proinflammatory cytokines depress cardiac efficiency by a nitric oxide-dependent mechanism. Am J Physiol 275:H1016-H1023, 1998

44. Petros A, Lamb G, Leone A, Moncada S, Bennett D, Vallance P: Effects of a nitric oxide synthase inhibitor in humans with septic shock. Cardiovasc Res 28:34–39, 1994

45. Sessa WC: The nitric oxide synthase family of proteins. J Vasc Res 31:131–143, 1994

46. Wang Y, Marsden PA: Nitric oxide synthases: Biochemical and molecular regulation. Curr Opin Nephrol Hypertens 4:12–22, 1995

47. Holm P, Kankaanranta H, Oja SS, Knowles RG, Moilanen E: No detectable NO synthesis from L-arginine or N(G)-hydroxy-L-arginine in fMLP-stimulated human blood neutrophils despite production of nitrite, nitrate, and citrulline from N(G)-hydroxy-L-arginine. J Leukoc Biol 66:127–134, 1999

48. Lewis DF, Watson E, Lake BG: Evolution of the cytochrome P450 superfamily: Sequence alignments and pharmacogenetics. Mutat Res 410:245–270, 1998

49. Baroni A, Ruocco V, De Paolis P, Cicatiello L, Esumi H, Tufano MA: Ketoconazole inhibits lipopolysaccharide-induced activation of the nitric oxide synthase gene in the murine macrophage cell line J774. Arch Dermatol Res 291:54–58, 1999

50. Bogle RG, Whitley GS, Soo SC, Johnstone AP, Vallance P: Effect of anti-fungal imidazoles on mRNA levels and enzyme activity of inducible nitric oxide synthase. Br J Pharmacol 111:1257–1261, 1994

51. Galley HF, Webster NR: Brain nitric oxide synthase activity is decreased by intravenous anesthetics. Anesth Analg 83:591–594, 1996

52. Kessler P, Kronemann N, Hecker M, Busse R, Schini-Kerth VB: Effects of barbiturates on the expression of the inducible nitric oxide synthase in vascular smooth muscle. J Cardiovasc Pharmacol 30:802–810, 1997

53. Fulco AJ: P450BM-3 and other inducible bacterial P450 cytochromes: Biochemistry and regulation. Annu Rev Pharmacol Toxicol 31:177–203, 1991

54. Baek KJ, Thiel BA, Lucas S, Stuehr DJ: Macrophage nitric oxide synthase subunits: Purification, characterization, and role of pros-

thetic groups and substrate in regulating their association into a dimeric enzyme. J Biol Chem 268:21120–21129, 1993

55. Conte A, Ottaviani E: Nitric oxide synthase activity in molluscan hemocytes. FEBS Lett 365:120–124, 1995

56. Heinzel B, John M, Klatt P, Bohme E, Mayer B: Ca^{2+}/calmodulin-dependent formation of hydrogen peroxide by brain nitric oxide synthase. Biochem J 281:627–630, 1992

57. Pou S, Pou WS, Bredt DS, Snyder SH, Rosen GM: Generation of superoxide by purified brain nitric oxide synthase. J Biol Chem 267:24173–24176, 1992

58. Mayer B, Heinzel B, Klatt P, John M, Schmidt K, Bohme E: Nitric oxide synthase-catalyzed activation of oxygen and reduction of cytochromes: Reaction mechanisms and possible physiological implications. J Cardiovasc Pharmacol 20(Suppl 12):S54–S56, 1992

59. Evans T, Carpenter A, Cohen J: Purification of a distinctive form of endotoxin-induced nitric oxide synthase from rat liver. Proc Natl Acad Sci USA 89:5361–5365, 1992

60. Stuehr DJ, Gross SS, Sakuma I, Levi R, Nathan CF: Activated murine macrophages secrete a metabolite of arginine with the bioactivity of endothelium-derived relaxing factor and the chemical reactivity of nitric oxide. J Exp Med 169:1011–1020, 1989

61. Cho HJ, Xie QW, Calaycay J, Mumford RA, Swiderek KM, Lee TD, Nathan C: Calmodulin is a subunit of nitric oxide synthase from macrophages. J Exp Med 176:599–604, 1992

62. Abu-Soud HM, Stuehr DJ: Nitric oxide synthases reveal a role for calmodulin in controlling electron transfer. Proc Natl Acad Sci USA 90:10769–10772, 1993

63. Bredt DS, Ferris CD, Snyder SH: Nitric oxide synthase regulatory sites: Phosphorylation by cyclic AMP-dependent protein kinase, protein kinase C, and calcium/calmodulin protein kinase: Identification of flavin and calmodulin binding sites. J Biol Chem 267:10976–10981, 1992

64. Michel T, Li GK, Busconi L: Phosphorylation and subcellular translocation of endothelial nitric oxide synthase. Proc Natl Acad Sci USA 90:6252–6256, 1993

65. Cobb JP: Use of nitric oxide synthase inhibitors to treat septic shock: The light has changed from yellow to red (Editorial). Crit Care Med 27:855–856, 1999

66. Westendorp RG, Langermans JA, Huizinga TW, Elouali AH, Verweij CL, Boomsma DI, Vandenbroucke JP: Genetic influence on cytokine production and fatal meningococcal disease. Lancet 349:170–173, 1997

67. Tan TQ, Smith CW, Hawkins EP, Mason EO Jr, Kaplan SL: Hematogenous bacterial meningitis in an intercellular adhesion molecule-1-deficient infant mouse model. J Infect Dis 171:342–349, 1995

Gilbert Blaise, M.D.

The Endothelium at Rest

2

ANATOMY OF THE VASCULAR WALL

The arterial wall is composed of several layers.[1,2] The outermost, the adventitia, is composed mainly of nerves and fibrotic tissue (fibroblasts, collagen bundles, and a loose network of thin elastic fibers). The second layer, the media, is made up of several sheets of long, branching smooth muscle interspersed with laminae of elastin, occasional fibroblasts, collagen fibers, and extracellular matrix. The media is separated from the innermost layer, the intima, by the internal elastic membrane. The intima lines the vessel lumen and is in direct contact with blood cells. It is composed of endothelial cells supported by extracellular matrix and loose connective tissue. This connective tissue layer contains some fibroblasts and smooth muscle cells as well as collagenous and elastic fibers. As the size of the vessels decreases from the central circulation (arteries) to the periphery (arterioles and capillaries), the thickness of the medial smooth muscle layer also diminishes. At the capillary level, the media is no longer present.

The blood is carried from the capillary networks back to the heart by the veins. In progressing toward the heart, the veins gradually increase in caliber and their walls progressively thicken; their walls nonetheless remain thinner, more supple, and less elastic than those of the arteries. This explains their appearance in cross section, where the lumen frequently collapses and appears slit-like and irregular. Three layers are present in the venous walls: the tunica intima, the tunica media,

The Relationship Between Coagulation, Inflammation, and Endothelium, edited by
Bruce Spiess, Lippincott Williams & Wilkins, Baltimore © 2000.

and the tunica adventitia. The three are not always readily distinguishable because their boundaries are frequently indistinct. The tunica media, in particular, is often difficult to detect. The muscular and elastic tissue is not nearly as well developed in the veins as in the arteries, whereas the connective tissue component is much more prominent.

If we consider the endothelium to be an organ, it would certainly be the largest organ in the body: if we put all of the vessels together (arteries, arterioles, capillaries, veins, and lymphatics), they would stretch to a length of 600 miles, and their endothelial lining would weigh 1.5 kg. The endothelial cells alone would cover an area equivalent to an entire football field.

THE ULTRASTRUCTURE OF VASCULAR ENDOTHELIAL CELLS

Endothelial cells of the intima are polygonal and measure 10 to 15 μm in width and 25 to 50 μm in length. Their long axis is oriented longitudinally in the vessel, and adjacent cells are attached by simple occluding junctions and occasional gap junctions. The cells possess all the common organelles in limited numbers, and these organelles are usually located in the thicker region of the cytoplasm around the flattened nucleus. Under normal conditions, the endothelium is a very slowly renewing tissue with cells rarely found in the cell division cycle. Their plasmalemma have numerous vesicles opening onto both the lumen and the extravascular space. These vesicles seem to be involved in transendothelial transport of water, electrolytes, and macromolecules. Short, blunt processes occasionally extend from the base of the endothelial cells through fenestrae in the elastica interna to establish communicating junctions with smooth muscle cells in the media. Rod-like cytoplasmic inclusions, called Weibel-Palade bodies, are present in arterial endothelial cells; von Willebrand factor (vWF), some adhesion molecules, and tissue-type plasminogen activator (tPA)[3] are stored in these inclusions.

At the capillary level, the capillary wall consists of a basal lamina, a sparse network of reticular fibers, and a layer of extremely attenuated endothelial cells. In cross sections of small capillaries, a single endothelial cell may extend all around the lumen. In larger capillaries, the wall may be made up of portions of two or three cells. The nucleus of capillary endothelial cells is greatly flattened and appears elliptical in cross section. The thicker nuclear region of the cells bulges into the lumen. The peripheral portion of the cell is extremely thin, with the adluminal and abluminal portions separated by a layer of cytoplasm of only 0.2 to 0.4 μm. The Golgi complex is small, and relatively few mitochondria are found in the juxtanuclear region. Lysosomes are rare, but multivesicular bodies are not uncommon. In the blood vessels irrigating muscle, nerves, and connective tissue, the vascular endothelium forms a thin, uninterrupted layer around the entire surface of the capillary; these are designated as continuous or "muscle-type capillaries." In vessels of the pancreas, intestine, and endocrine glands, the endothelium varies in thickness and some regions are interrupted by circular fenestrations 80 to 100 nm in diameter. These pores are closed by a thin diaphragm with a punctured central thickening. In these fenestrated (visceral type) capillaries, only a fraction of the vessel wall typically contains pores, with the remainder resembling the endothelium of muscle-type capillaries.

FUNCTION OF THE VASCULAR ENDOTHELIUM

The vascular endothelium has historically been considered a passive tissue, a layer of nucleated cellphane functioning solely as a barrier between the bloodstream and the vessel wall. More recently, however, important physiological and pharmacological roles are emerging for this tissue. We shall review these roles, particularly in the areas of endothelial control of vascular tone, endothelial involvement in the processes of inflammation and coagulation, and endothelial control of vascular plasticity and growth.

The endothelium releases an array of factors that can act to either contract or relax adjacent vascular smooth muscle. Relaxing factors include prostacyclin (PGI_2), nitric oxide (NO), endothelium-derived hyperpolarizing factor (EDHF), and purines. Constricting factors include endothelin (ET), angiotensin II, thromboxane A_2 (TXA_2), and reactive oxygen species (ROS).

PRODUCTION OF PROSTANOIDS BY ENDOTHELIAL CELLS

Physical stimuli, such as sheer force,[4,5] and chemical stimuli acting on endothelial cell receptors increase intracellular calcium $[Ca^{2+}]_i$ and activate calcium-dependent phospholipase A_2 (PLA_2). This, in turn, hydrolyzes phosphatidylcholine and, to a lesser extent, phosphatidylethanolamine and phosphatidylinositol, which yields free arachidonic acid (AA) and lysophospholipid.[6,7] Agonists that produce these effects include hormones, neurotransmitters, growth factors, and cytokines (ie, thyrotropin-releasing hormone, antidiuretic hormone, bradykinin, serotonin, glutamate, angiotensin II, fibroblast-derived growth factor, platelet-derived growth factor, epidermal growth factor, and interferons).[8–18]

Another less important pathway leading to the production of AA involves phosphatidylinositol; upon activation of guanine-binding G-protein–coupled receptors, phosphatidylinositol is cleaved by phospholipase C (PLC), which produces diacylglycerol (DAG). The metabolism of DAG by DAG lipases yields free AA and glycerol. PLA_2 binds directly to G-proteins, which causes a reduction in the PLA_2 requirement for free calcium,[19,20] thereby activating the enzyme. This binding can occur in the absence of receptor activation. Even if calcium is not required for the activation of some isoforms of PLA_2, calcium will still play an indirect potentiating role by facilitating translocation of the enzyme from the cytosol to the membrane[14] where its phospholipid substrate and a G-protein component[21,22] are available. In endothelial cells, AA can be metabolized by the enzyme cyclooxygenase, which catalyzes the oxidation of AA at the C_9, C_{11}, and C_{15} positions to form the cyclic endoperoxide prostaglandin G_2 (PGG_2). Subsequent reduction of the C_{15} peroxide of PGG_2 to a hydroxyl group yields PGH_2 (peroxidase activity).[23,24] The endoperoxides that produce PGH_2 are metabolized by tissue-specific enzymes (isomerases, synthases, and reductases). In endothelial cells from the large arteries, synthases convert PGH_2 principally to PGI_2,[25-28] whereas in platelets, the predominant synthase product is TXA_2. PGE_2 is the major cyclooxygenase product in macrophages, and prostaglandin $F_{2\alpha}$ is the major cyclooxygenase product in the uterine endometrium.[29] AA can also be metabolized through the lipoxygenase pathway in leukocytes to produce leukotrienes and through the P-450 epoxygenase pathways in endothelial cells.

The eicosanoids mediate a remarkable diversity of physiological responses, which is not surprising given the multiplicity of receptor subtypes specific for each eicosanoid and the many different subtypes of G-protein, each coupled to diverse second messenger pathways.[30] In platelets, PGI_2 receptors are coupled to the G_s subtype of G-protein, which activates the enzyme adenylate cyclase and thereby increases intracellular cyclic adenosine monophosphate (cAMP). Platelet activation by TXA_2, on the other hand, occurs via a subtype of G-protein that is coupled to the enzyme PLC. PLC stimulates the hydrolysis of membrane phosphatidylinositol 4,5 bisphosphate (PIP_2) and produces two second messengers: inositol 1,4,5 triphosphate (IP_3) and 1,2 DAG. IP_3 stimulates calcium release from intracellular stores into the cytoplasm,[31] and DAG activates protein kinase C, which, in turn, phosphorylates and activates several proteins.[32] These processes ultimately lead to platelet activation, aggregation, and secretion.

Eicosanoids, especially the lipoxygenase products, can act as intracellular second messengers and play a significant role in the regulation of ion channels, modulation of endothelial barrier function, and Na^+/K^+ adenosine triphosphatase (ATPase) activity.[33,34] Leukotrienes can also modify cellular shape and stiffness by myosin light chain kinase-mediated polymerization of G-actin to F-actin.[35,36] In endothelial cells, this effect of leukotriene C_4 on cytoskeletal structure can effectively increase the gap between adjacent endothelial cells, thereby increasing vascular permeability. Endothelial cells do not themselves have the lipoxygenase enzyme and are therefore unable to synthesize leukotrienes, but it is common for intermediates of the lipoxygenase pathways to be transferred from circulating leukocytes to the adjacent vascular endothelium where they can be further metabolized.[37] This an example of the cross talking between endothelial cells and circulating cells.

PRODUCTION OF EDRF/NO BY ENDOTHELIAL CELLS

In 1980, Furchgott and Zavadski[38] discovered a novel vasodilator that was released by endothelial cells in response to acetylcholine (ACh) stimulation. This endothelial-derived relaxing factor (EDRF) was soon shown by a number of other groups to be released in response to a plethora of vasoactive compounds and physical stimuli. In 1987, Ignarro et al[39] suggested that EDRF could be NO, and this was confirmed by Palmer et al in 1987.[40] Interestingly, NO is the active moiety of several long-established nitrovasodilators such as nitroglycerine. In 1998, Furchgott, Ignarro, and Murrad were awarded the Nobel prize for their work on the biological role of NO.[41]

NO is produced not only by vascular endothelial cells but also by most of the cells of the body, and it seems to play an important role in the physiology and pharmacology of most organs. Stimulation of endothelial cells by a number of agonists whose receptors are coupled to the G_i subtype of G-protein leads to NO production. These agonists include serotonin, α_2-adrenergic agonists, leukotrienes, and thrombin. Likewise, some G_q-coupled receptors stimulate NO production, including those for bradykinin and adenosine diphosphate. NO is synthesized by nitric oxide synthase (NOS), which transforms L-arginine and oxygen into NO and L-citrulline.[42] Several cofactors, such as NADPH, flavine mononucleotide, flavin dinucleotide, and tetrahydrobiopterin, are required for the synthesis of NO. Three isoforms of NOS have been cloned.[43] The neuronal and endothelial types (nNOS and eNOS, respectively) are mainly found in neurons and endothelial cells, as their names imply. They are constitutively expressed, are calcium-dependent, and produce NO cyclically in picomolar concentrations when the cells are stimulated by chemical or physical stimuli that increase free $[Ca^{2+}]_i$.

Endothelial cells secrete NO in response to substances released from autonomic and sensory nerves (eg, ACh, norepinephrine, ATP, and substance P), circulating hormones (eg, catecholamines, vaso-pressin, angiotensin II, and insulin), coagulation derivatives, platelet products (eg, serotonin, ADP, and thrombin), and autacoids produced by endothelium and vascular smooth muscle cells (eg, bradykinin, purines, angiotensins, and endothelin [ET]).[44,45] The inducible form of NOS (iNOS) can be induced mainly in smooth muscle cells, endothelial cells, cardiomyocytes, and inflammatory cells by various stimuli, including bacterial toxins and cytokines.[43,46,47] Once induced, iNOS is calcium-independent and produces nanomolar concentrations of NO in a continuous manner. nNOS, eNOS, and macrophage-specific iNOS have been sequenced and cloned,[48-51] and the deduced amino acid sequence of eNOS reveals 57% and 50% homology with nNOS and macrophage iNOS, respectively.[50] eNOS, unlike other sequenced NOS isoforms, contains an N-myristoylation consensus sequence that is responsible for its membrane localization,[52] particularly its targeting to membrane caveolae,[42,53,54] which are small invaginations in the plasma membrane that are characterized by the presence of transmembrane regulating protein calveolin.[53,55-57] G-protein–coupled receptors are targeted to caveolae upon agonist stimulation.[42] The presence within caveolae of these receptors may facilitate the activation of NOS by establishing local caveolae domains in which NOS-coupled signaling molecules are in propinquity. eNOS acylation by saturated myristate acid (myristoylation) is required for NOS binding to caveolae[52] and Golgi apparatus[58]; the stabilization of eNOS association with plasmalemma requires eNOS palmitoylation, which is specific for the eNOS isoform.[59-62] Contrary to myristoylation, palmitoylation of eNOS is reversible; agonists acting on $G_s\alpha$ proteins such as bradykinin promote eNOS palmitate turnover. De-palmitoylation represents a plausible mechanism for the release of signaling proteins from the membrane in response to agonist stimulation. Plasmalemmal caveolae are highly enriched in cholesterol and sphingolipids and contain virtually no phospholipids.[55-57] Alterations in cellular lipid composition may profoundly affect caveolae structure and function. A recent publication has shown the opposing effect of cholesterol and ROS on caveolae function and endothelial NO synthase.[63] Bradykinin can stimulate eNOS in endothelial cells through two main pathways. Stimulation of bradykinin B_2 receptors either increases the $[Ca^{2+}]_i$ following receptor–G-protein coupling or increases ceramid (a product of the activation of the "sphingomyelin pathway": hydrolysis of shygomyelin to ceramide) in the caveolae. Ceramid can stimulate eNOS in a calcium-independent manner.[64] The function of eNOS can be regulated not only by calcium, its interaction with caveolae, and Golgi apparatus but also by phosphorylation of serine residues of eNOS. For example, phosphorylation of Ser1177 by phosphotidylinositol-3-OH kinase and the downstream serine/threonine kinase Akt/protein kinase

B by shear stress or by vascular endothelial growth factor (VEGF) induces a prolonged production of NO that is calcium independent.[65,66] The Akt-mediated increase in eNOS activity might represent a major determinant of vessel physiology and architecture and explain the effect of Akt on apoptosis, cell attachment, and cell proliferation.[67,68] Both the inducible and the constitutive NOSs are homodimers with dimer molecular weights of 130 kD and 150 kD, respectively.[48,50] The primary sequence of these enzymes demonstrates that the monomers are composed of an oxygenase and a reductase domain.[48,69] The combination of these two domains on one protein makes this family of enzymes a unique class of P-450 enzyme. Both inducible and constitutive isoforms contain flavins, bound tetrahydrobiopterin, a proton-transferring component, and a heme moiety[50,69–71] and must be composed as homodimers to be functional.

NOS enzymes use NADPH to oxidize L-arginine in a stepwise manner, forming NO and citrulline as primary products.[48,69] The initial step in NO synthesis is NADPH and oxygen-dependent hydroxylation of arginine to form N-hydroxyarginine. Finally, one atom of oxygen is incorporated into NO and one into L-citrulline in a process involving five electron reductions.[72–75]

INHIBITION OF NOS

Analogues of L-arginine, in which a substitution is made at one of the guanidino nitrogen atoms, are competitive antagonists of NOS.[76] These include N^G-monomethyl-L-arginine acetate (L-NMMA), N^G-nitro-L-arginine methyl ester (L-NAME), and N^5(1-iminoethyl)-L-ornithine (L-NIO).[77,78] These arginine analogues are effective inhibitors of both the constitutive and the inducible forms of NOS. Aminoguanidine is another inhibitor and is highly selective for iNOS.[79] Methylene blue inhibits NO activity, presumably via its inhibition of soluble guanylate cyclase[80–82]; alternatively, its inhibitory effects may be mediated by oxygen-derived free radical production or by inhibition of NOS.[83,84] NO itself can inhibit NOS and have a negative feedback on its own production. NO binding to NOS right after its production may keep most of the NOS enzyme (70%–90%) in an inactive, autoinhibiting form.[85] High oxygen concentrations, too, exert an inhibitory effect on NO, probably via production of ROS.

NO METABOLISM

NO interacts avidly with superoxide at diffusion-controlled rates to produce peroxynitrite,[86–89] which rapidly inactivates NO; therefore, reactions between oxygen and NO could be considered negative regulation of NO.[90,91] Superoxide can be produced either by NOS itself,[92,93] the endothelial xanthine,[94] and NADPH oxidase[95] as well as by various metabolic pathways.[96] peroxynitrite itself can produce a variety of effects by behaving as an NO donor[97,98] or by causing various modifications of proteins, including nitration of tyrosine,[99] cysteine residue formation of thiyl radicals and notrosothiols,[100] and inactivation of iron sulfur proteins.[101] The protonated form of peroxynitrite (pK_a 6.8) is rapidly converted to stable nitrate. However, in certain circumstances the concentration of peroxynitrite may become high enough to locally produce damaging species (hydroxyl radical, nitrogen dioxide, and NO_2^+ [nitronium icon]). These may initiate a cascade of events leading to cytotoxicity.[102] Elimination of superoxide by intracellular superoxide dismutase and interaction of peroxynitrite with thiols and functional alcohol groups are powerful detoxication mechanisms in cells. The regulation of superoxide dismutase activity, which controls cellular superoxide levels, is therefore thought to be important for the regulation of NO activity. NO can bind to oxygen and directly form different nitrogen oxide (nitrogen species) that are in different oxidation states.[103] NO can bind to thiol groups in proteins and modify their function. With albumin and hemoglobin, NO forms S-nitrosoalbumin[104] or S-nitrosohemoglobin,[105] which could be a storage form of NO and explain why it can have effects that are distant from the site of production. NO can also be sequestered in molecules composed of proteins combined to dinitro iron complexes to form dinitrosyl-iron complexes (DNIC), another form of NO storage.[89,106] NO binds with high affinity to the heme group of hemoglobin and is metabolized to nitrite, nitrate, and nitric acid.[107,108]

MECHANISMS OF NO ACTIVITY

NO that is produced in endothelial cells is released abluminally and acts upon neighboring smooth muscle and intraluminally, which affects circulating cells and NO-carrying proteins.

The main mechanism of NO action is the activation of soluble guanylate cyclase and ensuing production of cGMP.[109,110] Soluble guanylate cyclases are a family of heterodimers that consist of a 70-kD protein (α subunit) and an 82-kD protein (β subunit);[111,112] each subunit contains a heme of the ferroprotoporphyrin 1X family.[75,113] NO binds to the heme moiety, which causes dislocation of the heme-iron moiety and a subsequent conformational change that permits access to the catalytic site.[52] The physiological functions of cGMP are diverse.[75,78,113] It has direct effects on at least three classes of protein: cGMP-dependent protein kinases, cyclic nucleotide-binding phosphodiesterases, and ion channel proteins.[114,115] cGMP kinases are most abundant in smooth muscle, platelets, cerebellum, cardiac myocytes, and leukocytes.[116] These kinases mediate the cGMP-induced decrease in $[Ca^{2+}]_i$ in vascular smooth muscles by several mechanisms. First, they can activate calcium-dependent ATPase, which leads to the reuptake of calcium from the cytoplasm into the sarcoplasmic reticulum and its extrusion through the plasmalemma.[116,117] cGMP kinase phosphorylates both phospholamban (a regulatory protein of calcium-dependent ATPases in the sarcoplasmic reticulum)[118,119] and the IP_3 receptor on the sarcoplasmic reticulum, which causes a decrease in calcium release from the sarcoplasmic reticulum.[116,117] cGMP also activates potassium channels in smooth muscle cell membranes, which causes cell hyperpolarization and a decrease in $[Ca^{2+}]_i$.[69,120,121] In addition, cGMP potentiates Na^+/Ca^{2+} exchange, thereby decreasing $[Ca^{2+}]_i$ and inducing relaxation.[122] cGMP may also decrease smooth muscle $[Ca^{2+}]_i$ by inhibiting G-protein function[123–125] and PLC activation.[126] In platelets, cGMP reduces $[Ca^{2+}]_i$ by inhibiting PLC.[127] In neutrophils, cGMP mediates agonist-induced chemotaxis and degranulation. These effects are independent of calcium; they are mediated by phosphorylation of the intermediate filament cytoskeleton protein vimentin by a cGMP-dependent kinase.[128] Additional mechanisms of cGMP effects include direct gating of ion channels and interaction with cGMP-binding phosphodiesterase, which modulates the intracellular level of cyclic nucleotides.[116,117,129]

NO has several actions that are not mediated through activation of soluble guanylate cyclase. NO as a free radical can activate ADP ribosyltransferase[130] and inhibit a number of enzymes, including mitochondrial aconitase, electron transport chain complexes I and II, ribonucleotide reductase,[131–133] and protein kinases.[134] Many of the protein/enzyme interactions of NO seem to be caused by its ability to form complexes with iron, both in the presence and absence of a heme group.[135] One example is the previously described binding of NO to the heme group of NOS, which provides negative feedback control of NO synthesis.[136] In addition, NO can modify the function of many proteins via its nitrosylating or nitrating actions. NO also plays an important role in gene regulation. It directly activates several DNA- and RNA-binding factors and induces DNA mutation through deamination, oxidation, and cross-linking.[89,137]

ENDOTHELIAL CELLS AND ENDOTHELIUM-DEPENDENT HYPERPOLARIZATION

While NO and eicosanoids are clearly important endothelium-derived factors with hyperpolarizing and relaxant effects on vascular smooth muscle, not all endothelium-dependent relaxation can be explained by these factors. In 1984, Bolton et al[138] demonstrated that a muscarinic agonist elicited endothelium-dependent hyperpolarization and relaxation of vascular smooth muscle. This phenomenon has since been confirmed in various blood vessels from different species[139–142] and is partially or totally resistant to inhibitors of cyclooxygenase or NOS.[143–145] Hyperpolarization of smooth muscle induces relaxation by reducing the open probability of the voltage-dependent calcium channel, thereby decreasing calcium influx.[146] Additionally, hyperpolarization may reduce the intracellular phosphatidylinositol turnover stimulated by agonist-induced receptor activation.[147] Endothelium-dependent hyperpolarization may involve electrical coupling through myoendothelial junctions; however, although this seems to occur at the microcirculatory level where myoendothelial junctions are numerous, it is unlikely to play an important role in large vessels.[148–151] Because at least part of the endothelium-dependent hyperpolarization is resistant to inhibitors of NOS and cyclooxygenase, it has been attributed to an as-yet unidentified substance known as endothelial derived relaxing factor (EDHF). It has been postulated that EDHF is a short-lived metabolite of AA derived from the P-450 epooxygenase pathway[152–156] or anandamide,[157–159] a cannabinoid derivative of AA.[160–162] These metabolites may be hyperpolarizing factors in some experimental preparations, but it seems unlikely that they represent the major EDHF. Other small, short-lived molecules such as carbon monoxide, hydroxyl radicals, and hydrogen peroxide are all candidates for EDHF because they are produced by the vascular endothelium and induce hyperpolarization of vascular smooth muscle.[140,163]

Endothelium-dependent hyperpolarization induces relaxation by opening potassium channels on smooth muscle cells. The amplitude of the hyperpolarization is inversely related to the extracellular concentration of potassium ions and it disappears if the potassium concentration is higher than 25 mM.[164–166] Inhibitors of calcium-activated potassium channels, such as tetraethylammonium, tetrabutylammonium, apamin, or the combination of apamin plus charybdotoxin, prevent endothelium-dependent hyperpolarization.[165,167,168] Potassium channels are also expressed on endothelial cells where they control potassium efflux. Endothelial cells, therefore, represent a potential source of potassium in the extravascular space, which could induce hyperpolarization of neighboring vascular smooth muscle by activating the inwardly rectifying potassium channel[169] and the Na^+/K^+ pump in rat cerebral arteries as shown by Edwards et al.[169,170] However, this mechanism has not been found to be important in guinea-pig carotid and porcine coronary arteries by Quignard et al.[171]

ENDOTHELIAL-DERIVED CONSTRICTING FACTORS

Endothelial cells release several constricting factors, including angiotensin II, ET, TXA_2, PGH_2, and oxygen-derived free radicals. The precursor, angiotensinogen, is produced by the liver and metabolized by renin to angiotensin I.[172] Angiotensin I is cleaved by angiotensin-converting enzyme (ACE) to become angiotensin II, the active peptide. In vascular smooth muscle, angiotensin II initiates numerous cellular and intercellular signaling events that ultimately lead to vasoconstriction and arterial structural changes.[173] Angiotensin II has two known specific receptors. AT_2 receptor activation induces endothelium-dependent vasodilation and apoptosis and inhibits smooth muscle growth. AT_1 receptor activation causes endothelium-dependent relaxation by a bradykinin-dependent mechanism[174–176] and induces vasoconstriction, cellular growth, sodium and water retention, vascular and cardiac hypertrophy, reduction in renal blood flow, and production of oxygen-derived free radicals.[173,177] Angiotensin II stimulates the generation of superoxide via NADH/NADPH oxidase in vascular smooth muscle and can thereby inactivate NO, with concomitant loss of its relaxant effects.[91,95,177] It also induces the expression and secretion of ET-1 in vascular smooth muscle cells, thereby exacerbating vasoconstriction.[178] Angiotensin II interacts with presynaptic receptors on adrenergic nerves to enhance catecholamine release and can also facilitate catecholamine-induced activation of vascular smooth muscle.[45] Angiotensin II promotes DNA synthesis by activation of mitogenic protein kinases.[173,178–180] In addition, angiotensin II induces the expression of growth factors such as platelet-derived growth factor, insulin-like growth factor, basic fibroblast growth factor, and heparin-binding epidermal growth factor.[173] The stimulation of proliferation induced by angiotensin II may lead to a phenotypically altered population of smooth muscle cells with reduced responsiveness to vasodilators. ACE inhibitors are commonly used to decrease blood pressure and act by several mechanisms. Because they inhibit the conversion of angiotensin to its active form, they effectively decrease angiotensin II levels, with a concomitant decrease in angiotensin-dependent vasoconstriction. Angiotensin II-dependent smooth muscle cell proliferation is also decreased, which seems to maintain smooth muscle cell responsiveness to the relaxant effects of NO. Because ACE is also involved in the metabolism of bradykinin and other kinins, its inhibition enhances the effects of these substances. Bradykinin stimulates NO production in endothelial cells, which, in turn, dilates blood vessels. Inhibition of ACE also decreases ROS production and increases NO activity.

ET exists in three isoforms that are encoded by three different genes ET peptides are generated through several steps.[181,182] ET-1 is the most important peptide. The ET-1 gene codes for a 212-amino acid prepropeptide. Prepro-ET is cleaved by an endopeptidase to form a 38-amino acid intermediate peptide called big ET-1. Big ET-1 is then cleaved between Trp^{21}-Val^{22} by endothelin-converting enzyme, which yields the

21-amino acid ET-1. ET-1 binds to ET-A and ET-B receptors. Vascular tone is normally maintained at a low level and is constantly regulated by the balance between relaxing and contracting factors. Constricting factors can be released from endothelial cells (eg, EDCF), inflammatory cells (eg, platelet-derived growth factor [PDGF]), and nerve terminals (eg, norepinephrine and purines) and may also be circulating hormones (eg, epinephrine and vasopressin).

ENDOTHELIAL DYSFUNCTION

Most arterial diseases are characterized by a deterioration of vasodilator function of the vascular endothelium and smooth muscle layers. Endothelial dysfunction is manifested by either a decrease in secretion of vasodilators or an increase in production of vasoconstrictors.[183–185] For its part, the smooth muscle may have increased sensitivity to these constrictors and/or decreased sensitivity to vasodilators. Thus, the normal balance of dilating and constricting activity is altered, leading to either a "vasodilating state," as in the case of sepsis,[118,186] or a "vasoconstricting state," as seen with atherosclerosis,[177,187] hypercholesterolemia, a high-fat diet, cigarette smoking,[188–190] hypertension,[173] diabetes,[187–191] old age,[192] and male gender.[193] When the endothelium is functionally imbalanced toward the constricting state, the endothelium-derived NO pathway is impaired. This impairment can be caused by downregulation of receptors or signal pathways,[184,185,194] which leads to a decrease in NO production, or by endogenous production of asymmetric methylarginine, an inhibitor of NO synthesis.[195–198] Alternatively, NO activity can be inhibited via interaction with the superoxide anion.[89,91,173,177,199,200] In sepsis, on the other hand, the imbalance of the vessel wall favors a relaxing state because of the induction of an inducible NOS and the production of large amounts of NO by smooth muscle and endothelial cells.[118,186] Exercise training,[201,202] vasodilator medications like ACE inhibitors[203–205] and calcium antagonists,[203,206] and certain foods like fish, fish oil,[207–209] red wine,[210–212] small amounts of alcohol,[213–215] vitamins C and E,[216–218] antioxidants,[219,220] arginine,[189,221,222] and aspirine[223] all interfere with NO production or efficacy, as do hormones such as insulin,[224,225] estrogens,[226] and androgens.[227] The effect of estrogens on vascular function is complex and concentration-dependent, and they vasodilate by both endothelium-dependent and endothelium-independent mechanisms. Estrogens enhance endothelium-dependent relaxation, possibly via an increase in basal or agonist-stimulated production of endothelium-derived relaxing factors such as prostacyclin and NO. Estrogens potentiate the expression of eNOS and scavenge superoxide, thereby enhancing the expression and biological half-life of NO.[228–230] Following cigarette smoking, infection, or inflammation, the endothelium-dependent relaxation is abolished or reduced for several hours because of the release of tumor necrosis factor-α (TNF-α).[231] Aging induces a reduction of endothelium-dependent relaxation; in humans, however, it is difficult to separate the effects of normal aging from those of age-related pathological processes such as hypertension and atherosclerosis.[232-234] In arteries from aging rats, the endothelium-dependent relaxation in response to adenine nucleotides is impaired because of an increase in production of endoperoxides.[235] ET-1–induced endothelium-dependent release of NO and EDHF is absent in old rats, which leaves the potent vasoconstrictor action of ET-1 unopposed at low concentrations.[236] In regenerated endothelium, endothelial cells lose their ability to release NO when challenged by aggregated platelets, thrombin, serotonin, or $_3\alpha_2$-adrenergic receptor agonists.[237-239] Endothelium-dependent relaxation that is induced by these agonists is pertussis toxin sensitive, indicating that their receptors recruit G α_i-proteins for signal transduction coupling.[184,185,194,240] On the other hand, agonists whose receptors are not coupled to G α_i (eg, bradykinin and ADP) maintain their ability to stimulate the release of vasodilators in a regenerated endothelium.[184,185,194] Elevated plasma levels of low-density lipoprotein and cholesterol are major risk factors for atherosclerosis and coronary artery disease. In the porcine model, endothelium-dependent relaxation to serotonin and catecholamines is impaired by hypercholesterolemia. The signal transduction mechanism of endothelial $5HT_{1D}$ serotoninergic and α_2-adrenergic receptors are coupled to pertussis toxin-sensitive G α_i proteins.[184,185,241-243] In humans, hypercholesteremia induces impairment of endothelium-dependent relaxation to ACh, which is pertussis toxin-dependent.[244] In animal models combining endothelial denudation and hypercholesterolemia, the affected arteries first lose pertussis toxin-sensitive endothelium-dependent relaxation; with time, however, all the endothelium-dependent vasodilator mechanisms are reduced.[238-242]

Lysophosphatidylcholine and oxidized lipoproteins, which are important atherogenic mediators, acutely reduce the release of NO and EDHF in vitro.[245] Oxidized low-density lipoproteins downregulate the expression of eNOS.[246] Endothelial dysfunction facilitates the vasoconstrictor and growth-stimulating actions of platelet-derived products, ET-1, and angiotensin II. Together with an increased production of vasoconstrictor prostaglandins and reactive oxygen species, the reduced production or action of NO incapacitates the endothelium to resist to the adhesion and aggregation of platelets as well as leukocytes activation and transendothelial migration, which leads to an inflammatory process that characterizes atherosclerosis.[247,248] As disease progresses, the smooth muscle response to NO and endothelium-dependent hyperpolarization are also impaired; endothelium-dependent hyperpolarization is also impaired in regenerated endothelium.[249] In hypertension, endothelium-dependent vasodilation is reduced.[45,173] The mechanisms underlying endothelial dysfunction vary between different forms of hypertension. In the aorta from spontaneously hypertensive rats, ET induces cyclooxygenase-related contraction of the underlying smooth muscle in response to ACh, purine nucleotides, serotonin, AA, and ET-1.[173,184] There is an increased endothelium-dependent release of PGH_2 by ACh in the aorta of spontaneously hypertensive rats. This is associated with an enhanced expression of cyclooxygenase I, which is primarily expressed in smooth muscle.[250] Perhaps endothelial cells send a signal to the smooth muscle that either induces the secretion of endoperoxides by vascular smooth muscle or facilitates the action of endoperoxides that are basally released. The latter interpretation is favored because of the observation of an increased sensitivity of the smooth muscle to the vaso-constrictive action of PGH_2.[250] Products of cyclooxygenase and the activation of endoperoxide and TXA_2 receptors all seem to be involved in endothelial dysfunction and the associated vascular complications of essential hypertension. Indeed, blunted endothelium-dependent vasodilation to ACh observed in the forearm of human essential hypertensives is partially restored by indomethacin.[232]

In cardiac failure, high peripheral resistance is caused by the impairment of endothelium-dependent vascular relaxation. This, in turn, is because of a reduction of endothelial NO production[251,252] or action by interaction with ROS[199,253] and the release of potent vasoconstrictors such as catecholamines, angiotensin II,[203,254,255] and ET-1.[256,257] ACE inhibitors can not only reduce vasoconstriction but can also partially restore endothelial function.[203,255] Both angiotensin-converting enzyme inhibitor and β-blockers upregulate eNOS activity in the myocardium.[258]

ENDOTHELIUM AND CIRCULATORY CELLS

Under normal conditions, the endothelium maintains the vessels patent by releasing three potent vasodilators that not only increase the lumen diameter but also decrease the shear stress of circulating cells on the vessel wall. NO and prostacyclin have a negative synergistic effect on platelet and leukocyte activation and aggregation; in normal conditions, circulating cells such as leukocytes and platelets do not adhere to the endothelium as they circulate in the most central part of the vessel lumen because adhesion molecules and their corresponding ligands are not expressed on the surface of platelets, leukocytes, and endothelial cells. Following the initialization of inflammatory processes secondary to the local or systemic release of exogenous or endogenous toxins, several cytokines are secreted by vascular and inflammatory cells. Platelet-activating factor and adhesion molecules are expressed on endothelial cells, leukocytes, and platelets.[259] The two most important types of adhesion molecules involved in the interaction between endothelial cells, platelets, and leukocytes are the selectins (P, L, and E), which bind to their ligands on endothelial cells, platelets, and leukocytes and the integrins (CD11 a,b,c/CD18), which are expressed on leukocytes and bind to intercellular adhesion molecule (ICAM) and vascular cell adhesion molecule (VCAM) on endothelial cells. After activation of leukocytes and platelets and expression of adhesion molecules, these cells begin bouncing and rolling along the endothelium because of the tethering action of the selectins. This reversible adhesion greatly reduces the speed of the circulating cells. Irreversible firm adhesion of leukocytes and platelets to the endothelium is then accomplished when the integrins and activated leukocytes release a host of inflammatory mediators, including enzymes (elastase, collagenase, and oxidase), ROS, and leukotrienes.[260–263] Leukocytes also produce pseudopods between endothelial cells and thereby invade the vessel wall. Activated platelets adhere to each other, to leukocytes, and to the vascular wall. This interaction can lead to clot formation and vascular obstruction, which is further exacerbated by the vasoconstriction induced by serotonin and TXA_2 (released by platelets) and leukotrienes (released by leukocytes). The normal vascular endothelium releases NO, prostacyclin, and adenosine, which act synergistically to inhibit platelet and leukocyte activation. The effect of NO on platelet function has been studied extensively[264,265]; it inhibits platelet aggregation, secretion, adhesion, and binding to fibrinogen via the GpIIb/IIIa receptor. The inhibitory effect of NO on platelets is mediated by cGMP protein kinase, which can phosphorylate receptors coupled to G-proteins, particularly the TXA_2 receptor.[266] NO inhibits leukocyte adhesion as well as ROS expression and activity. NO also attenuates leukocyte rolling by non–cGMP-dependent mechanisms: it inhibits P-selectin expression in Weibel-Palade bodies and platelet α granules. NO also attenuates firm leukocyte adhesion by inhibiting GPIIb/IIIa, ICAM-1, and VCAM-1 expression.[267,268] The mechanism for this action is via nuclear factor-κB (NF-κB) inhibition and subsequent reduction of mRNA expression for these adhesion molecules. NF-κB is a group of heterodimer proteins, consisting of a p65 subunit and a p50 subunit, that regulate transcription of a host of genes by binding to specific recognition sequences in the 5′ promoter region of the gene. In unstimulated cells, NF-κB is bound to two proteins in the cell cytoplasm, I-κB α and I-κB β, which sequester it and inhibit its activity by preventing translocation to the nucleus. When NF-κB is stimulated, I-κB is phosphorylated and rapidly breaks down, which releases NF-κB and permits NF-κB–mediated gene transcription for several hours.[269–271] Through inhibition of NF-κB by I-κB, NO and other drugs decrease the expression of proinflammatory substances such as cytokines, chemokines, platelet-activating factor, tissue factor (TF), and others. NO may inhibit NF-κB by three cGMP-independent mechanisms: (1) Scavenging of superoxide which reduces hydrogen peroxide-induced stimulation of NF-κB activity; (2) Increased mRNA expression of I-κB; and (3) Reduction of degradation of the I-κB/NF-κB complex. Some other actions of NO may also mediate its antiinflammatory effects. For example, NO decreases superoxide production by leukocytes and monocytes. Its vasodilator action reduces shear stress and the chances of contact between endothelial cells and circulating inflammatory cells, while increasing washout of procoagulant and proinflammatory compounds. Prostacyclin and adenosine[272] (acting on the A_2 receptor) increase cAMP and activate cAMP-dependent protein kinase, which is a second important pathway of cell regulation. These two compounds have antiinflammatory properties and have a synergistic effect with NO.

ENDOTHELIUM AND COAGULATION

The normal endothelium maintains the vessels patent by several mechanism[273,274]: it dilates them by producing several vasodilators, it inhibits platelet and leukocyte activation, and it has anticoagulant properties. The generation of thrombin to produce fibrin is critical for hemostasis. Thrombin is formed from its inactive zymogen prothrombin by the action of the prothrombinase complex.[275,276] This complex is composed of activated factor X (FXa), calcium, and activated factor V (FVa), which are all bound on a phospholipid surface. The principal initiating pathway of coagulation in vivo is the extrinsic system. A critical component of this system, TF, is a transmembrane glycoprotein that is present on the surface of all cell types that are not normally in contact with the circulation. This cell surface glycoprotein consists of two immunoglobulin-like domains associated through an extensive interdomain, interface region. In addition to the 219-residue extracellular domain, TF consists of a 23-residue transmembrane domain and a 21-residue intracellular domain. The extracellular domain binds to FVII/VIIa . Deletion of the cytoplasmic and transmembrane domains produces a truncated, soluble tissue factor that can be measured. Vascular endothelial cells are the only cells that do not produce TF under normal conditions.[277] After vascular damage, however, TF is expressed and exposed to blood. TF synthesis is induced by endotoxins, interleukin-1 (IL-1), and TNF.[278] Endothelial cells stimulated in vitro by lipopolysaccharide (LPS), thrombin, IL-I, and TNF express TF on their surface. These inflammatory mediators may also induce the production of TF by the endothelium in vivo and induce intravascular coagulation.

Endothelial cells also constitutively express a TF pathway inhibitor (TFPI), which binds to FXa. The complexed TFPI:Xa then goes on to inactivate the complex TF:FVIIa. The endothelium produces glycosaminoglycans (heparan sulfate) and antithrombin III, which combine to inhibit the activity of circulating thrombin. Endothelial cells produce ADPase, which inactivates ADP by dephosphorylation to adenosine monophosphate and subsequently to adenosine and inosine. ADP is released from platelets; its primary role is platelet recruitment by activation of circulating platelets. Endothelial cells express thrombomodulin, a cellular receptor for thrombin. The complex of thrombomodulin and thrombin activates protein C, which is then a cofactor for protein S in inactivating factors Va and VIIIa. Protein C and protein S are naturally occurring anticoagulants and fibrinolytic agents. tPA is produced by endothelial cells and induces fibrinolysis. Besides its multiple pathways for the inhibition of coagulation, endothelial cells synthesize vWF (a cofactor for platelet adhesion), plasminogen activator inhibitor 1 (an inhibitor of tPA), and platelet-activating factor, which increases platelet and leukocyte adhesion to the endothelium. NO and ET have opposing effects on coagulation[278]: the former is one of the most potent inhibitors of platelet activation and coagulation, and the latter is capable of creating a hypercoagulable state. ET can shorten partial thromboplastin time, increase FVIII activity, and decrease antithrombin level, effects that are not induced by other vasoconstrictors such as angiotensin II or norepinephrine. ET suppresses thrombin-stimulated tPA release from endothelial cells with little effect on the tPA inhibitor. These data suggest that ET not only induces a procoagulable state but is also an antifibrinolytic factor.

The endothelium is involved in a wide range of homeostatic processes, including the maintenance of blood fluidity, the control of vascular tone, and the transfer of nutrients and cells between blood and underlying tissue.[279,280] Hemostasis is mediated by a balance of inducible coagulant and anticoagulant forces. Under normal conditions, a delicate balance between the anticoagulant and procoagulant activities of the endothelium is achieved by a series of regulatory linking mechanisms. The temporal and spatial nature of these regulatory mechanisms endows the hemostatic system with tremendous flexibility and is responsible to the specific phenotype of the different vascular bed. What are the mechanisms responsible for generating and maintaining vascular bed–specifc phenotypes? Both extracellular signals and cell-subtype–specific signaling pathways are involved in vascular bed–specific response. Extracellular signals include growth factors, cytokines, mechanical forces, circulating lipoproteins, coagulation factors, components of the extracellular matrix, and neighboring cells.[281–289] Endothelial cells from various vascular beds have different responses to the same signal. For example, increases in blood flow lead to an upregulation of NOS mRNA in the endothelium of the aorta but not in the endothelium from the pulmonary artery.[290] In the heart, only some of the microvascular endothelial cells in the myocardium express the gene for vWF.[284] The restricted distribution of this protein is governed by a signaling pathway mediated by cardiomyocite-dependent, PDGF-αβ heterodimer. Endothelial cells that have receptors for PDGF-α can transduce the signal, whereas neighboring endothelial cells without receptors for PDGF-α lack this ability.

ENDOTHELIUM AND VASCULAR GROWTH

Growth-promoting and growth-inhibiting factors are produced by the endothelium.[291,292] Angiogenesis, the growth of new blood vessels, is a complex process that occurs during wound healing, collateral formation, vascularization of solid tumors, and atherosclerosis.[293,294] This process involves a concerted sequence of events, including degradation of the basement membrane, directional migration and proliferation of endothelial cells, and canalization of solid endothelial cords penetrating the tissue (tube formation). Several factors released by the endothelium stimulate angiogenesis, including fibroblast growth factor, vascular permeability factor, transforming growth factor-α (TGF-α), angiogenin, TGF-β, TNF-α, and insulin-like growth factor. Many of these factors induce NO production by endothelial cells; NO stimulates angiogenesis by cGMP-dependent mechanisms. Angiogenesis is negatively regulated by the combination of heparin and cortisone as well as by thrombospondin, platelet factor, and interferon. A central regulator of angiogenesis is vascular endothelial growth factor (VEGF).[295–300] VEGF exists in different isoforms, and its production is stimulated by hypoxia, oncogenes, and cytokines. VEGF binds to cell surface heparin-sulfate proteoglycans where it can activate its specific receptors. Two receptor subtypes (VEGFR1 and VGEFR2) have been identified on endothelial cells, and both are linked to tyrosine kinase pathways. VEGFR2 has recently been shown to be required for endothelial cell differentiation and for movement of primitive precursors of endothelial cells from the posterior primitive streak to the yolk sac, a precondition for the subsequent formation of blood vessels. VEGFR2 also stimulates endothelial cell division, whereas activation of VEGFR1 induces endothelial cell migration. VEGF stimulates the production of prostacyclin and NO, the latter by prolonged upregulation of eNOS expression.

Clinical trials suggest that VEGF effectively stimulates angiogenesis and collateral circulation in patients suffering from coronary and peripheral artery diseases. Caution in its use for atherosclerosis is warranted, however, as neovascularization may, in fact, favor the growth of atherosclerotic plaques by providing them with nutrients and circulating growth factors.

Normally, smooth muscle cells in the vessel wall (VSMC) are relatively refractory to growth stimuli. The endothelium is important for maintenance of this smooth muscle phenotype: endothelium removal permits initiation of the mitogenic response, and regrowth of normal endothelium inhibits further proliferation.

Heparin and other glycosaminoglycans inhibit VSMC mitogenesis and migration. Heparin is able to reduce neointimal proliferation if administered during the first three days after vascular injury.

The normal endothelium inhibits VSMC growth by secreting growth-inhibitory factors such as NO and transforming growth factor (TGF). In smooth muscle, enhancement of cGMP by NO is growth-inhibitory.[297,301] The effects of TGF include both a direct effect on smooth muscle growth and an indirect effect via alteration of the autocrine production of growth factors (ie, PDGF). TGF can also affect the composition of the extracellular matrix. Glycosaminoglycans and other matrix components are growth-inhibitory for VSMC, as is heparin. In disease states such as atherosclerosis and hypertension, endothelial cells secrete several factors with known smooth muscle mitogenic effects. These include PDGF, insulin-like growth factor 1, IL-1, fibroblast growth factor, and ET.

Vascular structure and remodeling are the result of a balance between cell growth and cell death. Cell death can be either a programmed event (apoptosis) or an accidental one (necrosis). Apoptosis is an active process that involves activation of the caspase family of proteases.[302–305] Activation of the caspase family triggers a cascade of specific biochemical events and morphological changes, which leads to cell death via proteolytic degradation of a number of important proteins, eg, lamin, actin, and poly(ADP-ribose)polymerase.[306–310] Necrotic cell death, on the other hand, is a passive process that results in disruption of the cell membrane and cell death without a series of programmed events.[302]

TGF-β1 can induce endothelial cell apoptosis, whereas it prevents VSMC death.[311] This cell-specific effect is modulated by cell-matrix interactions mediated by β1 integrins. While ROS play a role in cell necrosis via the formation of highly reactive intermediates such as hydroxyl radical,[302] their role in apoptosis is unclear. It seems that the induction of cell death by ROS is a function not only of the cellular concentration of superoxide and hydroxyl radical, but also of the redox status of the cells. Low levels of ROS (superoxide) coupled with a low pH (high H^+ level), known as reductive stress, induce apoptosis; on the other hand, a high level of ROS and high pH, known as oxidative stress, induce necrosis. The role of NO and cGMP in apoptosis and/or necrosis is controversial. Indeed, it has been shown that NO can have proapoptotic or antiapoptotic properties.[312] The antiapoptotic properties are because of NO induction of cytoprotective stress proteins,[313] inhibition of apoptotic signal transduction,[314–316] suppression of caspase activity,[316–318] inhibition of cytochrome *c* release,[319,320] and the induction of protective pathways through the induction of hemeoxygenase[321] or cyclooxygenase pathways.[322] Most of the studies using NO donors or other cGMP-elevating agents report blockade of cell cycle progression and apoptosis.[323–326] Scavenging the endogenous production of NO from epithelial or mesothelial cell lines blocks cell cycle progression in the late S and G_2/M phases, which suggests that NO is required for completion of the cell cycle.[326] In neuronal cells, NO can elicit either necrosis or apoptosis. High concentrations of NO produce a large amount of peroxynitrite upon reaction with superoxide, which damages neurons and causes necrosis.[327,328] Lower concentrations of NO, on the other hand, can interfere with mitochondrial function and lead to apoptosis. Mitochondrial enzymes such as cytochrome oxidase and complexes I–III,[329] in particular, seem to play a role in determining whether NO causes necrosis or apoptosis.[328] The redox status and the balance between NO and ROS could determine NO action on cells death; reductive stress potentiates NO-induced apoptosis and oxidative stress potentiates NO-induced necrosis.[302,330–333] NO could also convert apoptosis into necrosis by S-nitrosylating active site cysteine residues in some of the important effectors of apoptosis, particularly caspases and tissue transglutaminase.[318,334] NO also inhibits the DNA-binding activity of both NF-κB[335–337] and apoptosis protein-1,[338] two transcription factors that are implicated in apoptosis.[339,340]

ENDOTHELIUM AND VASCULAR PERMEABILITY

Endothelial cells interfere with vascular cell permeability. Prostacyclin has been shown to reduce microvascular hydraulic permeability[341–343] at plasma concentrations below those causing vasodilatation.[344] The effect of NO on vascular permeability is more complex. There are studies showing that both NO and cGMP can either decrease[345–347] or increase[348,349] vascular permeability depending on the NO concentration. In normal conditions or after stimulation with bradykinin, endothelial NO or exogenous NO attenuates capillary permeability.[347,350] In sepsis, however, there is a large amount of NO release through the induction of iNOS in different inflammatory cells and endothelium, and smooth muscle cell blockade of NO synthesis decreases vascular permeability.[351] The mechanism of how vascular cells alter permeability via the endothelial derived vasoactive substances is not completely established. However, vasodilatation through an increase in cAMP (stimulation by prostacyclin) or through an increase in cGMP (stimulation by NO) reduces the intraendothelial microfilament tension and the intercellular space.[352] Conversely, vasoconstrictors such as leukotriene-B4 that stimulate the cytoskeleton in the endothelial cells and the intercellular space increase the permeability. cAMP and cGMP also interfere with leukocyte and platelet adhesion to endothelial cells and the inflammatory process. Endothelial cells also regulate the matrix composition.[353,354] Other mechanisms by which endothelial cells can interfere with vascular permeability include effects on cell-to-cell adhesion, interstitial matrix composition, cell and matrix interaction, and the electrical loading of endothelial cells and plasma proteins.[352,355]

CONCLUSION

This chapter reviewed the important role of the endothelium in vascular physiology and the pharmacology of the vascular wall as well as the role of different regulatory mediators released by endothelial cells in normal and pathological conditions. In particular, this chapter focussed on the role of NO because it has been extensively studied and because NO is often an unavoidable step in the action of medications or intermediates that interfere with vascular homeostasis. Furthermore, the role of NO is complex and could have both beneficial and detrimental effects in the same pathology. For example, if NO-induced apoptosis is effective at reducing restenosis after balloon coronary angioplasty, NO produced by the iNOS could induce apoptosis of smooth muscle cells in coronary atherosclerotic plaque. The disparition of smooth muscles could weaken the plaque, which could then rupture and induce platelet aggregation and thrombosis, causing unstable angina or myocardial i nfarction.[356]

References

1. Blood and Lymph Vascular Systems. In: Fawcett DW. A Textbook of Histology. 11th ed. Philadelphia: WB Saunders Company, 1986: 367–405
2. Majno G, Joris I: Endothelium 1977: A Review. AdV Exp Med Biol 1978; 104:169–225, 481–526
3. Rosnoblet C, Vischer UM, Gerard RD, Irminger JC, Halban PA, Kruithof EK: Storage of tissue-type plasminogen activator in

Weibel-Palade bodies of human endothelial cells. Arterioscler Thromb Vasc Biol 19:1796–1803, 1999

4. Karwatowska-Prokopczuk E, Ciabbattoni G, Wennmalm A: Effects of hydrodynamic forces on coronary production of prostacyclin and purines. Am J Physiol 256:H1532-H1538, 1989

5. Koller A, Sun D, Kaley G: Role of shear stress and endothelial prostaglandins in flow-and viscosity-induced dilatation of arterioles in vitro. Circ Res 72:1276–1284, 1993

6. Lister MD, Deems RA, Watanabe U, Ulevitch R, Dennis EA: Kinetic analysis of the Ca^{2+}-dependent, membrane- bound, macrophage phospholipase A_2 and the effects of arachidonic acid. J Biol Chem 263:7506–7513, 1988

7. Ulevitch TJ, Watanabe Y, Sano M, Lister MD, Deems RA, Denis EA: Solubilization, purification, and characterization of a membrane-bound phospholipase A_2 from the P388D1 macrophage-like cell line. J Biol Chem 263:3079–3085, 1988

8. Judd AM, MacLeao RM: Thyrotropin-releasing hormone and lysine-bradykinin stimulate arachidonate liberation from rat anterior pituitary cells through different mechanisms. Endocrinology 131:1251–1260, 1992

9. Garcia-Perez A, Smith WL: Apical-basolateral membrane asymmetry in canine cortical collecting tubule cells: Bradykinin, arginine vasopressin, prostaglandin E_2 interrelationships. J Clin Invest 74: 63–74, 1984

10. Felder CC, Kanterman RY, Ma AL, Axelrod J: Serotonin stimulates phospholipase A_2 and the release of arachidonic acid in hippocampal neurons by a type 2 serotonin receptor that is independent of inositolphospholipid hydrolysis. Proc Natl Acad Sci USA 87: 2187–2191, 1990

11. Aramori I, Nakanishi S: Signal transduction and pharmacological characteristics of a metabotropic glutamate receptor, MGluR1, in transfected CHO cells. Neuron 8:757–765, 1992

12. Fafeur V, Jiang ZP, Bohlen P: Signal transduction by bFGF, but not TGFb1, involves arachidonic acid metabolism in endothelial cells. J Cell Physiol 14:277–283, 1991

13. Bonventre JV, Weber PC, Gronich JH: PAF and PDGF increase cytosolic $[Ca^{2+}]$ and phospholipase activity in mesangial cells. Am J Physiol 254:F87–F94, 1988

14. Channon JY, Leslie CC: A calcium-dependent mechanism for associating a soluble arachidonoyl-hydrolyzing phospholipase A_2 with membrane in the marcophage cell ligne RAW 264.7. J Biol Chem 265:5409–5413, 1990

15. Hannigan GE, Williams BR: Signal transduction by interferon-α through arachidonic acid metabolism. Science 251:204–207, 1991

16. Ponzoni M, Montaldo PG, Cornaglia-Ferraris P: Stimulation of re-

ceptor-coupled phospholipase A_2 by interferon-γ. FEBS Lett 310: 17–21, 1992

17. Dennis EA: Regulation of eicosanoid production: Role of phospholipases and inhibitors. Biotechnology 5:1294–1300, 1985

18. Neufeld EJ, Majerus PW: Arachidonate release and phosphatidic acid turnover in stimulated human platelets. J Biol Chem 258: 2461–2467, 1983

19. Nakashima S, Nagata KI, Ueeda K, Nozawa Y: Stimulation of arachidonic acid release by guanine nucleotide in saponin-permeabilized neutrophils: Evidence for involvement of GTP-binding protein in phospholipase A_2 activation. Arch Biochim Biophys 261:375–383, 1988

20. Axelrod J, Burch RM, Jelsema CL: Receptor-mediated activation of phospholipase A_2 via GTP-binding proteins: Arachidonic acid and its metabolites as second messengers. Trends Neurosci 11:117–123, 1988

21. Cantiello HF, Patenaude CR, Codina J, Birnbaumer L, Ausiello DA: Gα i-3 regulates epithelial Na$^+$ channels by activation of phospholipase A_2 and lipoxygenase pathways. J Biol Chem 265:21 624–21628, 1990

22. Christ-Hazelhof E, Nugteren DH: Prostacyclin is not a circulating hormone. Protaglandins 22:739–746, 1981

23. Ohki S, Ogino N, Yamamoto S, Hayaishi O: Prostaglandin hydroperoxidase, an integral part of prostaglandin endoperoxide synthetase from bovine vesicular gland microsomes. J Biol Chem 254:829–836, 1979

24. Pagels WR, Sachs RJ, Marnett LJ, DeWitt DL, Day JS, Smith WL: Immunochemical evidence for the involvement of prostaglandin H synthase in hydroperoxide-dependent oxidations by ram seminal vesicle microsomes. J Biol Chem 258:6517–6523, 1983

25. DeWitt DL, Day JS, Sonneburg WK, Smith WL: Concentrations of prostaglandin endoperoxide synthase and prostaglandin I_2 synthase in the endothelium and smooth muscle of bovine aorta. J Clin Invest 72:1882–1888, 1983

26. Ingerman-Wojenski C, Silver MJ, Smith JB, Macarak E: Bovine endothelial cells in culture produce thromboxane as well as prostacyclin. J Clin Invest 67:1292–1296, 1981

27. Gerritsen ME, Cheli CD: Arachidonic acid and prostaglandin endoperoxide metabolism in isolated rabbit and coronary microvessels and isolated and cultivated coronary microvessel endothelial cells. J Clin Invest 72:1658–1671, 1983

28. Goldsmith JC, Needleman SW: A comparison study of thromboxane and prostacyclin release from ex vivo and cultured bovine vascular endothelium. Prostaglandins 24:173–178, 1982

29. Huslig RL, Fogwell RL, Smith WL: The prostaglandin forming

cyclooxygenase of ovine uterus: Relationship to luteal function. Biol Reprod 21:589–600, 1979

30. Crooke ST, Mong S, Sarau HM, Winkler JD, Vegesna VK: Mechanism of regulation of receptors and signal transduction pathways for the peptidyl leukotrienes. Ann NY Acad Sci 524:153–161, 1991

31. Brass LF, Shaller CC, Belmonte J: Inositol 1,4,5-triphosphate-induced granule secretin in platelets. J Clin Invest 79:1269–1275, 1987

32. de Chaffoy de Courcelles D, Roevens P, Van Belle H, Kennis L, Somers Y, DeClerck F: The role of endogenously formed diacylglycerol in the propagation and termination of platelet activation: A biochemical and functional analysis using the novel diacyglycerol kinase inhibitor R59 949. J Biol Chem 264:3274–3285, 1989

33. McGiff JC: Cytochrome P-450 metabolism of arachidonic acid. Annu Rev Pharmacol Toxicol 31:339–369, 1991

34. Freeman EJ, Terrian DM, Dorman RV: Presynaptic facilitation of glutamate release from isolated hippocampal mossy fiber nerve endings by arachidonic acid. Neurochem Res 15:743–750, 1990

35. Wysolmerski RB, Lagunoff D: Involvement of myosin light-chain kinase in endothelial cell retraction. Proc Natl Acad Sci USA 87:16–20, 1990

36. Wysolmerski RB, Lagunoff D: Regulation of permeabilized endothelial cell retraction by myosin phosphorylation. Am J Physiol 261:C32–40, 1991

37. Fein SJ, Cannon PJ: Endothelial cell leukotriene C_4 synthesis results from intercellular transfer of leukotriene A_4 synthesized polymorphonuclear leukocytes. J Biol Chem 261:16466–16472, 1986

38. Furhgott RF, Zawadzki JV: The obligatory role of endothelial cells in the relaxation of arterial smooth muscle by acetylcholine. Nature 280:373–376, 1980

39. Ignarro LJ, Buga GM, Wood KS, Byrns RE, Chaudhuri G: Endothelium-derived relaxing factor produced and released from artery and vein is nitric oxide. Proc Natl Acad Sci USA 84:9265–9569, 1987

40. Palmer RM, Ferrige AG, Moncada S: Nitric oxide release accounts for the biological ativity of endothelium-derived relaxing factor. Nature 327:524–526, 1987

41. Murad Furad: Nitric oxide leads to prized NObility: Background to the work of Ferid Murad. Texas Heart Institute J 26:1–5, 1999

42. Michel T, Feron O: Nitric oxide synthases: Which, where, how and why? J Clin Invest 100:2146–2152, 1997

43. Nathan C: Induce nitric oxide synthase: What difference does it make? J Clin Invest 100:2417–2423, 1997

44. Bassenge E, Heuch G: Endothelial and neurohumoral control of coronary blood flow in health and disease. Rev Physiol Biochem Pharmacol 116:79–163, 1990
45. Vanhoutte PM: Endothelium and control of vascular function: State of the art lecture. Hypertension 13:658–667, 1989
46. Busse R, Mulsch A: Induction of nitric oxide synthase by cytokines in vascular smooth muscle cells. FEBS 275:87–90, 1990
47. Nathan C: Nitric oxide as a secretory product of mammalian cells. FASEB J 6:3051–3064, 1992
48. Bredt DS, Hwang PM, Glatt CE, Lowenstein C, Reed RR, Snyder SH: Cloned and expressed nitric oxide synthase structurally resembles cytochrome P-450 reductase. Nature 351:714–718, 1991
49. Janssens SP, Shimouchi A, Quertermous T, Bloch DB, Bloch KD: Cloning and expression of a cDNA encoding human endothelium-derived relaxing factor/nitric oxide synthase. J Biol Chem 267:14519–14522, 1992
50. Sessa WC, Harrison JK, Barber CM, Zeng D, Durieux ME, D'Angelo DD, Lynch KR, Peach MJ: Molecular cloning and expression of a cDNA encoding endothelial cell nitric oxide synthase. J Biol Chem 267:15274–15276, 1992
51. Xie QE, Cho HJ, Calaycay J, Mumford RA, Swiderek KM, Lee TD, Ding A, Troso T, Nathan C: Cloning and characterization of inducible nitric oxide synthase from mouse macrophages. Science 256:225–228, 1992
52. Busconi L, Michel T: Endothelial nitric oxide synthase: N-terminal myristoylation determines subcellular localization. J Biol Chem 268:8410–8413, 1993
53. Feron O, Belhassen L, Kobzik L, Smith TW, Michel T: Endothelial nitric oxide synthase targeting to caveolae: Specific interactions with caveolin isoforms in cardiac myocytes and endothelial cells. J Biol Chem 271:22810–22814, 1996
54. Shaul PW, Smart EJ, Robinson LJ, German Z, Yuhanna IS, Ying Y, Anderson RG, Michel T: Acylation targets endothelial nitric-oxide synthase to plasmalemmal caveolae. J Biol Chem 271:6518–6522, 1996
55. Anderson RG: Caveolae: Where incoming and outgoing messengers meet. Prot Natl Acad Sci USA 90:10909–10913, 1993
56. Parton RG: Caveolae and caveolins. Curr Opin Cell Biol 8:542–548, 1996
57. Couet J, Li S, Okamato T, Scherer PE, Lisanti MP: Molecular and cellular biology of caveolae. Trends Cardiovasc Med 4:103–110, 1997
58. Sessa WC, Garcia-Cardena G, Liu J, Keh A, Pollock JS, Bradley J, Thiuri S, Braverman IM, Desai KM: The Golgi association of endothe-

lial nitric oxide synthase is necessary for the efficient synthesis of nitric oxide. J Biol Chem 270:17641–17644, 1995

59. Robinson LJ, Michel T: Mutagenesis of palmitoylation sites in endothelial nitric oxide synthase identifies a novel motif for dual acylation and subcellular targeting. Proc Natl Acad Sci USA 92: 11776–11780, 1995

60. Shaul PW, Smart ET, Robinson L, German Z, Yuhanna IS, Ying Y, Anderson RG, Michel T: Acylation targets endothelial nitric-oxide synthase to plasmalemmal caveolae. J Biol Chem 271:6518–6522, 1996

61. Garcia-Cardeba G, Oh P, Liu J, Schnitzer JE, Sessa WC: Targeting of nitric oxide synthase to endothelial cell caveolae via palmitoylation: Implications for nitric oxide signaling. Proc Natl Acad Sci USA 96:6448–6453, 1996

62. Liu J, Garcia-Cardeba G, Sessa WC: Biosynthesis and palmitoylation of endothelial nitric oxide synthase: Mutagenesis of palmitoylation sites, cysteines-15 and/or -26, argues against depalmitoylation-induced translocation of the enzyme. Biochemistry 34: 12333–12340, 1995

63. Peterson TE, Poppa V, Ueba H, Wu a, Yan C, Berk BC: Opposing effects of reactive oxygen species and cholesterol on endothelial nitric oxide synthase and endothelial cell caveolae. Circ Resp 85: 29–37, 1999

64. Igarashi J, Thatte H, Prabhakar P, Golan DE, Michel T: Ceramide and Ca^{2+}-independent activation of endothelial no synthase. Acta Physiol Scand 167:6, 1999

65. Fulton D, Gratton JP, McCabe TJ, Fontana J, Fujio Y, Walsh K, Franke TF, Papapetropoulos A, Sessa WC: Regulation of endothelium-derived nitric oxide production by the protein kinase Akt. Nature 399:597–601, 1999

66. Dimmeler S, Fleming I, Fisslthaler B, Hermann C, Busse R, Zeiher AM: Activation of nitric oxide synthase in endothelial cells by Akt-dependent phosporylation. Nature 399:601–605, 1999

67. Khwaja A, Rodriquez-Viciana P, Wennström S, Warne, PH, Downward J: Matrix adhesion and ras transformation both activate a phosphoinositide 3-OH kinase and protein kinase B/Akt cellular survival pathway. Embo J 16:2783–2793, 1997

68. Kuffmann-Zeh A et al: Suppression of c-Myc-induced apoptosis by Ras signalling through PI(3)K and PKB. Nature 385:544–548, 1997

69. White KA, Marletta MA: Nitric oxide synthase is a cytochrome P-450 type hemoprotein. Biochemistry 130:319–322, 1992

70. Hevel JM, Marletta MA: Macrophage nitric oxide synthase: Relationship between enzyme-bound tetrahydrobiopterin and synthase activity. Biochemistry 31:7160–7165, 1992

71. Hevel JM, Marletta MA: Macrophage nitric oxide synthase: Tetrahydrobiopterin decreases sthe NADPH stoichiometry. Adv Exp Med Biol 338:285–288, 1993

72. Know NS, Nathan CF, Gilker C, Griffith OW, Matthews DE, Stuehr DJ: L-citrulline production from L-arginine by macrophage nitric oxide synthase: The ureido oxygen derives from dioxygen. J Biol Chem 265:13442–13445, 1990

73. Moncada S: The L-arginine: Nitric oxide pathway. Acta Physiol Scand 145:201–227, 1992

74. Rengasamy A, Johns RA: Characterization of EDRF/NO synthase from bovine cerebellum and mechanism of modulation by high and low oxygen tensions. J Pharmacol Exp Ther 259:310–316, 1991

75. Schmidt HH, Lohmann SM, Walter U: The nitric oxide and cGMP signal transduction system: Regulation and mechanism of action. Biochim Biophys Acta 1178:153–175, 1993

76. Rees D, Palmer RMJ, Hodson HF, Moncada S: A specific inhibitor of nitric oxide formation from L-arginine attenuates endothelium-dependent relaxation. Br J Pharmacol 96:418–424, 1989

77. Johns RA, Peach MJ, Linden J, Tichotsky A: N^G-monomethyl-L-arginine inhibits endothelium-derived relaxing factor-stimulated cyclic GMP accumulation in cocultures of endothelial and vascular smooth muscle cells by an action specific to the endothelial cell. Circ Res 67:979–985, 1990

78. Moncada S, Palmer RM: Nitric oxide: Physiology, pathophysiology, and pharmacology. Pharmacol Rev 88:134–138, 1991

79. Misko TP, MooreWM, Kasten TP, Nickols GA, Corbett JA, Tilton RG, McDaniel ML, Williamson JR, Currie MG: Selective inhibition of the inducible nitric oxide synthase by aminoguanidine. Eur J Pharmacol 233:119–125, 1993

80. Yu P, Robin J, Pattison CW: Reversal of refractory hypotension with single-dose methylene blue after coronary artery bypass surgery. J Thorac Cardiovasc Surg 118:195–196, 1999

81. Deutsch SI, Rosse RB, Mastropaolo J: Behavioral approaches to the functional assessment of NMDA-mediated neural transmission in intact mice. Clin Neuropharmacol 20:375–384, 1997

82. Iadecola C, Li J, Ebner TJ, Ebner TJ, Xu X: Nitric oxide contributes to functional hyperemia in cerebellar cortex. Am J Physiol 268:R1153-R1162, 1995

83. Mayer B, Brunner F, Schmidt K: Inhibition of nitric oxide synthesis by methylene blue. Biochem Pharmacol 45:367–374, 1993

84. Volke V, Wegener G, Vasar E, Rosenberg R: Methylene blue inhibits hippocampal nitric oxide synthase activity in vivo. Brain Research 826:303–305, 1999

85. Dewanjee MK: Molecular biology of nitric oxide synthases: Re-

duction of complications of cardiopulmonary bypass from platelets and neutrophils by nitric oxide generation from L-arginine and nitric oxide donors. ASAIO J 43:151–159, 1997

86. Beckman JS, Koppenol WH: Nitric oxide, superoxide and peroxynitrite: The good, the bad and ugly. Am J Physiol 271:C1424–C1437, 1996

87. Szabo C: The role of peroxynitrite in the pathophysiology of shock, inflammation and ischemia-reperfusion injury. Shock 6:79–88, 1996

88. Szabo C, Billiar TR: Novel roles of nitric oxide in hemorrhagic shock. Shock 12:1–9, 1999

89. Stoclet JC, Troncy E, Mulleer B, Brua C, Kleschyov AL: Molecular mechanisms underlying the role of nitric oxide on the cardiovascular system. Exp Opin Invest Drugs 7:1769–1779, 1998

90. Langenstroer P, Pieper GM: Regulation of spontaneous EDRF release in diabetic rat aorta by oxygen free radicals. Am J Physiol Heart Circ Physiol 263:H257–H265, 1992

91. Koh KK, Bui MN, Hathaway L, Csako G, Waclawiw MA, Panza JA, Cannon RO III: Mechanism by which quinapril improves vascular function in coronary artery disease. Am J Cardiol 83:327–31, 1999

92. Xia Y, Dawson VL, Dawson TM, Snyder SH, Zweier JL: Nitric oxide synthase generates superoxide and nitric oxide in arginine-depleted cells leading to peroxynitrite-mediated cellular injury. Proc Natl Acad Sci USA 93:6770–6774, 1996

93. Xia Y, Zweier JL: Superoxide and peroxynitrite generation from inducible nitric oxide synthase in macrophages. Proc Natl Acad Sci USA 94:6957–6958, 1997

94. Tan LR, Xaxman K, Clark L, Eloi L, Chhieng N, Miller B, Young A: Superoxide dismutase and allopurinol improve survival in a animal model of hemorrhagic shock. Am Surg 59:797–800, 1993

95. Warnholtz A, Nickenig G, Schulz E, Macharzina R, Brasen JH, Skatchkov M, Heitzer T, Stasch JP, Griendling KK, Harrison DG, Bohm M, Meinertz T, Munzel T: Increased NADH-oxidase-mediated superoxide production in the early stages of atherosclerosis: Evidence for involvement of the renin-angiotensin system. Circulation 99:2027–2033, 1999

96. Nohl H: Generation of superoxide radicals as hyproduct of cellular respiration. Ann Biol Clin 52:199–204, 1994

97. Moro MA, Darley-Usmar VM, Lizasoain I, Su Y, Knowles RG, Radomski MW, Moncada S: The formation of nitric oxide donors from peroxynitrite. Br J Pharmacol 116:1999–2004, 1996

98. Moro Ma, Darley-Usmar VM, Goodwin DA, Read NG, Zamora-Pino R, Feelisch M, Radomski MW, Moncada S: Paradoxical fate

and biological action of peroxynitrite on human platelets. Proc Natl Acad Sci USA 91:6702–6706, 1994

99. Ischiropoulos H: Biological tyrosine nitration: A pathophysiological function of nitric oxide and reactive oxygen species. Arch Biochem Biophys 356:1–11, 1998

100. Scorza G, Minetti M: One-electron oxidation pathway of thiols by peroxynitrite in biological fluids: Bicarbonate and ascorbate promote the formation of albumin disulphide dimers in human blood plasma. Biochem J 329:405–413, 1998

101. Bouton G, Hirling H, Drapier JC: Redox modulation of iron regulatory proteins by peroxynitrite. J Biol Chem 272:19969–19975, 1997

102. Beckman JS, Beckman TW, Chen J, Marshall PA, Freeman BA: Apparent hydroxyl radical production by peroxynitrite: Implications for endothelial injury from nitric oxide and superoxide. Proc Natl Acad Sci USA 87:1620–1624, 1990

103. van der Vliet A, Eiserich JP, Shigenaga MK, Cross CE: Reactive nitrogen species and tyrosine nitration in the respiratory tract. Am J Resp Crit Care Med 160:1–9, 1999

104. Gow AJ, Luchsinger BP, Pawloski JR, Singel DJ, Stamler JS: The oxyhemoglobin reaction of nitric oxide. Proc Natl Acad Sci USA 96:9027–9032, 1999

105. Jia L, Bonaventura C, Bonaventura J, Stamler JS: S-nitrosophaemoglobin: A dynamic activity of blood involved in vascular control. Nature 380:221–226, 1996

106. Muller B, Kleschyov AL, Stoclet JC: Evidence for N-acetylcysteine-sensitive nitric oxide storage as dinitrosyl-iron complexes in lipopolysaccaharide-treated rat aorta. Br J Pharmacol 119:1281–1285, 1996

107. Frostell C, Fratacci MD, Wain JC, Jones R, Zapol WM: Inhaled nitric oxide: A selective pulmonary vasodilator reversing hypoxic pulmonary vasoconstriction. Circulation 83:2038–2047, 1991

108. Gibson QH, Roughton FJ: The kinetics of equilibria of the reactions of nitric oxide with sheep hemoglobin. J Physiol (London) 136:507–526, 1957

109. Mayer B, Pfeiffer S, Schrammel A, Koesling D, Schmidt K, Brunner F: A new pathway of nitric oxide/cyclic GMP signaling involving S-nitrosoglutathione. J Biol Chem 273:3264–3270, 1998

110. Rapoport R, Murad F: Endothelium-dependent and nitrovasodilator-induced relaxation of vascular smooth muscle: Role of cyclic GMP. J Cyclic Nucleotide Prot Phos Res 9:281–296, 1983

111. Koesling D, Bohme E, Shultz G: Guanylyl cyclases: A growing family of signal-transducing enzymes. FASEB J 5:2785–2791, 1991

112. Nakane M, Saheki S, Kuno T, Ishii K, Murad F: Molecular cloning

of a 70 kilodalton subunit of soluble guanylate cyclase from rat lung. Biochem Biophys Res Commun 157:1139–1147, 1988

113. Waldman SA, Murad F: Cyclic GMP synthesis and function. Pharm Rev 39:163–196, 1987

114. Bredt DS, Snyder SH: Nitric oxide, a novel neuronal messenger. Neuron 8:3–11, 1992

115. Garland CJ, McPherson GA: Evidence that nitric oxide does not mediate the hyperpolarization and relaxation to acetylcholine in the rat small mesenteric artery. Br J Pharmacol 105:429–435, 1992

116. Lincoln TM, Cornwell TL: Intracellular cyclic receptor proteins. FASEB J 7:328–338, 1993

117. Lincoln TM: Cyclic GMP and mechanisms of vasodilatation. Pharmacol Ther 41:479–502, 1989

118. Kilbourn RG, Griffith OW: Overproduction of nitric oxide in cytokine-mediated and septic shock. J Natl Cancer Inst 342:762–766, 1992

119. Michel T, Li GK, Busconi L: Phosphorylation and subcellular translocation of endothelial nitric oxide synthase. Proc Natl Acad Sci USA 90:6252–6256, 1993

120. Chen XL, Rembold CM: Cyclic nucleotide-dependent regulation of Mn^{2+} influx, $[Ca^{2+}]_i$, and arterial smooth muscle relaxation. Am J Physiol 263:C468-C473, 1992

121. Forstermann U, Pollock JS, Schmidt HH, Heller M, Murad F: Calmodulin-dependent endothelium-derived relaxing factor/nitric oxide synthase activity is present in the particulate and cytoscolic fractions of bovine aortic Ecs. Proc Natl Acad Sci USA 88:1788–1792, 1991

122. Furukawa K-I, Ohshima N, Tawada-Iwata Y, Shigekawa M: Cyclic GMP stimulates Na^+/Ca^{2+} exchange in vascular smooth muscle cells in primary culture. J Biol Chem 266:12337–12341, 1991

123. H, Ikebe T, Murad FHirata M, Kohse KP, Chang CH, Ikebe T, Murad F: Mechanism of cyclic GMP inhibition of inositol phosphate formation in rat aorta segments and cultured bovine aortic smooth muscle cells. J Biol Chem 265:1268–1273, 1990

124. Holzmann S: Endothelium-induced relaxation by acetylcholine associated with larger rises in cyclic GMP in coronary arterial strips. J Cyclic Nucleotide Res 8:409–419, 1982

125. Light DB, Corbin JD, Stanto BA: Dual ion-channel regulation by cyclic GMP and cyclic GMP-dependent protein kinase. Nature 344:336–339, 1990

126. Rapoport RM: Cyclic guanosine monophosphate inhibition of contraction may be mediated through inhibition of phosphatidylinositol hydrolysis in rat aorta. Circ Res 58:407–410, 1986

127. Radomski MW, Palmer RM, Moncada S: Glucocorticoids inhibit the

expression of an inducible, but not the constitutive, nitric oxide synthase in vascular ECs. Proc Natl Acad Sci USA 87:10043– 10047, 1990

128. Wyatt TA, Lincoln TM, Pryzwansky KB: Vimentin is transiently colocalized with and phosphorylated by cyclic GMP-dependent protein kinase in formyl-peptide stimulated neutrophils. J Biol Chem 266:21274–21280, 1991

129. Ono K, Trauwein W: Potentiation by cyclic GMP of β-adrenergic effect on Ca^{2+} current in guinea-pig ventricular cells. J Physiol 443:387–404, 1991

130. Bruce B, Lapetina EG: Activation of a cytosolic ADP-ribosyltrasferase by nitric oxide-generating agents. J Biol Chem 264:8455– 8458, 1989

131. Harbrecht BG, Stadler J, Billiar TR, et al: Inhibition of glutathione metabolism decreases hepatocyte nitric oxide synthesis. FASEB J 5:A371-ABS#4364, 1991

132. Lancaster JE Jr, Hibbs JB Jr: EPR demonstration of iron-nitrosyl complex formation by cytotoxic activated macrophages. Proc Natl Acad Sci USA 87:1223–1227, 1990

133. Mayer B, Heinzel B, Klatt P, John M, Schmidt K, Bohme E: Nitric oxide synthase-catalyzed activation of oxygen and reduction of cytochromes: Reaction mechanisms and possible physiological implications. J Cardiovasc Pharmacol 20(Suppl 12):S54-S56, 1992

134. Gopalakrishna R, Chen ZH, Guidimeda U: Nitric oxide and nitric oxide-generating agents induce a reversible inactivation of protein kinase C activity and phorbol ester binding. J Biol Chem 268: 27180–27185, 1993

135. McDonald CC, Philips WO, Mower HF: An electron spin resonance study of some complexes of iron, nitric oxide and amionic ligands. J Am Chem Soc 87:3319–3326, 1965

136. Rengasamy A, Johns RA: Regulation of nitric oxide synthase by nitric oxide. Mol Pharmacol 44:124–128, 1993

137. Nathan C, Xie Q: Nitric oxide synthases: Roles, tolls, and controls. Cell 78:915–918, 1994

138. Bolton TB, Lang RJ, Takewaki T: Mechanism of action of noradrenaline and carbochol on smooth muscle of guinea-pig anterior mesenteric artery. J Physiol 351:549–572, 1984

139. Feletou M, Vanhoutte PM: Endothelium-dependent hyperpolarization of canine coronary smooth muscle. Br J Pharmacol 93: 515–524, 1988

140. Feletou M, Vanhoutte PM: Endothelial dysfunction: A novel therapeutic Target. The alternative: EDHF. J Mol Cell Cardiol 31:15–22, 1999

141. Chen G, Suzuki H, Weston AH: Acetylcholine releases endothelium-

derived hyperpolarizing factor and EDRF from rat blood vessels. Br J Pharmacol 95:1165–1174, 1988

142. Brayden JE: Membrane hyperpolarization is a mechanism of endothelium-dependent cerebral vasodilatation. Am J Physiol 259:H668-H673, 1990

143. Cowan CL, Cohen RA: Two mechanisms mediate relaxation by bradykinin of pig coronary artery: NO-dependent and independent responses. Am J Physiol 261:H830-H835, 1991

144. Mügge A, Lopez JAG, Piegors DJ, Breese KR, Heistad DD: Acetylcholine-induced vasodilatation in rabbit hindlimb in vivo is not inhibited by analogues of L-arginine. Am J Physiol 260:H242-H247, 1991

145. Suzuki H, Chen G, Yamamoto Y, Niwa K: Nitro-arginine-sensitive and insensitive components of the endothelium-dependent relaxation in the guinea-pig carotid artery. Jpn J Physiol 42:335–347, 1992

146. Nelson MT, Patlak JB, Worley JF, Stanben NB: Calcium channels, potassium channels, and voltage dependence of arterial smooth muscle tone. Am J Physiol 259:C3-C18, 1990

147. Itoh T, Seki N, Suzuki S, Ito S, Kajikuri J, Kuriyama H: Membrane hyperpolarization inhibits agonist-induced synthesis of inositol 1,4,5-trisphosphate in rabbit mesenteric artery. J Physiol 451: 307–328, 1992

148. Marchenko SM, Sage SO: Electrical properties of resting and acetylcholine-stimulated endothelium in intact rat aorta. J Physiol 462:735–751, 1993

149. Beny J-L, Gribi F: Dye and electrical coupling of endothelial cells in situ. Tissue Cell 21:797–802, 1989

150. Beny J-L, Paccica C: Bidirectional electrical communication between smooth muscle and endothelial cells in the pig coronary artery. Am J Physiol 266:H1465-H1472, 1994

151. Beny JL, Chabaud F: Kinins and Endothelium-Dependent Hyperpolarization in Porcine Coronary Arteries. In: Vanhoutte PM, ed, Endothelium-Derived Hyperpolarization Factor. Amsterdam: Harwood Academic Publishers, 1996:41–51

152. Komori K, Vanhoutte PM: Endothelium-derived hyperpolarization factor. Blood Vessels 27:238–245, 1990

153. Rubanyi GM, Vanhoutte PM: Nature of endothelium-derived relaxing factor: Are there two relaxing mediators? Circ Res 61(Suppl II):II61-II67, 1987

154. Campbell WB, Harder DR: Endothelium-derived hyperpolarizing factors and vascular cytochrome P450 metabolites of arachidonic acid in the regulation of tone. Circ Res 84:484–488, 1999

155. Thollon C, Bidouard JP, Cambarrat C, Delescluse I, Villeneuve N,

Vanhoutte PM, Vilaine JP: Alteration of endothelium-dependent hyperpolarization in porcine coronary arteries with regenerated endothelium. Circ Res 84:371–377, 1999

156. Campbell WB, Gebremedhin D, Pratt PF, Harder DR: Identification of eposyeicosatrienoic acids as endothelium-derived hyperpolarizing. Circ Res 78:415–423, 1996

157. Randall MD, McCulloch AI, Kendall DA: Comparative pharmacology of endothelium-derived hyperpolarizing factor and anandamide in rat isolated mesentery. Eur J Pharmacol 33:191–197, 1997

158. Randall MD, Kendall DA: Involvement of a cannabinoid in endothelium-derived hyperpolarizing factor-mediated coronary vasorelaxation. Eur J Pharmacol 335:191–197, 1997

159. Randall MD, Kendall DA: Evidence for the involvement of potassium channels in anandamide-induced and EDHF-mediated vasorelaxations in rat isolated mesentery. Br J Pharmacol (In press)

160. Devane WA, Hanus L, Breuer A, Pertwee RG, Stevenson LA, Griffin G, Gibson D, Mandelbaum A, Etinger A, Mechoulam R: Isolation and structure of a brain constituent that binds to the cannabinoid receptor. Science 258:1946–1949, 1992

161. Di Marzo V, Fontana A, Cadas H, Schinelli S, Cimino G, Schwartz JC, Piomelli D: Formation and inactivation of endogenous cannabinoid anandamide in central neurons. Nature 372:686–691, 1994

162. Niederhoffer N, Szabo B: Involvement of CB_1 cannabinoid receptors in the EDHF-dependent vasorelaxation in rabbits. Br J Pharmacol 126:1383–1386, 1999

163. Mombouli J-V, Vanhoutte PM: Endothelium-derived hyperpolarizing factor(s): Updating the unknown. Trends Pharmacol Sci 18:252–256, 1997

164. Chen G, Suzuki H: Some electrical properties of the endothelium-dependent hyperpolarization recorded from rat arterial smooth muscle cells. J Physiol 410:91–106, 1989

165. Nagao T, Vanhoutte PM: Characterization of endothelium-dependent relaxations resistant to nitro-L-arginine in the porcine coronary artery. Br J Pharmacol 107:1102–1107, 1992

166. Corriu C, Feletou M, Canet E, Vanhoutte PM: Inhibitors of the cytochrome P450-monooxygenase and endothelium-dependent hyperpolarization in the guinea-pig isolated carotid artery. Br J Pharmacol 117:607–610, 1996

167. Chataingeau T, Feletou M, Duhault J, Vanhoutte PM: Epoxyeicosatrienoic acids, potassium channel blockers and endothelium-dependent hyperpolarization in the guinea-pig carotid artery. Br J Pharmacol 123:574–580, 1998

168. Chen G, Yamamoto Y, Miwa K, Suzuki H: Hyperpolarization of arterial smooth muscle induced by endothelial humoral substances. Am J Physiol 260:H1888-H1892, 1991

169. Edwards FR, Hirst GD, Silverberg GD: Inward rectification in rat cerebral arterioles, involvement of potassium ions in autoregulation. J Physiol (London) 404:455–466, 1988

170. Edwards G, Dora KA, Gardener MJ, Garland CJ, Weston AH: K$^+$ is an endothelium-derived hyperpolarizing factor in rat arteries. Nature 396:269–272, 1998

171. Quignard JF, Félétou M, Thollon C, Vilaine JP, Duhault J, Vanhoutte PM: Potassium ions and endothelium-derived hyperpolarizing factor in guinea-pig carotid and porcine coronary arteries. Br J Pharmacol 127:27–34, 1999

172. Johnston CI, Risvanis J: Preclinical pharmacology of angiotensin II receptor antagonists: Update and outstanding issues. Am J Hypertens 10:306S–310S, 1997

173. Gibbons GH: Cardioprotective mechanisms of ACE inhibition: The angiotensin II-nitric oxide balance. Drugs 54:(Suppl 5):1–11, 1997

174. Seyedi N, Xu X, Nasjietti A, Hintze TH: Coronary kinin generation mediates nitric oxide release after angiotensin receptor stimulation. Hypertension 26:164–170, 1995

175. Li P, Chappell MC, Brosnihan KB: Angiotensin-(1–7) augments bradykinin-induced vasodilatation by competing with ACE and releasing nitric oxide. Hypertension 29:394–400, 1997

176. Gohlke P, Pees C, Unger T: AT2 receptor stimulation increases aortic cyclic GMP in SHRSP by a kinin-dependent mechanism. Hypertension 31:349–355, 1998

177. Harrison DG: Endothelial function and oxidant stress. Clin Cardiol 20(Suppl 5):42–47, 1997

178. Griendling KK, Ushio-Fukai M, Lassegue B, Alexander RW: Angiotensin II signaling in vascular smooth muscle: New concepts. Hypertension 29:366–373, 1997

179. Seewald S, Seul C, Kettenhofen R, Bokemeyer D, Ko Y, Vetter H, Sachinidis A: Role of mitogen-activated protein kinase in the angiotensin II-induced DNA synthesis in vascular smooth muscle cells. Hypertension 31:1151–1156, 1995

180. Inagami T, Kambayashi Y, Ichiki T, Tsuzuki S, Eguchi S, Yamakawa T: Angiotensin receptors: Molecular biology and signalling. Clin Exp Pharmacol Physiol 26:544–549, 1999

181. Inoue A, Yanagisawa M, Kimura S, Kasuya Y, Miyauchi T, Goto K, Masaki T: The human endothelin family: Three structurally and pharmacologically distinct isopeptides predicted by three separate genes. Proc Natl Acad Sci USA 87:2863–2867, 1989

182. Masaki T: Possible role of endothelin in endothelial regulation of vascular tone. Annu Rev Pharmacol Toxicol 35:235–255, 1995

183. Celermajer DS: Endothelial dysfunction: Does it matter? Is it reversible? J Am Coll Cardiol 30:325–333, 1997

184. Mombouli JV, Vanhoutte PM : Endothelial dysfunction: A novel therapeutic target. Endothelial dysfunction: From physiology to therapy. J Mol Cell Cardiol 31:61–74, 1999

185. Vanhoutte PM: Endothelial dysfunction and vascular disease: Endothelium, Nitric Oxide, and Atherosclerosis (8):79–95, 1999

186. Stoclet JC, Fleming I, Gray G, : Nitric oxide and entotoxemia. Circulation 87(Suppl V):77–80, 1993

187. Cooke JP, Dzau VJ: Derangements of the nitric oxide synthase pathway, L-arginine, and cardiovascular diseases. Circulation 96: 379–382, 1997

188. Newby DE, Wright RA, Labinjoh C, Ludlam CA, Fox KA, Boon NA, Webb DJ: Endothelial dysfunction, impaired endogenous fibrinolysis, and cigarette smoking: A mechanism for arterial thrombosis and myocardial infarction. Circulation 99:1411–1415, 1999

189. Campisi R, Czernin J, Schöder H, Sayre JW, Schelbert HR: L-Arginine normalizes coronary vasomotion in long-term smokers. Circulation 99:491–497, 1999

190. Mayhan WG, Sharpe GM: Chronic exposure to nicotine alters endothelium-dependent arteriolar dilatation: Effect of superoxide dismutase. J Appl Physiol 86:1126–1134, 1999

191. Cosentino F, Lüsher TF: Endothelial dysfunction in diabetes mellitus. J Cardiovasc Pharmacol 32:S54-S61, 1998

192. Imaoka Y, Osanai T, Kamada T, Mio Y, Satoh K, Okumura K: Nitric oxide-dependent vasodilator mechanism is not impaired by hypertension but is diminished with aging in the rat aorta. J Cardiovasc Pharmacol 33:756–761, 1999

193. Knot HJ, Lounsbury KM, Brayden JE, Nelson MT: Gender differences in coronary artery diameter reflect changes in both endothelial Ca^{2+} and ecNOS activity. Am J Physiol 276:H961-H969, 1999

194. Boulanger CM, Vanhoutte PM: G-Proteins and endothelium-dependent relaxations. J Vasc Res 34:175–185, 1997

195. Tsao PS, Cooke JP: Endothelial alterations in hypercholesterolemia: More than simply vasodilator dysfunction. J Cardiovasc Pharmacol 32:S48-S53, 1998

196. Ito A, Tsao PS, Adimoolam S, Kimoto M, Ogawa T, Cooke JP: Novel mechasnim for endothelial dysfunction: Dysregulation of dimethylarginine dimethylaminohydrolase. Circulation 99:3092–3095, 1999

197. Miyazaki H, Matsuoka H, Cooke JP, Usui M, Ueda S, Okuda S, Imaizumi T: Endogenous nitric oxide synthase inhibitor: A novel marker of atherosclerosis. Circulation 99:1141–1146, 1999

198. Leiper JM, Santa Maria J, Chubb A, MacAllister RJ, Charles IG, Whitley GS, Vallance P: Identification of two human dimethylarginine dimethylaminohydrolases with distinct tissue distributions and homology with microbial arginine deaminases. Biochem J 343:209–214, 1999

199. Bauersachs J, Bouloumie A, Fraccarollo D, Hu K, Busse R, Ertl G: Endothelial dysfunction in chronic myocardial infarction despite increased vascular endothelial nitric oxide synthase and soluble guanylate cyclase expression: Role of enhanced vascular superoxide production. Circulation 100:292–298, 1999

200. Wambi-Kiesse CO, Katusic ZS: Inhibition of copper/zinc superoxide dismutase impairs NO-mediated endothelium-dependent relaxations. Am J Physiol 276:H1043-H1048, 1999

201. Mombouli JV, Nakashima M, Hamra M, Vanhoutte PM: Endothelium-dependent relaxation and hyperpolarization evoked by bradykinin in canine coronary arteries: Enhancement by exercise-training. Br J Pharmacol 117:413–418, 1996

202. Clarkson P, Montgomery HE, Mullen MJ, Donald AE, Powe AJ, Bull T, Jubb M, World M, Deanfield JE: Exercise training enhances endothelial function in young men. J Am Coll Cardiol 33:1379–1385, 1999

203. Zhang X, Recchia FA, Bernstein R, Xu X, Nasjletti A, Hintze TH: Kinin-mediated coronary nitric oxide production contributes to the therapeutic action of angiotensin-converting enzyme and neutral endopeptidase inhibitors and amlodipine in the treatment in heart failure. J Pharmacol Exp Ther 288:742–751, 1999

204. Zhang X, Nasjletti A, Xu X, Hintze TH: Neutral endopeptidase and angiotensin converting enzyme inhibitors increase nitric oxide production in isolated canine coronary microvessels by a kinin-dependent mechanism. J Cardiovasc Pharmacol 31:623–629, 1998

205. Koh KK, Bui MN, Hathaway L, Csako G, Waclawiw MA, Panza JA, Cannon RO III: Mechanism by which quinapril improves vascular function in coronary artery disease. Am J Cardiol 83:327–331, 1999

206. Zhang X, Hintze TH: Amlodipine releases nitric oxide from canine coronary microvessels: An unexpected mechanism of action of a calcium channel-blocking agent. J Cardiovasc Pharmacol 31:623–629, 1998

207. Shimokawa H, Lam JY, Chesebro T, Bowie EJ, Vanhoutte PM: Effects of dietary supplementation with cod-liver oil on endothelium-dependent responses in porcine coronary arteries. Circulation 76:898–905, 1987

208. Nagao T, Nakashima M, Smart FW, Bond RA, Morrison KJ, Vanhoutte PM: Potentiation of endothelium-dependent hyperpo-

larization to serotonin by dietary intake of NC 020, a defined fish oil, in the porcine coronary artery. J Cardiovasc Pharmacol 26:679–681, 1995

209. Hornstra G, Barth CA, Galli C, Mensink RP, Mutanen M, Riemersma RA, Roberfroid M, Salminen K, Vansant G, Verschuren PM: Functional food science and the cardiovascular system. Br J Nutr 80:S113-S146, 1998

210. Fitzopatrick DF, Hirschfield SL, Coffey RG: Endothelium-dependent vasorelaxing activity of wine and other grape products. Am J Physiol 265:H774-H778, 1993

211. Wollny T, Aiello L, Di Tommaso D, Bellavia V, Rotilio D, Donati MB, de Gaetano G, Iacoviello L: Modulation of haemostatic function and prevention of experimental thrombosis by red wine in rats: A role for increased nitric oxide production. Br J Pharmacol 127:747–755, 1999

212. Andriambeloson E, Stoclet JC, Andriantsitohaina R: Mechanism of endothelial nitric oxide-dependent vasorelaxation induced by wine polyphenols in rat thoracic aorta. J Cardiovasc Pharmacol 33:248–254, 1999

213. Grenett HE, Aikens ML, Torres JA, Demissie S, Tabengwa EM, Davis GC, Booyse FM: Ethanol transcriptionally upregulates t-PA and u-PA gene expression in cultured human endothelial cells. Alcohol Clin Exp Res 22:849–853, 1998

214. Hendrickson RJ, Cahill PA, Sitzmann JV, Redmond EM: Ethanol enhances basal and flow-stimulated nitric oxide synthase activity in vitro by activating an inhibitory guanine nucleotide binding protein. J Pharmacol Exp Ther 289:1293–1300, 1999

215. Venkov CD, Myers PR, Tanner MA, Su M, Vaughan DE: Ethanol increases endothelial nitric oxide production through modulation of nitric oxide synthase expression. Thromb Haemost 81:638–642, 1999

216. Motayama T, Kawano H, Kugiyama K, Hirashima O, Ohgushi M, Yoshimura M, Ogawa H, Yasue H: Endothelium-dependent vasodilation in the brachial artery is impaired in smokers: Effect of vitamin C. Am J Physiol 273:H1644-H1650, 1997

217. Ting HH, Timini FK, Boles KS, Ganz P, Creager MA: Vitamin C improves endothelium-dependent vasodilatation in fore-arm resistance vessels of humans with hypercholesterolemia. Circulation 95:2617–2622, 1994

218. Gokce N, Keaney JF Jr, Frei B, Holbrook M, Olesiak M, Zachariah BJ, Leeuwenburgh C, Heinecke JW, Vita JA: Long-term ascorbic acid administration reverses endothelial vasomotor dysfunction in patients with coronary artery disease. Circulation 99:3234–3240, 1999

219. Kinlay S, Fang JC, Hikita H, Ho I, Delagrange DM, Frei B, Suh JH, Gerhard M, Creager MA, Selwyn AP, Ganz P: Plasma alpha-tocopherol and coronary endothelium-dependent vasodilator function. Circulation 100:219–221, 1999

220. Kugiyama K, Motoyama T, Doi H, Kawano H, Hirai N, Soejima H, Miyao Y, Takazoe K, Moriyama Y, Mizuno Y, Tsunoda R, Ogawa H, Sakamoto T, Sugiyama S, Yasue H: Improvement of endothelial vasomotor dysfunction by treatment with alpha-tocopherol in patients with high remnant lipoproteins levels. J Am Coll Cardiol 33:1512–1518, 1999

221. Cooke JP, Andon NA, Girerd XJ, Hirsch AT, Creager MA: Arginine restores cholinergic relaxation of hypercholesterolemic rabbit thoracic aorta. Circulation 115:1057–1062, 1995

222. Creager MA, Gallagher SJ, Girerd XJ, Coleman SM, Dzau VJ, Cooke JP: L-Arginine improves endothelium-dependent vasodilatation in hypercholesterolemic humans. J Clin Invest 90:1248–1253, 1992

223. Husain S, Andrews NP, Mulcahy D, Panza JA, Quyyumi AA: Aspirin improves endothelial dysfunction in atherosclerosis. Circulation 97:716–720, 1998

224. Kahn AM, Husid A, Allen JC, Seidel CL, Song T: Insulin acutely inhibits cultured vascular smooth muscle cell contraction by a nitric oxide synthase-dependent pathway. Hypertension 30:928–933, 1997

225. Schroeder CA Jr, Chen YL, Messina EJ: Inhibition of NO synthesis or endothelium removal reveals a vasoconstrictor effect of insulin on isolated arterioles. Am J Physiol 276:H815-H820, 1999

226. Mendelsohn ME, Karas RH: Mechanisms of disease: The protective effects of estrogen on the cardiovascular system. N Engl J Med 340:1801–1811, 1999

227. Herman SM, Robinson, JTC, McCredie RJ, Adams MR, Boyer MJ, Celermajer DS: Androgen deprivation is associated with enhanced endothelium-dependent dilatation in adult men. Arterioscler Tromb Vasc Biol 17:2004–2009, 1997

228. Jovanovic A, Jovanovic S: Estrogen and vascular system: More questions for the future. Cardiovasc Res 42:9–11, 1999

229. Kon Koh K, Cardillo C, Bui MN, Hathaway L, Csako G, Waclawiw MA, Panza JA, Cannon RO III: Vascular effects of estrogen and cholesterol-lowering therapies in hypercholesterolemic postmenopausal women. Circulation 99:354–360, 1999

230. Hugel S, Neubauer S, Lie SZ, Ernst R, Horn M, Schmidt HH, Allolio B, Reincke M: Multiple mechanisms are involved in the acute vasodilatory effect of 17β-estradiol in the isolated perfused rat heart. J Cardiovasc Pharmacol 33:852–858, 1999

231. Vallance P: Endothelium, inflammation and cardiovascular disease.Circulation 96:3042–3047, 1996
232. Taddei S, Virdis A, Mattei P, Salvetti A: Vasodilation to acetylcholine in primary and secondary forms of human hypertension. Hypertension 21:929–933, 1993
233. Taddei S, Virdis A, Mattei P, Ghiadoni L, Gennari A, Fasolo CB, Sudano I, Salvetti A: Aging and endothelial function in normotensive subjects and patients with essential hypertension. Circulation 91:1981–1987, 1995
234. Taddei S, Virdis A, Mattei P, Ghiadoni L, Fasolo GB, Sudano I, Salvetti A: Hypertension causes premature aging of endothelial function in humans. Hypertension 29:736–743, 1997
235. Moubouli JV, Vanhoutte PM: Purinergic endothelium-dependent and -independent contractions in rat aorta. Hypertension 22:577–583, 1993
236. Nakashima M, Vanhoutte PM: Age-dependent decrease in endothelium-dependent hyperpolarizations to endothelin-3 in the rat mesenteric artery. J Cardiovasc Pharmacol 22(Suppl 8): S352-S354, 1993
237. Shimokawa H, Aarhus LL, Vanhoutte PM: Porcine coronary arteries with regenerated endothelium have a reduced endothelium-dependent responsivenes to aggregating platelets and serotonin. Circ Res 61:256–270, 1987
238. Shimokawa H, Flavahan NA, Lorenz RR, Vanhoutte PM: Endothelium-dependent inbition of ergonovine-induced contraction is impaired in porcine coronary arteries with regenerated endothelium. Circulation 80:643–650, 1989
239. Shimokawa H, Flavahan NA, Vanhoutte PM: Natural course of the impairment of endothelium-dependent relaxations after ballon endothelium removal in porcine coronary arteries: Possible dysfunction of a pertussis toxin-sensitive G-protein. Circ Res 65:740–753, 1989
240. Shimokawa H, Flavahan NA, Vanhoutte PM: Loss of endothelial pertussis toxin-sensitive G-protein function in atherosclerotic porcine coronary arteries. Circulation 83:652–660, 1991
241. Shimokawa H, Vanhoutte PM: Impaired endothelium-depenent relaxation to aggregating platelets and related vasoactive substances in porcine coronary arteries in hypercholesterolemia and atherosclerosis. Circ Res 64:900–914, 1989
242. Shimokawa H, Vanhoutte PM: Porcine coronary arteries with regenerated endothelium have a reduced endothelium-dependent responsiveness to aggregating platelets and serotonin. Circ Res 13:1402–1408, 1989
243. Vanhoutte PM: Hypercholesterolemia, atherosclerosis, and re-

lease of endothelium-derived relaxing factor by aggregating plaelets. Eur Heart J 12(Suppl E):25–82, 1991

244. Gilligan DM, Guetta V, Panza JA, Garcia CE, Quyyumi AA, Cannon RO III: Selective loss of microvascular endothelial function in human hypercholesterolemia. Circulation 90:35–41, 1994

245. Eizawa H, Yoshiki Y, Inoue R, Kosuga K, Hattori R, Aoyama T, Sasayama S: Lysophosphatidylcholine inhibits endothelium-dependent hyperpolarization and N^{ω}-nitro-L-arginine/indomethacin-resistant endothelium-dependent relaxation in the porcine coronary artery. Circulation 92:3520–3526, 1995

246. Vidal F, Colome C, Martinez-Gonzalez J, Badimon L: Atherogenic concentrations of native low-density lipoproteins down-regulate nitric oxide synthase mRNA and protein levels in endothelial cells. Eur J Biochem 252:378–384, 1998

247. Kinlay S, Selwyn AP, Libby P, Ganz P: Inflammation, the endothelium, and the acute coronary syndromes. J Cardiovasc Pharmacol 32(Suppl 3):S62-S66, 1998

248. Russell R: Atherosclerosis: Mechanisms of disease. Ann N Engl J Med 340:115–126, 1999

249. Thollon C, Bidouard JP, Cambarrat C, Delescluse I, Villeneuve N, Vanhoutte PM, Vilaine JP: Alteration of endothelium-dependent hyperpolarizations in porcine coronary arteries with regenerated endothelium. Circ Res 84:371–377, 1999

250. Ge T, Hughes H, Junquero DC, Wu KK, Vanhoutte PM, Boulanger CM: Endothelium-dependent contractions are associated with both augmented expression of protaglandin H synthase-1 and hypersensitivity to protaglandin H2 in the SHR aorta. Circ Res 76:1003–1010, 1995

251. Katz SD, Khan T, Zeballos GA, Mathew L, Potharlanka P, Knecht M, Whelan J: Decreased activity of the L-arginine-nitric oxide metabolic pathway in patients with congestive heart failure. Circulation 99:2113–2117, 1999

252. Drexler H: Nitric oxide synthases in the failing human heart: A doubled-edged sword? Circulation 99:2972–2975, 1999

253. Münzel T, Harrison DG: Increased superoxide in heart failure: A biochemical baroreflex gone awry. Circulation 100:216–218, 1999

254. Kichuk MR, Zhang X, Oz M, Michler R, Kaley G, Nasjletti A, Hintze TH: Angiotensin-converting enzyme inhibitors promote nitric oxide production in coronary microvessels from failling explanted human hearts. Ann J Cardiol 80:137A–142A, 1997

255. Su J, Barbe F, Houel R, Guyene TT, Crozatier B, Hittinger L: Effects according to the renin-angiotensin system activation. Basic Res Cardiol 94:128–135, 1999

256. Zolk O, Quattek J, Sitzler G, Schrader T, Nickenig G, Schnabel P,

Shimada K, Takahashi M, Bohm M: Expression of endothelin-1, endothelin-converting enzyme, and endothelin receptors in chronic heart failure. Circulation 99:2118–2123, 1999

257. Yamauchi-Kohno R, Miyauchi T, Hoshino T, Kobayashi T, Aihara H, Sakai S, Yabana H, Goto K, Sugishita Y, Murata S: Role of endothelin in deterioration of heart failure due to cardiomyopathy in hamsters: Increase in endothelin-1 production in the heart and beneficial effect of endothelin-A receptor antagonist on survival and cardiac function. Circulation 99:2171–1276, 1999

258. Fukuchi M, Hussain SN, Giaid A: Heterogeneous expression and activity of endothelial and inducible nitric oxide synthases in end-stage human heart failure: Their relation to lesion site and β-adrenergic receptor therapy. Circulation 98:132–139, 1998

259. Celi A, Lorenzet R, Furie BC: Platelet-leukocyte-endothelial cell interaction on the blood vessel wall. Semin Hematol 34:327–335, 1997

260. Henricks PA, Nijkamp, FP: Pharmacological modulation of cell adhesion molecules. Eur J Pharmacol 344:1–13, 1998

261. Braum M, Pietsch P, Schör K, Baumann G, Felix SB: Cellular adhesion molecules on vascular smooth muscle cells. Cardiovasc Res 41:395–401, 1999

262. Zimmerman GA, McIntyre TM, Prescott SM: Adhesion and signaling in vascular cell-cell interactions. J Clin Invest 100(Suppl 11):S3-S5, 1997

263. Asimakopoulos G, Taylor KM: Effects of cardiopulmonary bypass on leukocyte and endothelial adhesion molecules. Ann Thorac Surg 66:135–144, 1998

264. Radomski MW, Palmer RM, Moncada S: The role of nitric oxide and cGMP in platelet adhesion to vascular endothelium. Biochem Biophys Res Commun 148:1482–1489, 1987

265. Moncada S, Palmer RM, Higgs EA: Relationship between prostacyclin and nitric oxide in the thrombotic process. Thromb Res Suppl 11:3–13, 1990

266. Wang G-R, Zhu Y, Halushka PV, Lincoln TM, Mendelson ME: Mechanism of platelet inhibition by nitric oxide: In vivo phosphorylation of thromboxane receptor by cyclic GMP-dependent protein kinase. Proc Natl Acad Sci USA 95:4888–4893, 1998

267. Lyons CR: Emerging roles of nitric oxide in inflammation. Hosp Pract (Off Ed) 31:69–73, 77–80, 85–86, 1996

268. Lefer DJ, Jones SP, Girod WG, Baines A, Grisham MB, Cockrell AS, Huang PL, Scalia R: Leukocyte-endothelial cell interactions in nitric oxide synthase-deficient mice. Am J Physiol 276:H1943-H1950, 1999

269. Li N, Karin M: Is NF-κB the sensor of oxidative stress? FASEB J 13:1137–1143, 1999

270. Barnes PJ, Karin M: Nuclear factor-κB: A pivotal transcription factor in chronic inflammatory diseases. N Engl J Med 336:1066–1071, 1997

271. Baldwin AS Jr: The NF-κB and I-κB proteins: New discoveries and insights. Annu Rev Immunol 14:649–683, 1996

272. Bouma MG, van den Wildenberg FA, Buurman WA: The anti-inflammatory potential of adenosine in ischemia-reperfusion injury: Established and putative beneficial actions of a retaliatory metabolic. Shock 8:313–320, 1997

273. Cardigan RA, Mackie IJ, Machin SJ: Hemostatic-endothelial interactions: A potential anticoagulant role of the endothelium in the pulmonary circulation during cardiac surgery. J Cardiothorac Vasc Anesth 11:329–336, 1997

274. Boyle EM Jr, Verrier ED, Spiess BD: Endothelial cell injury in cardiovascular surgery: The procoagulant response. Ann Thorac Surg 62:1549–1557, 1996

275. Rock G, Wells P: New concept in coagulation. Crit Rev Clin Lab Sci 34:475–501, 1997

276. Alessi MC, Juhan-Vague I: Endothelium, thrombose et fibrinolyse. Rev Prat 47:2227–2231, 1997

277. Holzmuller H, Moll T, Hofer-Warbinek R, Mechtcheriakova D, Binder BR, Hofer E: A transcriptional repressor of the tissue factor gene in endothelial cells. Arterioscler Thromb Vasc Biol 19:1804–1811, 1999

278. Iba T, Kidokoro, Yagi Y: The role of the endothelium in changes in procoagulant activity in sepsis. J Am Coll Surg 187:321–329, 1998

279. Rosenberg RD, Aird WC: Vascular-bed–specific hemostasis and hypercoagulable states. N Engl J Med 340:1555–1564, 1999

280. Cines DB, Pollak ES, Buck CA, Loscalzo J, Zimmerman GA, McEver RP, Pober JS, Wick TM, Konkle BA, Schwartz BS, Barnathan ES, McCrae KR, Hug BA, Schmidt AM, Stern DM: Endothelial cells in physiology and in the pathophysiology of vascular disorders. Blood 91:3527–3561, 1998

281. Conway EM, Rosenberg RD: Tumor necrosis factor suppresses transcription of the thrombomodulin gene in endothelial cells. Mol Cell Biol 8:5588–5592, 1988

282. Sawdey M, Podor TJ, Loskutoff DJ: Regulation of type 1 plasminogen activator inhibitor gene expression in cultured bovine aortic endothelial cells: Induction by transforming growth factor-β, lipopolysaccharide, and tumor necrosis factor-α. J Biol Chem 264:10396–10401, 1989

283. Conway EM, Bach R, Rosenberg RD, Konigsberg WH: Tumor necrosis factor enhances expression of tissue factor mRNA in endothelial cells. Thromb Res 53:231–241, 1989

284. Edelberg JM, Aird WC, Wu W, Rayburn H, Mamuya WS, Mercola M, Rosenberg RD: PDGF mediates cardiac microvascular communication. J Clin Invest 102:837–843, 1998

285. Malek AM, Jackman R, Rosenberg RD, Izumo S: Endothelial expression of thrombomodulin is reversibly regulated by fluid shear stress. Circ Res 74:852–860, 1994

286. Kawai Y, Matsumoto Y, Watanabe K, Yamamoto H, Satoh K, Murata M, Handa M, Ikeda Y: Hemodynamic forces modulate the effects of cytokines on fibrinolytic activity of endothelial cells. Blood 87:2314–2321, 1996

287. Lin MC, Almus-Jacobs F, Chen HH, Parry GC, Mackman N, Shyy JY, Chien S: Shear stress induction of tissue factor gene. J Clin Invest 99:737–744, 1997

288. Ziegler T, Silacci P, Harrison VJ, Hayoz D: Nitric oxide synthase expression in endothelial cells exposed to mechanical forces. Hypertension 32:351–355, 1998

289. Pinsky DJ, Liao H, Lawson CA, Yan SF, Chen J, Carmeliet P, Loskutoff DJ, Stern DM: Coordinated induction of plasminogen activator inhibitor-1 (PAI-1) and inhibition of plasminogen activator gene expression by hypoxia promotes pulmonary vascular fibrin deposition. J Clin Invest 102:919–928, 1998

290. Everett AD, Le Cras TD, Xue C, Johns RA: eNOS expression is not altered in pulmonary vascular remodeling due to increased pulmonary blood flow. Am J Physiol 274:L1058-L1065, 1998

291. Griendling KK, Alexander RW: Endothelial control of the cardiovascular system: Recent advances. FASEB J 10:283–292, 1996

292. Montrucchio G, Lupia E, De Martino A, Battaglia E, Arese M, Tizzani A, Bussolino F, Camussi G: Nitric oxide mediates angiogenesis induces in vivo by platelet-activating factor and tumor necrosis factor-α. Am J Pathol 151:557–563, 1997

293. Isner JM: Cancer and atherosclerosis: The broad mandate of angiogenesis. Circulation 99:1653–1655, 1999

294. Moulton KS, Heller E, Konerding MA, Flynn E, Palinski W, Folkman J: Angiogenesis inhibitors endostatin and TNP-470 reduce intimal neovascularization and plaque growth in apolipoprotein E-deficient mice. Circulation 99:1726–1732, 1999

295. Murohara T, Ashara T, Silver M, et al: Nitric oxide synthase modulates angiogenesis in response to tissue ischemia. J Biol Chem 101:2567–2578, 1998

296. Servos S, Zachary I, Martin JF: VEGF modulates NO production: The basis of a cytoprotective effect? Cardiovascular Research 41:509–510, 1999

297. Neufeld G, Cohen T, Gengrinovithch S, Polorak Z: Vascular en-

dothelial growth factor (VEGF) and its receptors. FASEB J 13:9–22, 1999

298. Scalia R, Booth G, Lefer DJ: Vascular endothelial growth factor attenuates leukocyte-endothelium interaction during acute endothelial dysfunction: Essential role of endothelial-derived nitric oxide. FASEB J 13:1039–1046, 1999

299. Gustafsson T, Puntschart A, Sundberg CJ, Jansson E: Related expression of vascular endothelial growth factor and hypoxia-inducible factor-1 mRNAs in human skeletal muscle. Acta Physiol Scand 165:335–336, 1999

300. Weltermann A, Wolzt M, Petersmann, Czerni C, Graselli U, Lechner K, Kyrle PA: Large amounts of vascular endothelial growth factor at the site of hemostatic plug formation in vivo. Arterioscler Tromb Vasc Biol 19:1757–1760, 1999

301. Sarkar R, Webb RC: Does nitric oxide regulate smooth muscle cell proliferation? A critical appraisal. J Vasc Res 35:135–142, 1998

302. Clement MV, Pervaiz S: Reactive oxygen intermediates regulate cellular response to apoptotic stimuli: An hypothesis. Free Radic Res 30:247–252, 1999

303. Alnemeri ES, Livingston DJ, Nicholson DW, Salvesen G, Thornebery NA, Wong WW, Yuan Y: Human ICE/CED-3 protease nomenclature. Cell 87:171, 1996

304. Nicholson DW, Ali A, Thornberry NA, Vaillancourt JP, Ding CK, Gallant M, Gareau Y, Griffin PR, Labelle M, Lazebnik YA, et al: Identification and inhibition of the ICE/CED-3 protease necessary for mammalian apoptosis. Nature 376:37–43, 1995

305. Ashkenazi A, Dixit VM: Death receptors: Signaling and modulation. Science 281:1305–1308, 1998

306. Takahachi A, Musy PY, Martins LM, Poirier GG, Moyer RW, Earnshaw WC: CrmA SPI-2 inhibition of an endogenous ICE-related protease responsible for lamin A cleavage and apoptic nuclear fragmentation. J Biol Chemistry 271:32487–32490, 1996

307. Villa P, Henzel W, Sensenbrenner M, Henderson C, Pettmann B: Calpain inhibitors, but not caspase inhibitors, prevent actin proteolysis and DNA fragmentation during apoptosis. J Cell Science 111:713–722, 1998

308. Yang F, Sun X, Beech W, Teter B, Wu S, Sigel J, Vinters HV, Frautschy SA, Cole GM: Antibody to caspase- cleaved actin detects apoptosis in differentiated neuroblastoma and plaque-associated neurons and microglia in Alzheimer's disease. Am J Pathol 152:379–389, 1998

309. Zhivotovsky B, Gahm A, Orrenius S: Two different proteases are involved in the proteolysis of lamin during apoptosis. Biochem Biophys Res Commun 233:96–101, 1997

310. Kaufmann SH, Desnoyers S, Ottaviano Y, Davidson NE, Poirier GG: Specific proteolytic cleavage of poly(ADP- ribose) polymerase: An early marker of chemotherapy-induced apoptosis. Cancer Res 53:3976–3985, 1993

311. Pollman MJ, Naumovski L, Gibbons GH: Vascular cell apoptosis: Cell type-specific modulation by transforming growth factor-β_1 in endothelial cells versus smooth muscle cells. Circulation 99:2019–2026, 1999

312. Kim YM, Bombeck CA, Billiar TR: Nitric oxide as a bifunctional regulator of apoptosis. Circ Res 84:253–256, 1999

313. Kim YM, de Vera ME, Watkins SC, Billiar TR: Nitric oxide protects cultured rat hepatocytes from tumor necrosis factor-α-induced apoptosis by inducing heat shock protein 70 expression. J Biol Chem 272:1402–1411, 1997

314. Genaro AM, Hortelano S, Alvarez A, Martinez C, Bosca L: Splenic B lymphocyte programmed cell death is prevented by nitric oxide release through mechanisms involving sustained Bcl-2 levels. J Clin Invest 95:1884–1890, 1995

315. Kim YM, Talanian RV, Billiar TR: Nitric oxide inhibits apoptosis by preventing increases in caspase-3-like activity via two distinct mechanisms. J Biol Chem 272:31138–31148, 1997

316. Mannick JB, Miao XQ, Stamler JS: Nitric oxide inhibits Fas-induced apoptosis. J Biol Chem 272:24125–24128, 1997

317. Kim YM, Talanian RV, Li J, Billiar TR: Nitric oxide prevents IL-1β and IFN-γ-inducing factor (IL-18) release from macrophages by inhibiting caspase-1 (IL-1β-converting enzyme). J Immunol 161:4122–4128, 1998

318. Melino G, Bernassola F, Knight RA, Corasaniti MT, Nistico G, Finazzi-Agro A: S-nitrosylation regulates apoptosis. Nature 388:432–433, 1997

319. Ashkenazi A, Dixit VM: Death receptors: Signaling and modulation. Science 281:1305–1308, 1998

320. Kim YM, Kim TH, Seol DW, Talanian RV, Billiar TR: Nitric oxide suppression of apoptosis occurs in association with an inhibition of Bcl-2 cleavage and cytochrome c release. J Biol Chem 273:31437–31441, 1998

321. Kim YM, Bergonia H, Lancaster JR Jr: Nitrogen oxide-induced autoprotection in isolated rat hepatocytes. FEBS Lett 374:228–232, 1995

322. von Knethen A, Brune B: Cyclooxygenase-2: An essential regulator of NO-mediated apoptosis. FASEB J 11:887–895, 1997

323. Dubey RK, Overbeck HW: Culture of rat mesenteric arteriolar smooth muscle cells: Effects of platelet-derived growth factor, angiotensin, and nitric oxide on growth. Cell Tissue Res 275:133–141, 1994

324. Lopez-Farre A, Sanchez de Miguel L, Caramelo C, Gomez-Macias J, Garcia R, Mosquera JR, de Frutos T, Millas I, Rivas F, Echezarreta G, Casado S: Role of nitric oxide in autocrine control of growth and apoptosis of endothelial cells. Am J Physiol 272:H760-H768, 1997

325. Sarkar R, Gordon D, Stanley JC, Webb RC: Cell cycle effects of nitric oxide on vascular smooth muscle cells. Am J Physiol 272: H1810-H1818, 1997

326. Janssen YM, Soultanakis R, Steece K, Heerdt E, Singh RJ, Joseph J, Kalyanaraman B: Depletion of nitric oxide causes cell cycle alterations, apoptosis, and oxidative stress in pulmonary cells. Am J Physiol 275:L1100-L1109, 1998

327. Lipton SA, Choi YB, Pan ZH, Lei SZ, Chen HS, Sucher NJ, Loscalzo J, Singel DJ, Stamler JS: A redox-based mechanism for the neuroprotective and neurodestructive effects of nitric oxide and related nitroso-compounds. Nature 364:626–632, 1993

328. Ankarcrona M, Dypbukt JM, Bonfoco E, Zhivotovsky B, Orrenius S, Lipton SA, Nicotera P: Glutamate-induced neuronal death: A succession of necrosis or apoptosis depending on mitochondrial function. Neuron 15:961–973, 1995

329. Lizasoain I, Moro MA, Knowles RG, Darley-Usmar V, Moncada S: Nitric oxide and peroxynitrite exert distinct effects on mitochondrial respiration which are differentially blocked by glutathione or glucose. Biochem J 314:877–880, 1996

330. MacLellan WR, Schneider MD: Death by design: Programmed cell death in cardiovascular biology and disease. Circ Res 81:137–144, 1997

331. Pollman MJ, Hall JL, Gibbons GH: Determinants of vascular smooth muscle cell apoptosis after balloon angioplasty injury: Influence of redox state and cell phenotype. Circ Res 84:113–121, 1999

332. Ing DJ, Zang J, Dzau VJ, Webster KA, Bishopric NH: Modulation of cytokine-induced cardiac myocyte apoptosis by nitric oxide, Bak, and Bcl-x. Circ Res 84:21–33, 1999

333. Gow AJ, Thom SR, Ischiropoulos H: Nitric oxide and peroxynitrite-mediated pulmonary cell death. Am J Physiol 274:L112-L118, 1998

334. Dimmeler S, Haendeler J, Nehls M, Zeiher AM: Suppression of apoptosis by nitric oxide via inhibition of interleukin-1β-converting enzyme (ICE)-like and cysteine protease protein (CPP)-32-like proteases. J Exp Med 185:601–607, 1997

335. Selzman CH, Shames BD, McIntyre RC Jr, Banerjee A, Harken AH: The NFκB inhibitory peptide, IκBα, prevents human vascular smooth muscle proliferation. Ann Thorac Surg 67:1227–1232, 1999

336. Erl W, Hansson GK, de Martin R, Draude G, Weber KS, Weber C:

Nuclear factor-κB regulates induction of apoptosis and inhibitor of apoptosis protein-1 expression in vascular smooth muscle cells. Circ Res 84:668–677, 1999

337. Matthews JR, Botting CH, Panico M, Morris HR, Hay RT: Inhibition of NF-κB DNA binding by nitric oxide. Nucleic Acids Res 24:2236–2242, 1996

338. Tabuchi A, Sano K, Oh E, Tsuchiya T, Tsuda M: Modulation of AP-1 activity by nitric oxide (NO) in vitro: NO- mediated modulation of AP-1. FEBS Lett 351:123–127, 1994

339. Lipton SA: Janus faces of NF-κB: Neurodestruction versus neuroprotection. Nat Med 3:20–22, 1997

340. Smeyne RJ, Vendrell M, Hayward M, Baker SJ, Miao GG, Schilling K, Robertson LM, Curran T, Morgan JI: Continuous c-fos expression precedes programmed cell death in vivo. Nature 363:166–169, 1993

341. Hirose T, Ikeda T, Aoki E, Hara N: The protective effect of PGI_2 On increased lung vascular permeability caused by endotoxin in dogs. Nippon Kyobu Shikkan Gakkai Zasshi 16:410–417, 1978

342. Jahr J, Ekelund U, Grande PO: In vivo effects of prostacyclin on segmental vascular resistances, on myogenic reactivity, and on capillary fluid exchange in cat skeletal muscle. Crit Care Med 23:523–531, 1995

343. Moller AD, Grande P: Role of prostacyclin and nitric oxide in regulation of basal microvascular hydraulic permeability in cat skeletal muscle. J Vasc Res 36:245–252, 1999

344. Moller AD, Grande PO: Low-dose prostacyclin has potent capillary permeability-reducing effect in cat skeletal muscle in vivo. Am J Physiol 273:H200-H207, 1997

345. Oliver JA: Endothelium-derived relaxing factor contributes to the regulation of endothelial permeability. J Cell Physiol 151:506–511, 1992

346. Kubes P: Nitric oxide-induced microvascular permeability alterations: A regulatory role for cGMP. Am J Physiol 265:H1909-H1915, 1993

347. Arnhold S, Antoine D, Blaser H, Bloch W, Andressen C, Addicks K: Nitric oxide decreases microvascular permeability in bradykinin stimulated and nonstimulated conditions. J Cardiovasc Pharmacol 33:938–947, 1999

348. Rumbaut RE, McKay MK, Huxley VH: Capillary hydraulic conductivity is decreased by nitric oxide synthase inhibition. Am J Physiol 268:H1856-H1861, 1995

349. Kubes P: Nitric oxide affects microvascular permeability in the intact and inflamed vasculature. Microcirculation 2:235–244, 1995

350. Dusting GJ: Nitric oxide in cardiovascular disorders. J Vasc Res 32:143–161, 1995

351. Filep JG, Delalandre A, Beauchamp M: Dual role for nitric oxide in the regulation of plasma volume and albumin escape during endotoxin shock in conscious rats. Circ Res 81:840–847, 1997
352. Clough G: Relationship between microvascular permeability and ultrastructure. Prog Biophys Mol Biol 55:47–69, 1991
353. Kim NN, Villegas S, Summerour SR, Villarreal FJ: Regulation of cardiac fibroblast extracellular matrix production by bradykinin and nitric oxide. J Mol Cell Cardiol 31:457–466, 1999
354. Myers PR, Tanner MA: Vascular endothelial cell regulation of extracellular matrix collagen: Role of nitric oxide. Arterioscler Thromb Vasc Biol 18:717–722, 1998
355. Lum H, Malik AB: Regulation of vascular endothelial barrier function. Am J Physiol 267:L223-L241, 1994
356. Cromheeke KM, Kockx MM, Knaapen MW, De Meyer GRY, Bosmans J, Vrints CJ, Bult H, Herman AG: The presence of inducible nitric oxide synthase and hemeoxygenase in microhemorrhages/thrombosis in human atherosclerosis. Acta Physiol Scand 167:13, 1999

Edward M. Boyle, Jr, M.D.
Elizabeth N. Morgan, M.D.
Edward D. Verrier, M.D.

The Endothelium Disturbed: The

3 Procoagulant Response

A number of abnormalities in coagulation occur in the perioperative period in heart surgery patients. Clinically these are manifested by an overall early tendency to bleed and later thrombose, and by abnormalities in the laboratory measurements of the coagulation system, such as the platelet count and the protime. Why this occurs, however, is not entirely understood; therefore, there are still substantial efforts to determine this in order to best develop and time the delivery of interventional agents in this setting. It seems increasingly apparent that there may be many factors that contribute to post cardiopulmonary bypass (CPB) bleeding and thombosis, and in particular, that these responses seem to be associated with an overall activation of the coagulation system, which result in part from changes that occur at the microvascular level.

Under resting conditions the vascular endothelium regulates coagulation through the constitutive expression and release of anticoagulant substances and the inducible expression of procoagulant substances. CPB dysregulates this process by activating endothelial cells, initially promoting bleeding and then thrombosis at the microvascular level.[1] The biologic events that lead to dysregulated endothelial cell function in the setting of CPB are becoming increasingly understood as new methods in vascular biology are being tested in the laboratory and the clinical setting. The role of the endothelium in activating coagulation in

The Relationship Between Coagulation, Inflammation, and Endothelium, edited by
Bruce Spiess, Lippincott Williams & Wilkins, Baltimore © 2000.

the setting of CPB is probably best appreciated by examining the factors that contribute to activated coagulation in this setting.

ACTIVATED COAGULATION

Coagulation can either be activated by the extrinsic or intrinsic pathways. Traditionally, it has been taught that activation of coagulation after CPB occurs secondary to activation of the intrinsic pathway via the contact systems. It is speculated that plasma proteins are instantaneously adsorbed onto the nonendothelial surfaces of the CPB circuit; plasma factor XII is cleaved into serine proteases; and platelets are activated to aggregate, adhere to adsorbed fibrinogen, and release granule contents. The subsequent activation of factor XII initiates coagulation by the intrinsic coagulation pathway and activates complement.[2] Evidence suggests, however, that this may not be entirely the source of activated coagulation in CPB patients. Patients congenitally deficient in factor XII are not protected from thrombin generation after CPB, which suggests that other mechanisms may be at play. Inhibiting the contact activation system has little effect on preventing thrombin and platelet activation in simulated CPB.[3] Furthermore, extensive efforts to limit the degree of contact activation by lining CPB circuits with heparin only minimally impacted the degree of bleeding and did not impact the generation of thrombin.[4] This, coupled with what has been learned regarding the role of the tissue of factor (TF) pathway in the initiation of coagulation in vivo, has led to an expanded investigation of the role of the extrinsic pathway of coagulation in heart surgery patients.

The extrinsic pathway was so named because its activation required contact with TF (also known as thromboplastin), which was usually found outside of the intravascular system. TF can be induced on intravascular cells, such as endothelial cells and monocytes, as well as the underlying parynchymal cells, such as smooth muscle cells and myocytes, in response to inflammatory activation.[5] Substantial accumulated evidence indicates that the tissue factor pathway (or the extrinsic pathway) plays a primary role in initiating blood coagulation in vivo.

TF is a cell surface transmembrane glycoprotein with an extracellular domain that is the functional receptor for the coagulation factor VII/VIIa.[6] This pathway begins by exposure of blood to TF and formation of the complex between TF and plasma factor VII/VIIa. When the TF/VIIa complex is formed, it then activates factors IX and X. Factor IXa thus generated can also activate factor X in the presence of calcium and factor VIIIa. Factor Xa, formed either through IXa/VIIIa or VIIa/TF, then converts prothrombin to thrombin. Thrombin, in turn, converts fibrinogen to the fibrin clot. When this occurs at the site of tissue injury, it can be lifesaving. When this occurs diffusely, as it may in patients exposed to extreme sources of systemic stress, it can dysregulate both the coagulation and inflammatory systems.

THE ENDOTHELIUM DISTURBED

The endothelium plays a major role in regulating membrane permeability, lipid transport, vasomotor tone, inflammation, vascular wall structure, and coagulation. These critical endothelial cell functions are extremely sensitive to injury in the form of hypoxia, exposure to cytokines, endotoxin, cholesterol, nicotine, surgical manipulation, or hemodynamic shear stress.[7] In response to injury, endothelial cells become disturbed, tipping the balance of endothelial-derived factors to disrupt barrier function, and enhance vasoconstriction, leukocyte adhesion, smooth muscle cell proliferation, and coagulation. Although these responses likely exist as protective mechanisms, if the stimuli are severe, the responses may become excessive. This results in damaged tissue, impaired organ function, an abnormal fibroproliferative response, bleeding, and thrombosis. Endothelial cell injury from hypertension, diabetes mellitus, hyperlipidemia, fluctuating shear stress, smoking, or transplant rejection disrupts normal endothelial cell function.[8] This causes the loss of the constitutive protective mechanisms and an increase in inflammatory, procoagulant, vasoactive, and fibroproliferative responses to injury. These changes promote vasospasm, intimal proliferation, and thrombus formation, all of which play a significant role in the initiation, progression, and clinical manifestations of atherosclerosis.[8] Thus, many of the patients that come to cardiovascular surgery have preexisting abnormalities in endothelial cell function. Furthermore, many of the components currently used to perform cardiovascular operations lead to systemic insults that result from CPB circuit-induced contact activation, circulatory shock, and resuscitation, and a syndrome similar to endotoxemia.[9] Experimental observations have demonstrated that these events have profound effects on activating endothelial cells to promote both fibrinolysis, initially, and later microvascular coagulation.[1]

We have been studying how changes at the endothelial cell level may contribute to the activation of coagulation in the setting of CPB. Normal endothelial cell function provides a nonthrombogenic surface to prevent intravascular coagulation. The endovascular surface is lined with thombomodulin and heparin-like molecules that prevent coagulation in the resting state. Thrombomodulin is a high-affinity thrombin receptor present on endothelial cell membrane that plays an important role as a natural anticoagulant. It acts as a cofactor of thrombin-catalyzed activation of protein C, and inhibits the procoagulant functions of thrombin. In response to injury, however, the endothelium acquires phenotypic properties that may promote coagulation. From our understanding to date, this can occur in one of three ways. First, the endothelium can become activated. In this paradigm, the natural anticoagulent proteins are downregulated or overwhelmed, and the procoagulant substances, such as TF, are upregulated or expressed. Second, the endothelium may be disrupted, which allows the serum proteins of the coagulation cascades to encounter subendothelial TF. Finally, recent evidence indicates that the endothelium may, in the process of being injured by stimuli such as hypoxia or endotoxin, undergo apoptosis. These apoptotic cells, in turn, become procoagulant.[10] The molecular mechanisms of how the various procoagulant changes occur in the context of CPB may help develop novel therapies to attenuate this process. What follows is a discussion of several recent findings in our laboratory and others in the effort to learn more about the role that the injured endothelium plays in the development of coagulation disturbances in heart surgery patients.

THE INITIAL ANTICOAGULANT EFFECT

The body possesses complex and redundant systems to suppress the overactivation of coagulation at the microvascular level. One pathway that has been more recently characterized is the endothelial derived "a" factor Xa-dependent inhibitor of TF/VIIa complex, the tissue factor pathway inhibitor (TFPI). Until 1993, this Xa-dependent inhibitor was referred to as lipoprotein-associated coagulation inhibitor or extrinsic pathway inhibitor. The primary site of TFPI synthesis is the endothelium, and to a lesser degree, platelets. TFPI directly inactivates coagulation factor Xa and produces feedback inhibition of the factor VIIa/TF catalytic complex, which is responsible for the initiation of coagulation. Animal studies have established that TFPI functions as a natural anticoagulant that protects rabbits from intravascular coagulation triggered by the exposure of blood to small amounts of TF.[11] Furthermore, studies in rabbits immunodepleted of TFPI suggest that, in contrast with the sensitization of TFPI-depleted rabbits to TF-induced coagulation, TFPI-depleted rabbits were not sensitized to coagulation initiated by factor Xa and phospholipid in the absence of TF. These data support a conclusion that the physiological function of TFPI in regulating TF-dependent coagulation stems primarily from its ability to inhibit factor VIIa/TF catalytic activity.[12]

Quantification of TFPI offers insight into the mechanisms of disseminated intravascular thrombin generation in CPB patients. We have found that there is a rapid rise in TFPI when patients are heparinized prior to CPB, and that this returns to baseline when the patients are given protamine (unpublished observations). Only recently has TFPI been studied clinically and in the laboratory setting. It seems that TFPI effectively shuts down the extrinsic pathway of coagulation during CPB and that this effect is almost completely gone at the end of the bypass run. It is likely that this response is protective in preventing blood clotting in the extracorporeal circuit; however, it is equally likely that this response contributes, at least in part, to intraoperative bleeding in CPB patients. The fact that thrombin levels remain high, even when TFPI levels are high, provides further evidence of the complexity of the response of the coagulation system to CPB.

TISSUE FACTOR EXPRESSION: ON OR UNDER THE ACTIVATED ENDOTHELIUM?

Ample evidence suggests that TF is activated on endothelial cells in vitro by many of the same conditions that are found during CPB.[5,13] Thus, we initially thought that TF was induced on endothelial cells in vivo. This has not held true in several small animal models, studied by us and others. For example, Erlich et al[14] performed a detailed analysis of TF induction in a rabbit model of endotoxemia to better understand the cell types that may contribute to local fibrin deposition and disseminated intravascular coagulation in the setting of systemic inflammation. Northern blot analysis demonstrated that lipopolysaccharide (LPS) increased TF expression in the brain, lung, and kidneys. In situ hybridization showed that TF mRNA expression was increased in cells identified morphologically as epithelial cells in the lung and as astrocytes in the brain. In the kidney, in situ hybridization experiments and immunohistochemical analysis showed that TF mRNA and protein expression was increased in renal glomeruli and induced in tubular epithelium. Dual staining for TF and von Willebrand factor failed to demonstrate TF expression in endothelial cells in LPS-treated animals.[14] Likewise, in a similar study with this same group, we examined the cellular source of TF after cardiac ischemia-reperfusion in a rabbit model to determine its location and its functional significance. We found that TF is dramatically upregulated in the cardiomyocytes in response to ischemia-reperfusion injury, but again, not on the endothelial cells. The role of induced TF in ischemia-reperfusion injury was examined using an inhibitory anti-TF monoclonal antibody. Treatment with this antibody reduced infarct dramatically. Thus, just as in the endotoxemia models, endothelial cells were not identified as upregulating TF either because of oxidative stress in the setting of myocardial ischemia-reperfusion injury. In both of these models, however, inhibiting TF is protective, which suggests that something is occurring at the microvascular level that exposes the coagulation factors to the upregulated TF that ultimately triggers the initiation of coagulation in the small vessels. The mechanism by which the coagulation factors might be exposed to TF are unknown. In vivo and ex vivo models of cardiac ischemia and reperfusion have demonstrated physical and physiological disruption of the endothelial barrier. Studies using several species show that endothelium is not structurally intact following cardiac ischemia-reperfusion injury. Ample data also suggests that even when structurally intact by electron microscopy, the coronary vascular endothelium in rabbits and other animals loses its barrier function and becomes significantly more permeable even after brief periods of ischemia.

Because inhibiting TF is protective in animal models, it seems reasonable to pursue the mechanisms further in heart surgery patients. Kappelmayer et al assayed for TF upregulation on monocytes in a simulated extracorporeal circulation model.[15] They found that TF significantly increased between 2 and 6 hours of simulated extracorporeal circulation. In particular, procoagulant activity increased from 21 to 776pg TF/10^6 monocytes and was blocked 99.6% by preincubation of cells with a mixture of monoclonal antibodies to TF. We have found similar findings in our lab, and showed an increase in both TF expression and activity in monocytes exposed to an in vitro CPB circuit. It may be that the CPB circuit contributes to TF expression, at least on circulating monocytes. The ability to initiate a TF-induced increase in procoagulant activity in an in vitro model of CPB is an excellent model to screen potential therapeutic interventions to address this response clinically. Barstad et al[16] found that heparin coating of the extracorporeal circuit reduced induction of adherent cell TF-procoagulant activity by 70%.

We duplicated these findings in our lab, and showed an increase in both TF expression and activity in monocytes exposed to the CPB circuit. As depicted in Figure 3–1, TF activity increases over time and manifests as a reduction in the time-to-clot formation. Correspondingly, TF expression quantified as picograms per monocyte also increases over time. Therefore, these studies show that the CPB circuit alone serves as a stimulus for the inducible expression of TF in circulating monocytes. We are currently working to further understand the transcriptional regulation of this event by examining the role of the transcription factor, NF-κB in the setting of CPB. Because these strategies can also prevent endothelial cell activation, we anticipate that targeting transduction of the signals that activate cells in the setting of CPB may be a useful technique to reduce this response clinically.

At this point, however, the ultimate proof that TF is implicated in the microvascular dysfunction seen in heart surgery patients will

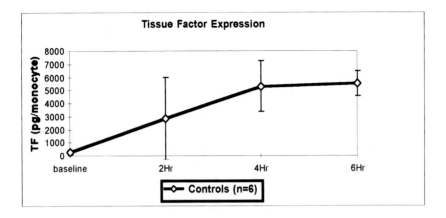

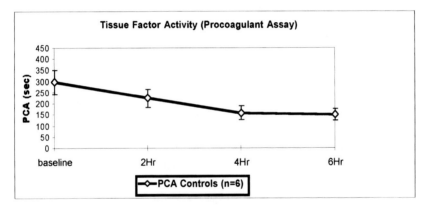

FIGURE 3–1. Tissue factor (TF) expression, expressed as picograms per monocyte, increases progressively as whole blood from normal donors is circulated through a cardiopulmonary bypass circuit. TF activity, assessed by a procoagulant assay (PCA) that measures the time to clot formation, demonstrates a corresponding decrease in clotting time, which represents an increase in TF activity.

come from examining tissue and blood samples directly before and after bypass clinically. In part this is because of the difficulty of measuring TF because it is a cell-based glycoprotein. Whether TF is expressed on the endothelium, monocytes, the pericardium, or on the exposed underlying parenchyma is of concern only because it may help direct the timing and delivery of anti-TF oriented therapies in the setting of CPB.

ENDOTHELIAL APOPTOSIS

Another mechanism by which endothelial cells may contribute to the procoagulant response is by becoming apoptotic in response to the types of inflamamtory stimuli encountered in heart surgery patients. In general, endothelial cells are relatively resistant to apoptosis. With ongoing exposure to stimuli such as oxidative stress, however, endothelial cells will undergo programmed cell death. For example in an in vitro model, Stempien-Otero et al[17] found that human umbilical vein endothelial cells (HUVEC) were initially resistant to hypoxia-induced cell death with only a 2% reduction in viability at 24 hours; however, by 48 hours, there was a 45% reduction in viability because of apoptosis. Bombeli et al[10] investigated whether apoptotic endothelial cells contribute to the development of a prothrombotic state. As assessed by flow cytometric determination of annexin V binding (a marker of apoptosis), HUVECs undergoing cell death typically exhibited a more rapid exposure of membrane phosphatidylserine, which corresponded with an increase in procoagulant activity. Although apoptotic cells did not show antigenic or functional TF activity, when preactivated with LPS, TF procoagulant activity increased by 50% to 70%. At 8 hours after apoptosis induction, antigenic thrombomodulin, heparan sulfates, and TFPI decreased by about 83%, 80%, and 59%, respectively. The functional activity of these components was reduced by about 36%, 52%, and 39%, respectively. Moreover, the presence of apoptotic HUVECs led to a significant increase in thrombin formation in recalcified citrated plasma. Thus, apoptotic HUVECs, either adherent or in suspension, become procoagulant by increased expression of phosphatidylserine and the loss of anticoagulant membrane components.[10]

Bombeli et al[18] also investigated whether apoptotic endothelial cells attracted nonactivated platelets. Under normal conditions, unactivated platelets do not adhere to quiescent endothelium. However, when platelets are activated, they bind avidly to endothelium, which is mediated by a GpIIb/IIIa-dependent briding mechanism involving platelet-bound adhesive proteins and the endothelial cell receptors intracellular adhesion molecule $\alpha\beta_3$-integrin, and, to a lesser extent, $GpIb_\alpha$. Because there is accumulating evidence that endothelial cells may become apoptotic under certain proinflammatory or prothrombotic conditions, they investigated whether endothelial cells undergoing apoptosis may become proadhesive for nonactivated platelets. HUVECs were induced to undergo apoptosis by staurosporine, a nonspecific protein kinase inhibitor, or by culture in suspension with serum-deprivation. After treatment of HUVEC or platelets with different receptor antagonists, nonactivated, washed human platelets were allowed to adhere to HUVEC for 20 minutes. Independent of the method of apoptosis induction, there was a marked increase in platelet binding to apoptotic HUVEC. Adhesion assays after blockade of different platelet receptors showed only involvement of β_1-integrins. Platelet binding to apoptotic HUVEC was inhibited by more than 70% when platelets were treated with blocking anti-β_1 antibodies. Treatment of apoptotic HUVEC with blocking antibodies to different potential platelet receptors, including known ligands for β_1-integrins, did not affect platelet binding.[19] These data provide further evidence that endothelial cells undergoing apoptosis may contribute to thrombotic events. Thus, endothelial cells becoming apoptotic may contribute to an overall procoagulant state by attracting unactivated platelets diffusely, which makes platelets less available at sites of surgical injury.

CONCLUSION

It is increasingly apparent that the endothelium plays a critical role in the regulation of the events that contribute to coagulation abnormalities in heart surgery patients. If this occurs because endothelial cells become activated to express certain procoagulant proteins, are disrupted or become apoptotic is an area of increasing investigation (Figure 3–2). As the overall understanding grows of how coagulation is activated in re-

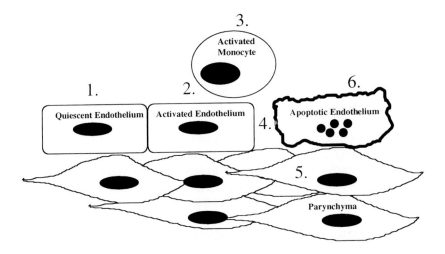

FIGURE 3–2. Possible sources of procoagulant activity in the setting of microvascular inflammation. The quiescent endothelium (1) can become activated (2) by inflammatory stimuli, such as TNF, Il-1, LPS, oxidative stress, and shear stress, to express tissue factor. Activated endothelial cells can adhere to activated monocytes (3) expressing tissue factor. Also, the endothelium may become disrupted (4), exposing underlying parynchymal tissue (5) where tissue factor is upregulated. Finally, apoptotic endothelial cells (6) have been shown to be procoagulant and adhesive to platelets.

sponse to CPB, it may be possible to apply these principles to what we know about the disturbed endothelium in heart surgery patients. Because the endothelium is at the centerpoint of this response, it is imperative that we continue to study the impact that CPB has an altering the quiescent endothelium so that we can better evaluate therapeutic interventions to try to prevent this potentially dangerous responses.

Acknowledgments

Funded, in part, by the Thoracic Surgery Foundation for Research and Education and the Bayer Corporation Grant for the Study of Blood Conservation in Thoracic Surgery. The authors thank Nigel Mackman, Ph.D., Richard Santucci, M.D., J. Craig Kovacich, and Jonathan Erlich, M.D., Ph.D. at the Scripps Research Institute for their expert collaboration on the subject of tissue factor, and Angela Farr, Louise Soltow, and Ellen Collins for their expert technical assistance.

References

1. Boyle EM Jr, Verrier ED, Spiess BD: Endothelial cell injury in cardiovascular surgery: The procoagulant response. Ann Thorac Surg 62: 1549–1557, 1996.
2. Edmunds LH Jr: Blood-surface interactions during cardiopulmonary bypass. J Card Surg 8: 404–10, 1993.
3. Wachtfogel YT, Bischoff R, Bauer R, Hacke CE, Nuijens JH, Kucich U, Niewiarowski S, Edmunds LH Jr, Colman RW: Alpha 1-antitrypsin inhibits the contact pathway of intrinsic coagulation and alters the release of human neutrophil elastase during simulated extracorporeal circulation. Thromb Haemost 72: 843–897, 1994.
4. Gorman RC, Ziats N, Rao AK, Gikakis N, Sun L, Khan MM, Stenach N, Sapatnekar S, Chouhan V, Gorman JH III, Niewiaroski S, Colman RW, Anderson JM, Edmunds LH Jr: Surface-found heparin fails to reduce thrombin formation during clinical cardiopulmonary bypass. J Thorac Cardiovasc Surg 111: 1–11; discussion 11–12, 1996.
5. Mackman N: Regulation of the tissue factor gene. Faseb J 9: 883–889, 1995.
6. Edgington TS, Mackman N, Brand K, Ruf W: The structural biology of expression and function of tissue factor. Thromb Haemost 66: 67–79, 1991.
7. Verrier ED, Boyle EM Jr: Endothelial cell injury in cardiovascular surgery. Ann Thorac Surg 62: 915–922, 1996.
8. Boyle EM Jr, Lille ST, Allaire E, Clowes AW, Verrier ED: Endothe-

lial cell injury in cardiovascular surgery: Atherosclerosis. Ann Thorac Surg 63: 885–894, 1997.

9. Boyle EM Jr, Pohlman TH, Johnson MC, Verrier ED: Endothelial cell injury in cardiovascular surgery: The systemic inflammatory response. Ann Thorac Surg 63: 277–284, 1997.

10. Bombeli T, Karsan A, Tait JF, Halan JM: Apoptotic vascular endothelial cells become procoagulant. Blood 89: 2429–2442, 1997.

11. Warn-Cramer BJ, Maki SL, Rapaport SI: Heparin-releasable and platelet pools of tissue factor pathway inhibitor in rabbits. Thromb Haemost 69: 221–226, 1993.

12. Warn-Cramer BJ, Rapaport SI: Studies of factor Xa/phospholipid-induced intravascular coagulation in rabbits: Effects of immunodepletion of tissue factor pathway inhibitor. Arterioscler Thromb 13: 1551–1557, 1993.

13. Mackman N: Regulation of tissue factor gene expression in human monocytic and endothelial cells. Haemostasis 26(Suppl 1): 17–19, 1996.

14. Erlich J, Fearns C. Mathison J, Ulevitch RJ, Mackman N: Lipopolysaccharide induction of tissue factor expression in rabbits. Infect Immun 67: 2540–2546, 1999.

15. Kappelmayer J, Bernabei A, Edmunds LH Jr, Edgington TS, Colman RW: Tissue factor is expressed on monocytes during simulated extracorporeal circulation. Circ Res 72: 1075–81, 1993.

16. Barstad RM, Ovrum E. Ringdal MA, Oystesc R, Hamers MJ, Veiby OP, Rolfsen T, Stephens RW, Sakariassen KS: Induction of monocyte tissue factor procoagulant activity during coronary artery bypass surgery is reduced with heparin-coated extracorporeal circuit. Br J Haematol 94: 517–525, 1996.

17. Stempien-Otero A, Karsan A, Cornejo CJ, Xiang H, Eunson T, Morrison RS, Kay M, Winn R, Harlan J: Mechanisms of hypoxia-induced endothelial cell death: Role of p53 in apoptosis. J Biol Chem 274: 80-39–8045, 1999.

18. Bombeli T, Schwartz BR, Harlan JM: Adhesion of activated platelets to endothelial cells: Evidence for a GPIIbIIIa-dependent bridging mechanism and novel roles for endothelial intercellular adhesion molecule 1 (ICAM-1), $\alpha\beta_3$ integrin, and GPIb$_3$. J Exp Med 187:329–339, 1998.

19. Bombeli T, Schwartz BR, Harlan JM: Endothelial cells and undergoing apoptosis become proadhesive for nonactivated platelets. Blood 93: 3831–3838, 1999.

Jerrold H. Levy, M.D.

The Relationships Between Coagulation, Inflammation, and Endothelium:
4 | Inflammation Responds

The activation of coagulation is closely linked to inflammatory responses via a complex network of both humoral and cellular components, which includes proteases of the clotting and fibrinolytic cascades.[1-4] Hemostatic initiation, contact activation, and other pathways amplify inflammatory responses to collectively produce end-organ damage as part of host defense mechanisms. Coagulation is activated as a central element of both local and systemic responses to inflammation.[5-7] Several of the key coagulation components and their products have proinflammatory effects, including thrombin and factor Xa. Thrombin also has a direct chemoattractant activity for polymorphonuclear leukocytes and monocytes and is a potent activator of mast cells.[8-10] Factor Xa also interacts with receptors on mast cells and causes degranulation through a variety of different mechanisms that include receptor activation.[11] Activation of monocytes and macrophages results in the release of interleukin-1 (IL-1), tumor necrosis factor (TNF), and other chemotactic factors that recruit additional leukocytes into the lesion. Mast cells, therefore, may play a pivotal role in linking coagulation and inflammation.[11-20]

THROMBIN

Thrombin is an important mediator in signaling inflammatory processes. After endothelial damage, tissue factor is expressed and

The Relationship Between Coagulation, Inflammation, and Endothelium, edited by Bruce Spiess, Lippincott Williams & Wilkins, Baltimore © 2000.

thrombin is formed from its precursor prothrombin. Thrombin can induce a variety of cellular responses involved in inflammation. Thrombin is chemotactic for monocytes and neutrophils via multiple mechanisms that include (1) increasing cytokine mediated neutrophil chemotaxis; (2) acting as a potent mitogen of a variety of cell types; and (3) stimulating endothelial cell activation by binding to thrombomodulin.[1-9] Thrombin may have variable vasoactive properties (vasoconstriction or dilation) depending upon the state of endothelial function. Thrombin is capable of inducing cytokine expression through stimulation of a variety of cell types. When generated at a site of injury, thrombin may further amplify inflammation. Thrombin receptor activation on leukocytes increases the release of chemotactic and inflammatory cytokines.[21-25]

INFLAMMATORY CELLS

Vascular cells and polymorphonuclear leukocytes, as part of their complex host immunosurveillance properties, can initiate and amplify coagulation via multiple, receptor-mediated processes. Leukocytes also have the ability to generate thrombin as part of their role in modulating inflammatory responses. The inflammatory response induced by factor Xa includes the prominent perivascular accumulation of activated and partially degranulated mast cells.[11] Although the neutrophils play central roles in acute inflammation, findings have also identified a direct role of clotting and fibrinolytic proteases in intracellular signal transduction and modulation of inflammatory cell responses.

Mast cells are the key cells of type I hypersensitivity reactions; however, their ubiquitous distribution throughout perivascular spaces makes their "pharmacopoeia" of mediators available to a spectrum of cell types, which include vascular endothelial cells, inflammatory cells, and vascular smooth muscle.[15] Mast cells have been suggested to play important roles in a series of inflammatory and proliferative disorders. The release of mast cell mediators by multiple stimuli may play a pivotal role in host defense. Mast cell–derived mediators can produce multiple proinflammatory effects. Histamine enhances both fibroblast proliferation and collagen synthesis; tryptase and chymase can digest multiple cellular components, and cytokines such as TNF, IL-4, and growth factors have effects on multiple cell types.[15] Mast cells will be considered in more detail later.

FACTOR Xa

Factor Xa can produce acute inflammatory response by recruiting mast cells to release vasoactive mediators, as judged by the prominent perivascular accumulation of activated and partially degranulated mast cells.[10,11] As a target of factor Xa, mast cells are ideally positioned to initiate and amplify a broad range of vascular and inflammatory cell responses, which include acute angioedema or urticaria.[11–15] Mast cell release of inflammatory mediators such as histamine, serotonin, leukotrienes (LT), platelet activating factor, and cytokines triggers increased vascular permeability, enhanced leukocyte activation, upregulation of β-integrin function, and increased leukocyte rolling and adherence to endothelium, which further exacerbates tissue injury and disruption of the endothelial cell monolayer.[14–18] A spectrum of molecular structures can degranulate mast cells by multiple complex pathways that may not be different than pathologic activation by immunoglobulin E (IgE).[19]

DISSEMINATED INTRAVASCULAR COAGULATION

Disseminated intravascular coagulation (DIC) is a syndrome that can be triggered by a multitude of stimuli related to the underlying disease processes including tissue factor released from injured tissues, endotoxin from Gram-negative bacteria, or excessive contact pathway-tissue factor–mediated activation related to extracorporeal circulation.[26,27] Although the initiating mechanisms may be different, activation of the coagulation cascade and thrombin generation are thought to be key events in the initiating process; kallikrein activation may be of key importance as well. It is interesting to note that despite the research effort in cardiopulmonary bypass (CPB), the basic triggering mechanism on coagulation and inflammation is still not known.

Tissue damage produces thrombin generation on the surface of injured endothelial cells in the microcirculation; this, in turn, activates the hemostatic cascade locally. There are a number of direct thrombin inhibitors (eg, antithrombin [ATIII]), indirect thrombin inhibitors (eg, protein C and protein S), and other hemostatic regulating molecules (eg, tissue plasminogen activator and α_2-antiplasmin) that circulate and prevent unbridled thrombin generation. In addition, heparan is bound to the surface of vascular endothelium, thereby providing an activation site for ATIII. In DIC, thrombin generation and activity releases free thrombin into the circulation to produce a more generalized fibrin formation and deposition in the microvasculature, occlusion of microcirculatory flow, and thrombosis, which leads to multiple organ failure. Plasmin is generated as well, which produces fibrino(geno)lysis and eventually restores vascular patency. A complex balance between anticoagulation and coagulation exists normally within the microvasculature that is altered in DIC and produces both thrombotic and hemorrhagic complications.

ATIII binds to heparan molecules on the surface of normal vascular endothelium, and the intact endothelium also expresses thrombomodulin molecules. If thrombin is generated, it is either inactivated by ATIII or binds to thrombomodulin. Bound thrombin is no longer capable of converting fibrinogen to fibrin or stimulating platelet activation. Therefore, the surface activity of ATIII and heparan together create a hemostatic mechanism for deactivating or limiting the procoagulant/inflammatory actions of thrombin. Furthermore, thrombomodulin-bound thrombin activates the protein C system, which also functions as an anticoagulant and inhibits factors V and VIII. When the endothelium is injured (after cytokine activation, sepsis, or other inflammatory insults), unbridled thrombin generation occurs, which triggers a spectrum of other pathways and contributes to the pathogenesis of DIC.

Consumption of the coagulation proteins and activation of the fibrinolytic system follow this initial thrombotic phase. Clinically, DIC manifests as a syndrome of consumptive coagulopathy with hemorrhage and microthrombi. Supportive laboratory evidence in the diagnosis of DIC include microangiopathic hemolytic anemia, with the appearance of red cell fragments and defects in the coagulation profile including thrombocytopenia, prolonged prothrombin time, activated partial thromboplastin time, and thrombin time, and decreased fibrinogen levels along with increased fibrin degradation products.[26,27] In DIC, ATIII is consumed, its activity is diminished, and levels below 50% to 60% predict poor outcome and death, while 100% mortality is observed in patients with levels below 20% activity.[26–28]

ATIII

In experimental models of DIC, the administration of ATIII either prophylactically or within 5 hours after infection in septicemic animals has been shown to correct abnormal coagulation profiles or significantly reduce mortality.[28] The experience with ATIII concentrate in patients with DIC is difficult to interpret because of variability in study design, the small number of patients evaluated, lack of homogeneity within and between study groups, diverse inclusion criteria, variable pretreatment ATIII levels, and response criteria. Most studies have demonstrated improvement in the coagulation parameters and shortened duration of DIC with the use of ATIII concentrate, but definitive clinical benefit has yet to be demonstrated. In a placebo-controlled, double-blind, randomized trial in patients with DIC that received ATIII concentrate, Fourrier et al[29] reported a trend toward reduction in overall mortality of 44%, and when analyzed in an intention-to-treat fashion, mortality was 18%. However, DIC is a term applied to a syndrome with a wide number of causes and a tremendous spectrum of individual responses. In many studies, a wide dose range has been used with the intention of increasing ATIII levels to near 100%.[29–32] However, it should be noted that DIC is a catch-all term for a syndrome with a wide number of causes and a large graduation of individual responses.

CPB AND SYSTEMIC INFLAMMATORY RESPONSE SYNDROME

CPB has often been compared to the pathophysiologic changes occurring in sepsis or systemic inflammatory response syndrome (SIRS). DIC occurs after SIRS and can also occur after CPB. In DIC, overactivation of thrombin and/or clotting leads to bleeding complications caused by depletion of coagulation proteins, platelets, and endothelial dysfunction to produce microvascular dysfunction and a thrombotic state. DIC is characterized by decreased platelet counts, low fibrinogen, increased prothrombin time and activated partial thromboplastin time, and elevated D-dimer levels, changes that can also occur in the pharmacologically naive patient who undergoes CPB.[32] Acquired ATIII deficiency in the perioperative cardiac surgical period may be related to the preoperative use of heparin, the effects of hemodilution, and/or CPB-related consumption. ATIII levels as low as 40% to 50% activity, which are similar to levels observed with heterozygous hereditary deficiency, are commonly seen during CPB.[33–35] Because the data in DIC suggest that ATIII may play a major role in reducing inflammation and/or end-organ dysfunction, we have further expanded this consideration to cardiac surgical patients and are investigating whether ATIII represents an important therapeutic intervention that alone, or in conjunction with other therapies, may further reduce the inflammatory sequelae.[36–38]

MAST CELLS

Most clinicians consider neutrophils to represent the major inflammatory cell of inflammatory responses during sepsis, system inflammatory responses, and CPB. Mast cells and basophils also play a pivotal role in inflammatory processes.[12–15] Basophils share several notable features with the polymorphonuclear leukocytes but are distinctly different cell types. Both mast cells and basophils contain dense metachromatic cytoplasmic granules that contain stored inflammatory mediators including histamine and other potent chemical mediators that have been implicated in a wide variety of inflammatory processes.[41-44] They also constitutively express plasma membrane receptors that bind with the Fc portion of IgE antibodies.[45,46] Mature basophils are differentiated circulating polymorphonuclear leukocytes that can infiltrate tissues during inflammatory processes.[41] Mature mast cells are fixed in the perivascular areas of certain tissues (eg, skin, heart, lung, and intestine).

Ultrastructurally, human mast cells appear as either round or elongated cells and contain cytoplasmic granules that are usually smaller, more numerous, and generally variable in appearance (Figure 4–1). The basophils also have metachromatic granules that contain mediators and comprise approximately 0.5% to 1.0% of total leukocytes. Mast cells are distributed throughout perivascular spaces and beneath epithelial surfaces that are exposed to the external environment, such as those of the respiratory system, the gastrointestinal system, and the skin.[47-53] The number of mast cells in tissue varies considerably according to the

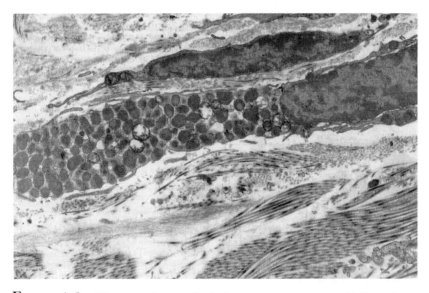

FIGURE 4–1. Electron micrograph of a human cutaneus mast cell. Note the electron dense granules that contain histamine, tryptase, and other preformed mediators. The cell outline is well preserved and the cytoplasmic granules are well delineated and demonstrate normal electron density. Note also the proximity to a probable vascular endothelial cell. Mast cells are present in the perivascular regions of the skin lung and intestine. Also note the collagen bundles in the micrograph. Magnification × 50,000. Reprinted with permission from Levy JH, Brister NW, Shearin WA, Ziegler JS, Hug CC, Adelson DM, Walker BF: Wheal and flare responses to opioids in humans. Anesthesiology 70:756–760, 1989.

anatomic site. Mast cells can also vary in their morphology, histochemistry, mediator content, response to drugs, and activation.[47-53] The different mast cell populations may be important for different functions.[15,40,41]

Mast Cell Mediators

Mast cells and basophils contain either stored mediators in the granules (eg, tryptase, histamine, heparin, serine proteases, carboxypeptidase A, and small amounts of sulfatases and exoglycosidases) or elaborate a diverse group of biologically active mediators that are synthesized on activation of the cell by antigen binding to immunospecific IgE (eg, arachidonic acid oxidation products synthesized via the cyclooxygenase or lipoxygenase pathways).[15,40-44] Cytokines are also mast cell and basophil mediators that can be preformed and stored in mast cells or can be newly synthesized by activated cells.[15] Human mast cells contain combinations of heparin and chondroitin sulfate proteoglycans.[41,43,50,54] Proteoglycans contained in mast cells and basophils bind histamine and proteases, which allows storage within the secretory granules. Tryptase is the major protease contained in the electron dense granules of human mast cells—a serine endopeptidase that exists in the granule in active form as a tetramer of 134,000 daltons that contains subunits of 31,000 to 35,000 daltons but does not exist in basophils. Mast cell tryptase levels are used to assess mast cell activation and acute anaphylaxis.[56-58] The exact role of tryptase is unclear, but it likely represents a proteolytic enzyme involved in initial host cell defenses against invading pathogens.

Mast cells or basophils activation also causes the synthesis of both prostaglandin and leukotrienes—lipid-derived cyclooxygenase and lipoxygenase metabolites of arachidonic acid that have potent inflammatory activities and modulate cell activation.[40,41,54,56] Prostaglandin D_2 (PGD_2) is the major cyclooxygenase product of mast cells, and the major lipoxygenase products derived from mast cells and basophils are the sulfidopeptide LT: LTC4 and its peptidolytic derivatives, LTD4 and LTE4.[41,54,56] Lung and intestinal mast cells produce similar amounts of LTC4 and PGD_2. Cutaneus mast cells largely produce PGD_2, while basophils primarily generate LTC4.[41]

Mast Cells and Cytokines

Cytokines are a diverse group of small-molecular-weight polypeptides that are synthesized in response to inflammatory, stimuli thereby modulating and signaling inflammatory responses and other biologic processes. Cytokines upregulate the IgE responses (eg, IL-4 and IL-13), augment basophil recruitment (eg, TNF-α and IL-4), stimulate mediator production (eg, IL-4 and IL-13), promote eosinophil recruitment (eg, IL-5, IL-6 and IL-13), and promote monocyte and T cell recruitment (eg, IL-6, and certain chemokines).[41,55] Cytokines contribute to allergic-mediated inflammation by enhancing the recruitment of polymorphonuclear leukocytes. Cytokines such as TNF-α and IL-1 increase the expression of adhesion molecules, such as P-selectin and E-selectin, vascular cell adhesion molecule-1, and intercellular adhesion molecule-1, on vascular endothelial cells.[41,55,59,60] Mast cells and basophils can also modulate inflammatory responses by cytokine synthesis.[41,53,61] Mast cells can potentially synthesize a variety of cytokines, including TNF-α.[41] Human mast cells also seem to represent a potential source of many cytokines, which include TNF-α, basic fibroblast growth factor, IL-4, IL-5, IL-6, and IL-8, and IL-13.[41,65] Corticosteroids can inhibit cytokine production.[67] Human basophils can release IL-4 and IL-13 in response to activation that can be enhanced by exposure to IL-13.[1,3,4] Mast cell/basophil-derived cytokines may enhance IgE production or stimulate T-cell differentiation and promote immunoglobulin class switching.[41,55,69]

Role and Function of Mast Cells in Inflammation

Anaphylaxis is an immediate hypersensitivity reaction; the central role of the mast cell in the pathogenesis of this disorder has been well established.[40] An immediate hypersensitivity reaction is initiated by the interaction of antigen-specific IgE molecules on the surface of mast cells and/or basophils with an immunospecific antigen.[40] The end-organ effects are caused by the physiologic responses of target cells (vascular endothelial cells, vascular smooth muscle, bronchial smooth muscle, and inflammatory cells) to mediators released by activated mast cells and/or basophils.[40] Allergic reactions are usually accompanied by an increase in local levels of LTC4 and PGD_2 and by the liberation of histamine and tryptase.[41,43,54] Tryptase is thought to be mast cell derived, and its levels increase in anaphylaxis. Besides allergens, other mast cell stimuli, which include certain drugs (opioids, benzylisoquinoline-derived neuromuscular blocking agents, vancomycin, and protamine), complement anaphylatoxins, basic peptides, and peptide hormones, can also release mediators from mast cells independently of IgE to produce a spectrum of reactions that may mimic anaphylaxis.[43,56] Mast cells may also play a role in ischemia reperfusion injury. Kanwar et al[14] reported that that oxidant-induced mucosal mast cell degranulation is a key event in the granulocyte infiltration and tissue dysfunction associated with reperfusion of the ischemic intestine.

Galli et al[41] have formulated the hypothesis that a "mast cell–leukocyte cytokine cascade" critically contributes to the initiation and perpetuation of IgE-dependent inflammation via the activation of mast cells through the FcεRI to initiate the response. The activated mast cells then release TNF-α and other cytokines that can influence the recruitment and function of additional effector cells, thus amplifying the inflammatory response by providing additional sources of certain cytokines (that can also be produced by mast cells stimulated by ongoing exposure to allergen), as well as new sources of cytokines and other mediators that may not be produced by mast cells.[41,53,55,61] Mast cell activation may directly or indirectly promote the release of cytokines from certain cells, which include the alveolar macrophages, bronchial epithelial cells, vascular endothelial cells, fibroblasts, and epithelial cells. The cytokines released may contribute to the vascular and epithelial changes, including tissue remodeling, angiogenesis, and fibrosis, that are so prominent in many disorders associated with mast cell activation and leukocyte infiltration. At certain points in the natural history of these complex processes, cytokines derived from mast cells, or from eosinophils or other recruited cells, may also contribute to the downregulation of the response. In addition to their roles in allergic diseases, mast cell–leukocyte cytokine cascades may contribute to host defense, both in innate immunity to microbial infection, in which mast cells are activated independently of IgE, and in immune responses to parasites.[41]

SUMMARY

Complex interactions exist between inflammation and coagulation following the activation of thrombosis. Recent discoveries that explain the molecular basis of both crosstalk and amplification have been examined. Because of the complex variables, the cellular and humoral cascades involved, and the phenomenal humoral amplification that occurs in any injury process, understanding the pivotal role of any one mediator is still unclear. However, the ability under physiologic conditions to preserve the proinflammatory and antiinflammatory process when damage occurs and the importance of autoregulation via proteins such as ATIII are still being explored as potential therapeutic applications. The study of inflammation cannot be limited to the influence of single mediators or inflammatory cells but needs to include the complex influences of a broad spectrum of pathways that are initiated concomitantly or in a cascade. Mast cells may play a rather pivotal role in inflammatory responses. The role of specific mediators and their potential antagonists plays a never-ending role in our potential to block and decrease inflammatory injury and coagulation and ultimately improve patient outcomes. Future research will be directed at finding the unique pharmacologic and/or biologic agent(s) or combinations that may effectively attenuate these pathological responses.

References

1. Colvin RB, Johnson RA, Mihm MC, Dvorak HF: Role of the clotting system in cell-mediated hypersensitivity: I. Fibrin deposition in delayed skin reactions in man. J Exp Med 138:686–698, 1973
2. Tang L, Ugarova TP, Plow EF, Eaton JW: Molecular determinants of acute inflammatory responses to biomaterials. J Clin Invest 97: 1329–1334, 1996
3. Marcus, AJ: Thrombosis and inflammation as multicellular processes: Significance of cell-cell interactions. Semin Hematol 31: 261–269, 1994
4. Davie EW, Fujikawa K, Kisiel W: The coagulation cascade: Initiation, maintenance, and regulation. Biochemistry 30:10363–10370, 1991
5. Tordai A, Fenton JW, Anderson T, Gelfand EW: Functional thrombin receptors on human T lymphoblastoid cells. J Immunol 150: 4876–4886, 1993
6. Grandaliano G, Valente AJ, Abboud HE: A novel biologic activity of thrombin: Stimulation of monocyte chemotactic protein production. J Exp Med 179:1737–1741, 1994
7. Sower LE, Froelich CJ, Carney DH, Fenton JW, Klimpel GR: Thrombin induces IL-6 production in fibroblasts and epithelial cells: Evidence for the involvement of the seven transmembrane domain (STD) receptor for α-thrombin. J Immunol 155:895–901, 1995
8. Bar-Shavit R, Kahn A, Mudd MD, Wilner GD, Mann KG, Fenton JW: Localization of a chemotactic domain in human thrombin. Biochemistry 23:397, 1985
9. Bar-Shavit R, Kahn A, Wilner GD: Monocyte chemotaxis: Stimulation by specific exosite region in thrombin. Science 220:728, 1983
10. Struova SM, Dugina TN, Khgatian SV, Redkozubov AE, Redkozuba GP, Pinelis VG: Thrombin-mediated events implicated in mast cell activation. Semin Thromb Hemost 22:145, 1996
11. Cirino G, Cicala C, Bucci M, Sorrentino L, Ambrosini G, DeDominicis G, Altieri DC: Factor Xa as an interface between coagula-

tion and inflammation: Molecular mimicry of factor Xa association with effector cell protease receptor-1 induces acute inflammation in vivo. J Clin Invest 99:2446–2451, 1997

12. Galli SJ, Wershil BK: The two faces of the mast cell. Nature 381: 21–22, 1996

13. Tannenbaum S, Oertel H, Henderson W, Kaliner M: The biologic activity of mast cell granules: I. Elicitation of inflammatory responses. J Immunol 125:325–335, 1980

14. Kanwar S, Kubes P: Mast cells contribute to ischemia-reperfusion-induced granulocyte infiltration and intestinal dysfunction. Am J Physiol 267:G316–G321, 1994

15. Church MK, Levi-Schaffer F: The human mast cell. J Allergy Clin Immunol 99:155–160, 1997

16. Zimmerman GA, McIntyre TM, Prescott TM: Endothelial cell interactions with granulocytes: Tethering and signaling molecules. Immunol Today 13:93–100, 1992

17. Asako H, Kurose I, Wolf R, DeFrees S, Zheng ZL, Phillips ML, Paulson JC, Granger DN: Role of H1 receptors and P-selectin in histamine-induced leukocyte rolling and adhesion in postcapillary venules. J Clin Invest 93:1508–1515, 1994

18. Kubes P, Kanwar S: Histamine induces leukocyte rolling in postcapillary venules: A P-selectin-mediated event. J Immunol 152:3570–3577, 1994

19. Veien M, Holdin J, Szlam F, Yamaguchi K, Denson D, Levy JH: Mechanisms of non-immunological histamine and tryptase release from human cutaneous mast cells. In Review

20. Cirino G, Cicala C, Bucci M, Sorrentino L, Maragonore JM, Stone SR: Thrombin functions as an inflammatory mediator through activation of its receptor. J Exp Med 183:821–827, 1996

21. Ambrosini G, Altieri DC: Molecular dissection of effector cell protease receptor-1 recognition of factor Xa: Assignment of critical residues implicated in antibody reactivity and ligand binding. J Biol Chem 271:1243–1248, 1996

22. Nicholson AC, Nachman RL, Altieri DC, Summers BD, Ruf W, Edgington TS, Hajjar DP: Effector cell protease receptor-1 is a vascular receptor for coagulation factor Xa. J Biol Chem 271:28407–28413, 1996

23. Ambrosini G, Plescia J, Chu KC, High KA, Altieri DC: Activation-dependent exposure of the inter-EGF sequence Leu83-Leu88 in factor Xa mediates ligand binding to effector cell protease receptor-1. J Biol Chem 272:8340–8345, 1997

24. Cicala C, Cirino G: Linkage between inflammation and coagulation: An update on the molecular basis of the crosstalk. Life Sci 62:1817–1824, 1998

25. Altieri DC: Xa receptor EPR-1. FASEB J 9:860–865, 1995
26. Esmon CT: Cell mediated events that control blood coagulation and vascular injury. Annu Rev Cell Biol 9:1–26, 1993
27. Baglin T: Disseminated intravascular coagulation: Diagnosis and treatment. BMJ 312:683–687, 1996
28. Bick RL: Disseminated intravascular coagulation: Pathophysiological mechanisms and manifestations. Semin Thromb Hemost 24:3–18, 1998
29. Bucur SZ, Levy JH, Despotis GJ, Spiess BD, Hillyer CD: Uses of antithrombin III concentrate in congenital and acquired deficiency states. Transfusion 38:481–498, 1998
30. Fourrier F, Chopin C, Huart J, Runge I, Caron C, Goudemand J: Doubleblind, placebo-controlled trial of antithrombin III concentrates in septic shock with disseminated intravascular coagulation. Chest 104:882–888, 1993
31. Ostrovsky L, Woodman RC, Payne D, Teoh D, Kubes P: Antithrombin III prevents and rapidly reverses leukocyte recruitment in ischemia/reperfusion. Circulation 96:2302–2310, 1997
32. Okajima K, Uchiba M: The anti-inflammatory properties of antithrombin III: New therapeutic implications. Semin Thromb Hemost 24:27–32, 1998
33. Kalter RD, Saul CM, Wetstein L, Soriano C, Reiss RF: Cardiopulmonary bypass: Associated hemostatic abnormalities. J Thorac Cardiovasc Surg 77:427–435, 1979
34. Zaidan JR, Johnson S, Brynes R, Monroe S, Guffin AV: Rate of protamine administration: Its effect on heparin reversal and antithrombin recovery after coronary artery surgery. Anesth Analg 65:377–380, 1986
35. Hashimoto K, Yamagishi M, Sasaki T, Nakano M, Kurosawa H: Heparin and antithrombin III levels during cardiopulmonary bypass: Correlation with subclinical plasma coagulation. Ann Thorac Surg 58:799–805, 1995
36. Despotis GJ, Levine V, Joist JH, Joiner-Maier D, Spitznagel E: Antithrombin III during cardiac surgery: Effect on response of activated clotting time to heparin and relationship to markers of hemostatic activation. Anesth Analg 85:498–506, 1997
37. Montes FR, Levy JH: Can we alter heparin dose-responses with antithrombin III? (Abstract). Anesth Analg 82:SCA94, 1996
38. Fitch JCK, Smith MJ, Rinder CS, Smith BR: Supplemental antithrombin preserves platelet count and decreases platelet activation during in vitro bypass (Abstract). Anesth Analg 82:SCA3, 1996
39. Levy JH, Despotis GJ, Olson PJ, Weisinger A, Szlam F: Transgenically produced recombinant human ATIII enhances the an-

tithrombotic effects of heparin in patients undergoing cardiac surgery. Blood 90(Supp I):298A, 1997

40. Levy JH: Anaphylactic Reactions in Anesthesia and Intensive Care. 2nd ed. Boston: Butterworth-Heinemann, 1992

41. Costa JJ, Weller PF, Galli SJ: The cells of the allergic response: Mast cells, basophils, and eosinophils. JAMA 278:1815–1822, 1997

42. Kirshenbaum AS, Goff JP, Kessler SW, Mican JM, Zsebo KM, Metcalfe DD: Effect of IL-3 and stem cell factor on the appearance of human basophil and mast cells from CD34+ pluripotent progenitor cells. J Immunol 148:772–777, 1992

43. Enerback L: The differentiation and maturation of inflammatory cells involved in the allergic response: Mast cells and basophils. Allergy 52:4–10, 1997

44. Valent P, Bettelheim P: The human basophil. Crit Rev Oncol Hematol 10:327–352, 1990

45. Beaven MA, Metzger H: Signal transduction by Fc receptors. Immunol Today 14:222–226, 1993

46. Kinet J-P: The high-affinity receptor for IgE. Curr Opin Immunol 2:499–505, 1989

47. Galli SJ, Zsebo KM, Geissler EN: The kit ligand, stem cell factor. Adv Immunol 55:1–96, 1994

48. Galli SJ: New insights into "the riddle of the mast cells": Microenvironmental regulation of mast cell development and phenotypic heterogeneity. Lab Invest 62:5–33, 1990

49. Kitamura Y: Heterogeneity of mast cells and phenotypic changes between subpopulations. Annu Rev Immunol 7:59–76, 1989

50. Stevens RL, Austen KF: Recent advances in the cellular and molecular biology of mast cells. Immunol Today 10:381–386, 1989

51. Lane SJ, Lee TH: Mast cell effector mechanisms. J Allergy Clin Immunol 98:S67–S72, 1996

52. Marshall JS, Bienenstock J: The role of mast cells in inflammatory reactions of the airways, skin and intestine. Curr Opin Immunol 6:853–859, 1994

53. Gordon JR, Burd PR, Galli SJ: Mast cells as a source of multifunctional cytokines. Immunol Today 11:458–464, 1990

54. Holgate ST, Robinson C, Church MK: Mediators of Immediate Hypersensitivity. In: Middleton E Jr, Reed CE, Ellis EF, Adkinson NF, Yunginger JW, Busse WW, eds. Allergy: Principles and Practice. 4th ed. St Louis, MO: Mosby-Year Book Inc, 1993:267–301

55. Galli SJ, Costa JJ: Mast cell-leukocyte cytokine cascades in allergic inflammation. Allergy 50:851–862, 1995

56. Valone FH, Boggs JM, Goetzl EJ: Lipid Mediators of Hypersensitivity and Inflammation. In: Middleton E Jr, Reed CE, Ellis EF, Adkinson NF, Yunginger JW, Busse WW, eds. Allergy: Principles

and Practice. 4th ed. St Louis, MO: Mosby-Year Book Inc, 1993: 302–319

57. Bochner BS, Schleimer RP: The role of adhesion molecules in human eosinophil and basophil recruitment. J Allergy Clin Immunol 94:427–438, 1994

58. Bevilacqua MP: Endothelial-leukocyte adhesion molecules. Annu Rev Immunol 11:767–804,1993

59. Yong LC: The mast cell: Origin, morphology, distribution, and function. Exp Toxicol Pathol 49:409–424, 1997

60. Marone G, Casolaro V, Patella V, Florio G, Triggiani M: Molecular and cellular biology of mast cells and basophils. Int Arch Allergy Immunol 114:207–217, 1997

61. Galli SJ: New concepts about the mast cell. N Engl J Med 328:257–265, 1993

62. Wershil BK, Wang ZS, Gordon JR, Galli SJ: Recruitment of neutrophils during IgE-dependent cutaneous late phase reactions in the mouse is mast cell-dependent: Partial inhibition of the reaction with antiserum against tumor necrosis factor-α. J Clin Invest 87: 446–453, 1991

63. Enerback L: The differentiation and maturation of inflammatory cells involved in the allergic response: Mast cells and basophils. Allergy 52:4–10, 1997

64. Baggiolini M: Chemokines and leukocyte traffic. Nature 392:565–568, 1998

65. Bradding P, Holgate ST: The mast cell as a source of cytokines in asthma. Ann NY Acad Sci 796:272–281, 1996

66. Denburg JA: Hemopoietic progenitors and cytokines in allergic inflammation. Allergy 53(45 Suppl):22–26, 1998

67. Schleimer RP: Glucocorticosteroids: Their Mechanisms of Action and Use in Allergic Diseases. In: Middleton E Jr, Ellis EF, Adkinson NFJ, Yunginger JW, Busse WW, eds. Allergy: Principles and Practice. 4th ed. St Louis, MO: Mosby-Year Book Inc, 1993: 893–925

68. Wershil BK, Furuta GT, Lavigne JA, Choudhury AR, Wang ZS, Galli SJ: Dexamethasone or cyclosporin A suppresses mast cell-leukocyte cytokine cascades: Multiple mechanisms of inhibition of IgE- and mast cell-dependent cutaneous inflammation in the mouse. J Immunol 154:1391–1398, 1995

69. Gauchat JF, Henchoz S, Mazzei G, Aubry JP, Brunner T, Blasey H, Life P, Talabot D, Flores-Romo L, Thompson J, et al: Induction of human IgE synthesis in B cells by mast cells and basophils. Nature 365:340–343, 1993

70. Lin S, Ciccala C, Scharenberg AM, Kinet JP: The FcεRIb subunit functions as an amplifier of FcεRIγ-mediated cell activation signals. Cell 85:985–995, 1996

71. Dembo M, Goldstein B, Sobotka AK, Lichtenstein LM: Degranulation of human basophils: Quantitative analysis of histamine release and desensitization, due to a bivalent penicilloyl hapten. J Immunol 123:1864–1872, 1979
72. Conroy MC, Adkinson NF Jr, Lichtenstein LM: Measurement of IgE on human basophils. J Immunol 118:1317–1321, 1977
73. Stallman PJ, Aalberse RC, Bruhl PC, van Elven EH: Experiments on the passive sensitization of human basophils, using quantitative immunofluorescence microscopy. Int Arch Allergy Appl Immunol 54:364–373, 1977
74. Yamaguchi M, Lantz CS, Oettgen HC, Katona IM, Fleming T, Miyajima I, Kinet JP, Galli SJ: IgE enhances mouse mast cell FcεRI expression in vitro and in vivo: Evidence for a novel amplification mechanism in IgE-dependent reactions. J Exp Med 185:663–672, 1997
75. Yano K, Yamaguchi M, de Mora F, Lantz CS, Butterfield JH, Costa JJ, Galli SJ: Production of macrophage inflammatory protein-1α by human mast cells: increased anti-IgE-dependent secretion after IgE-dependent enhancement of mast cell IgE-binding ability. Lab Invest 77:185–193, 1997
76. MacGlashan DW Jr, Bochner BS, Adelman DC, Jardieu PM, Togias A, McKenzie-White J, Sterbinsky SA, Hamilton RG, Lichtenstein LM: Down-regulation of FcεRI expression on human basophils during in vivo treatment of atopic patients with anti-IgE antibody. J Immunol 158:1438–1445, 1997
77. Galli SJ, Wershil BK: The two faces of the mast cell. Nature 381: 21–22, 1996

Christine Stowe Rinder, M.D.

5 | Platelets and Their Interactions

Circulating hematopoietic cells have traditionally been thought to have largely nonoverlapping functions and to communicate only with cells of like lineage, ie, homotypic interactions. According to this scheme, leukocytes interact with other leukocytes for the purposes of immune surveillance and inflammatory response, platelets aggregate with other platelets for hemostasis, and erythrocytes are solely responsible for oxygen delivery. These homotypic interactions were felt to be flow independent, and largely identical in the arterial and venous circulations. All three cell types coexisted in the circulation, with communication between them limited to chance encounters with released soluble factors. New data have expanded this view of blood cell interactions.

Dynamic flow chambers have been developed that permit more realistic modeling of the different forces exerted on cells under different flow conditions. Homotypic interactions, particularly those of platelets, can no longer be viewed as uniform. Instead, the highly variable demands imposed by extremes of blood flow create a need for multiple adhesive strategies to achieve hemostasis under all conditions, while avoiding pathologic thrombus formation. This expanded repertoire of platelet-platelet interactions underscores the multiplicity of ways platelet function may be impaired. The first part of this chapter will discuss the homotypic interactions between platelets under varying flow forces, and in particular, the sequence of interactions that permit control of bleeding in the setting of high shear rates.

The Relationship Between Coagulation, Inflammation, and Endothelium, edited by Bruce Spiess, Lippincott Williams & Wilkins, Baltimore © 2000.

Identification of new classes of adhesion receptors in recent years that exclusively mediate interactions between *different* classes of cells (eg, heterotypic interactions) has forced a revision in the narrow scope of functions assigned to hematopoietic cells. Rather than merely coexisting in the circulation, platelets and leukocytes communicate via a highly conserved set of adhesive proteins and soluble mediators, which creates a role for platelets in inflammatory events and for leukocytes in thrombosis. Heterotypic cell interactions allow for functional cross-talk between coagulation and inflammatory pathways and produce a far more complex repertoire of physiology for hematopoietic cells than previously believed.[1] Platelets, in particular, have come to be recognized as critical participants in arterial inflammatory as well as thrombotic processes. Once viewed as relatively inert anucleate bodies serving as a framework on which clots are built, platelets are now seen as pivotal in the normal physiology of high shear stress, regulating thrombosis and leukocyte trafficking in the arterial circulation. The latter half of this chapter will discuss the emerging field of platelet-heterotypic cell interactions and their role in thrombosis and inflammation.

Platelet Homotypic Interactions

The arterial and venous circulations, with their widely disparate flow conditions, impose very different needs on the coagulation system. In the "pressurized" arterial system, relatively limited vascular damage can rapidly result in significant blood loss and hematoma formation, which creates the need for a coagulation system that can instantaneously arrest bleeding. Platelets specialize in this "rapid response" function, initially containing blood loss, then providing a surface on which to both localize and accelerate the fibrin formation that ultimately consolidates hemostasis. In the venous circulation, by contrast, the lesser flow rates diminish the need for speed, making platelets less critical, and indeed, the pivotal reaction controlling the balance of venous hemostasis is the rate of *thrombin* generation. These differences in arterial and venous blood flow are underscored by the anticoagulant agents used in these settings, ie, antiplatelet agents like aspirin to prevent coronary arterial thrombosis[2] in contrast to antithrombin-based interventions like coumadin for prophylaxis against deep venous thrombosis. The constraints imposed by arterial dynamic flow stresses make a sequence of interrelated platelet receptor-ligand interactions critical for initiating arterial hemostasis, and these comprise three major interactions. First, low-affinity but rapidly forming bonds allow for platelet adhesion to subendothelium at the leading edge of the platelet and, conversely, dissociation at the trailing edge. This on-off adhesion transforms platelet movement from high velocity flow to a slower rolling across the damaged subendothelium. Second, these adhesive events trigger transmembrane signaling, which produces platelet activation and formation of new high-affinity platelet-subendothelial and platelet-platelet bonds and yields an immobile platelet plug. Third, receptors exposed by platelet activation coordinate coagulation factor binding, which localizes the proteins in an orientation that facilitates enzyme complex assembly on the platelet membrane with kinetics several thousand-fold that of the unbound factors in plasma. This theme of rolling → firm adhesion → cell-specific action is one that is repeated for leukocyte adhesion under arterial flow conditions, as described in the second half of this chapter.

Platelet Adhesion Under High Shear

Significant mechanical stresses are created by the high flow velocities present in the arterial circulation. The interaction between the vessel wall and rapidly flowing blood, as shown on the left side of Figure 5–1, creates parallel planes of blood moving at different velocities, with blood near the wall moving more slowly than blood at the center of the

Platelet adhesion to von Willebrand factor

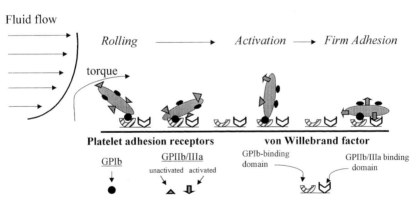

FIGURE 5–1. The evolution of adhesive interactions producing stable platelet attachment to subendothelial von Willebrand factor (vWF). The initial attachment between GpIb and its binding domain on vWF is rapidly formed but has a short half-life, which causes a rolling movement from torque generated by flowing blood. The vWF-GpIb interaction produces transmembrane signaling, thereby activating the platelet and transforming GpIIb/IIIa into a conformation capable of binding to the RGD domain on vWF. This secondary adhesion is essentially irreversible, thus anchoring the activated platelet to the exposed subendothelium.

vessel.[3] The different velocities of these moving layers of blood creates shear stress, which is greatest at the vessel wall and diminishes toward the center. This shear stress, expressed in inverse seconds (sec^{-1}), changes inversely with vessel diameter, with levels estimated to vary between 500 sec^{-1} in the larger arteries and 5,000 sec^{-1} in the smallest arterioles. Shear rates at the surface of atherosclerotic plaques of a modest 50% stenosis are in the range of 3,000 to 10,000 sec^{-1}, with even greater shear stress in tighter stenoses. The high velocity of blood flow in the arterial circulation strongly opposes any tendency to clot by limiting the time available for procoagulant reactions to occur and disrupting cells or proteins not tightly adherent to the vessel wall. However, when the vessel wall is damaged and bleeding occurs, these forces set in motion a sequence of hemostatic events designed to rapidly and decisively respond to the loss of endothelial integrity while simultaneously resisting the tendency to be swept downstream. One of the forces enhancing the state of hemostatic "readiness" in the arterial circulation is radial dispersion, or the tendency of larger cells, eg, erythrocytes and leukocytes, to stream in the center of the vessel where the shear is lowest; this effectively pushes the smaller platelets toward the vessel wall, and optimally positions them to respond to hemostatic challenges. This size-dependent cellular flow pattern may also explain the seemingly paradoxical tendency of arterial bleeding in the presence of severe anemia to decrease after red cell transfusions.[4] This effect also underscores the importance of platelets in arterial hemostasis; reductions in platelet number or function may be associated with catastrophic arterial hemorrhage. By contrast, the lesser shear forces experienced in the venous circulation permit more random cell movement and greater time for coagulation reactions to occur, which makes the minimum requirements for platelet number and function correspondingly less stringent. As such, the venous circulation is much more sensitive to defects in the soluble coagulation cascade, in which the kinetics of thrombin formation dictate the balance of procoagulant and anticoagulant forces.

Given the velocity of blood flow at an arterial bleeding site, platelets must activate and adhere to the injured vessel nearly instantaneously. Two molecules present in the subendothelium are critical for this process: von Willebrand factor (vWF) and collagen. Control of bleeding in vessels under the highest shear stresses is absolutely dependent on the action of vWF.[5] Large, multimeric forms of vWF that are immobilized by binding to exposed subendothelial collagen will bind to the receptor on the platelet surface known as glycoprotein Ib (GpIb) in response to the high shear stress (Figure 5–1). This is an extremely rapid but low-affinity adhesive event that markedly slows, but does not firmly anchor, the platelets to the subendothelium. With the platelet no longer streaming by but, instead, tumbling over the subendothelium, the high shear stress, itself, in tandem with transmembrane signaling produced by the GpIb-vWF interaction[6] results in platelet activation and loss of discoid shape (shape change).

One consequence of platelet activation is a conformational change in GpIIb-IIIa, the platelet receptor that is the target of a number of the newer antiplatelet agents.[7] Conformationally changed GpIIb-IIIa is able to bind either to fibrinogen or to the larger vWF multimers at a locus distinct from the GpIb binding epitope. This secondary adhesion to fibrinogen or vWF via GpIIb-IIIa is a higher-affinity interaction than the GpIb-vWF bond and serves to secure the platelet firmly to the subendothelium. At more moderate shear, a separate binding mechanism also occurs via subendothelial collagen, another adhesive moiety that is capable of arresting the platelet via binding to GpIa-IIa.[8] Thus, subendothelial vWF and collagen act cooperatively to initiate platelet adhesion, with the former predominating at higher shear. Collagen is unique in that it can act to both anchor platelets at one locus by binding to platelet GpIa-IIa and activate platelets at a second locus by binding to platelet GpVI.[9] The combined actions of subendothelial vWF and collagen producing platelet adhesion and activation are central to arresting blood loss through defects in the arterial wall. The rare congenital absence of either GpIb,[10] GpVI,[11] or GpIa-IIa[12] on the platelet can produce a significant hemostatic defect. Similarly, decreases in vWF or structural abnormalities impairing its adhesive capability can also predispose to bleeding.[13]

Platelet Activation and Formation of the Platelet Plug

Once a layer of adherent platelets is securely bound to the site of bleeding, they must next coordinate an array of interdependent processes that together are referred to as "activation." Ultimately, platelet activation has five major effects: (1) local release of ligands essential to a stable platelet-platelet matrix; (2) recruitment of additional platelets; (3) vasoconstriction of smaller arteries to slow bleeding; (4) localization and acceleration of platelet-associated fibrin formation; and (5) clot protection from fibrinolysis.

The basic building block of the platelet aggregate is a platelet-ligand-platelet matrix with fibrinogen or vWF serving as the bridging ligand. Both fibrinogen and vWF are stored in α granules inside the resting platelet and are released with activation. Both are capable of binding to a GpIIb-IIIa receptor on each of two platelets, thereby linking them. As mentioned above, GpIIb-IIIa is maintained in an inactive form on the resting platelet. Upon activation, GpIIb-IIIa undergoes a calcium-dependent conformational change that allows it to bind to a locus containing the amino acid sequence arginine-glycine-aspartate (RGD) on either fibrinogen or vWF. Each fibrinogen molecule has two RGD sites on its polar ends, and the larger vWF multimers have several RGD sites; all of the RGD sites are capable of binding to conformationally altered GpIIb-IIIa and creating the platelet-ligand-platelet matrix.[14] GpIIb-IIIa is the most abundant glycoprotein on the platelet surface, with approximately 50,000 copies on the *resting* platelet and additional receptors within a cytoplasmic pool that are mobilized to the surface as part of the activation process. The successful use of GpIIb-IIIa and RGD antagonists in patients at risk for coronary events reinforces the importance of this platelet receptor in hemostasis and thrombus formation in the arterial circulation.[15]

Additional platelets are recruited to the platelet plug by the release of platelet stimulants, or agonists, into the local microenvironment. One of these agonists is thromboxane A_2, which is formed in the platelet cytosol by a process initiated by cyclooxygenase cleavage of arachidonic acid and is ultimately released into the clot milieu.[16] Thromboxane A_2 is both a platelet agonist and a vasoconstrictor and is rapidly degraded to its inert by-product, thromboxane B_2. Cyclooxygenase activity is *irreversibly* inhibited by aspirin, thereby blocking thromboxane A_2 formation for the lifetime of that platelet. Other platelet agonists released by activation are located in the dense granule of the resting platelet and are liberated by fusion of the dense granule with the platelet canalicular membrane, which produces extrusion of granule contents. One of these dense granule constituents, serotonin, is also both an agonist and a vasoconstrictor.[17] The other constituent, ADP, acts purely as a platelet agonist with no known vasoactive properties. These agonists activate platelets in the immediate vicinity of the damaged vessel, thereby cementing the growing platelet plug. The importance of the thromboxane A_2-induced and serotonin-induced vasoconstriction is not entirely clear. However, vasoconstriction, by decreasing the vessel diameter, may increase shear stress, thus facilitating recruitment of platelets to the injured site. The importance of dense granule release to the maintenance of arterial hemostasis is manifested by the severe bleeding seen in congenital dense granule deficiency states, eg, Hermansky-Pudlak syndrome and storage pool disease.[18]

The Soluble Coagulation Cascade on the Platelet Surface

Chapter 6 will contain a more complete discussion of coagulation.

In the absence of platelets, activation and coordinated assembly of the soluble coagulation cascade proceeds relatively slowly. Under high flow conditions, these active serine proteases are easily diluted or displaced beyond the bleeding site. However, when platelets are bound to sites of injury, they serve to both localize and accelerate the coagulation cascade. In addition to providing an essential negative phospholipid surface for coagulation reactions, activated platelets provide specific receptors for factors Xa, IXa, and Va[19]; the latter factor is also released from the α granule of the activated platelet. Membrane association of these coagulation factors in their ideal spatial orientation with negatively charged, platelet-expressed phosphatidylserine accelerates procoagulant enzymatic reactions and simultaneously protects the activated factors from circulating inhibitors, which culminates in accelerated thrombin generation[20] (Figure 5–2). Cells that are not normally in contact with blood but may be exposed by vessel damage, eg, fibroblasts and myocytes, constitutively express tissue factor (also known as thromboplastin).[21,22] By contrast, cells in constant blood contact, eg, endothelial cells and monocytes, can synthesize and express tissue factor only after stimulation by factors such as endotoxin. Tissue factor binds to circulating factor VIIa and activates factor X to Xa and IX to IXa, both of which bind to receptors on the activated platelet membrane. The platelet Xa receptor is closely associated with platelet-bound factor Va. These factors, together with free calcium and platelet membrane phosphatidylserine, form the prothrombinase complex, thereby generating thrombin, albeit in relatively small amounts. This initially-formed thrombin is then able to activate factor VIII to VIIIa, which binds to membrane-bound factor IXa, and activates factor V to Va, which may already be bound to the platelet. Until this point in the cascade, the rate

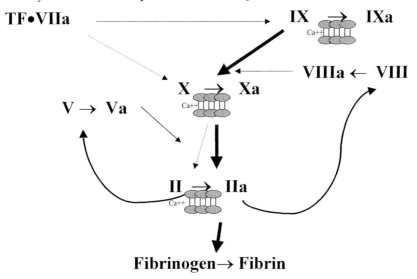

FIGURE 5–2. Acceleration of the coagulation cascade on the activated platelet surface. The key steps in the coagulation cascade are diagrammed, with those most accelerated by platelet membrane association represented by $_{Ca.++}$ The early, slower steps leading to thrombin generation are represented by *dotted arrows*, with the more accelerated later thrombin generation by the *heavier solid arrows*. See text for further explanation.

of Xa and thrombin generation formed is relatively slow. However, once an initial amount of thrombin can subsequently generate appreciable quantities of cofactors Va and VIIIa, the rate of both factor Xa and thrombin generation increases exponentially (heavy arrows in Figure 5–2).[23] With explosive thrombin generation, a fibrin matrix is formed that is integrated with the surface of the platelet plug. Factor XIIIa, which is produced by the action of thrombin on either plasma or platelet-released factor XIII, then crosslinks the fibrin chains and binds α_2-antiplasmin to the fibrin to protect it from plasmin-mediated dissolution.[24] Finally, the platelet plug undergoes clot retraction, which additionally protects the platelet-fibrinogen-platelet unit from lysis by plasmin.[25] These antilysis mechanisms, which are largely linked to platelet activation, may explain the relative resistance of platelet-rich clots to pharmacologic thrombolysis.

Endogenous Anticoagulants: Striking a Balance

In the intact circulation and at the perimeter of the newly-formed clot, a number of endogenous mechanisms operate to inhibit clotting and maintain blood in a liquid form. Different pathways are crucial in the arterial and venous circulation with, for reasons outlined above, antiplatelet activity predominating in the former and antithrombin activity in the latter. However, an intact endothelial cell barrier is fundamental to both processes. In the arterial circulation, total vessel occlusion by the growing clot is opposed by a number of mechanisms that operate to control the thrombus size. As described above, high-velocity blood flow dilutes and disperses coagulation factors. Antiplatelet factors are also part of the anticoagulant activity intrinsic to the healthy endothelial cell lining by limiting extension of the platelet plug past the area of endothelial damage. These include the following: (1) a net negative surface charge, which repels similarly charged platelets; (2) constitutive release of the vasodilators nitric oxide (also termed endothelial-derived relaxant factor or EDRF) and prostacyclin, which also inhibit platelet adhesion and aggregation; and (3) constitutive surface expression of an ADPase that inactivates platelet-released ADP,[26,27] thereby limiting recruitment of additional platelets. These naturally-occurring antiplatelet mechanisms, in addition to the arterial hemodynamic forces, work to maintain vessel patency and blood flow simultaneous with clot formation and vessel repair.

Once the platelet plug and associated fibrin deposition have halted the bleeding and covered any exposed endothelium, systems that rein in the coagulation system become dominant and are especially critical in the venous circulation. Many of these factors are bound to an extracellular matrix associated with neighboring intact endothelium and, like the analogous antiplatelet agents, prevent the clot from encroaching on areas of normal endothelium. Endothelial cells synthesize an endogenous heparin, heparan sulfate, in association with the extracellular matrix; heparan sulfate complexes with blood antithrombin and neutralizes locally developed thrombin. Thrombomodulin is similarly endothelial cell surface-associated; thrombin that escapes the above neutralization binds to thrombomodulin, and this complex activates protein C. Activated protein C then cleaves any non–platelet-associated factors Va and VIIIa, thereby downregulating thrombin formation.

These tonic anticoagulant and antiplatelet factors maintained by endothelial cells are a prime example of cells of one lineage modulating the behavior traditionally viewed as intrinsic to a different cell lineage. The second half of this chapter will discuss the ways in which platelets use a combination of soluble factors and adhesive interactions to modulate the activity of leukocytes in the circulation.

Platelet Heterotypic Interactions

Soluble Factors

As mentioned earlier, communication via soluble factors is a well-established mode of communication between activated platelets and other hematopoietic cells. Platelet activation produces fusion of the α granule with the surface membrane, which releases a combination of growth factors and cytokines into the surrounding environment. Table 5–1 lists some of the mediators in the α granule of the resting platelet that are released upon platelet activation. A number of these released mediators, such as the antiheparin agent platelet factor 4 and factor XIII, bind to the

TABLE 5–1. Platelet α-Granule Contents

Procoagulants	Platelet factor 4
	Factor V
Anticoagulants	Plasminogen
	α_2-antiplasmin
Growth factors	Transforming growth factor-β (TGF-β)
	Transforming growth factor-α (TGF-α)
	Platelet-derived growth factor (PDGF)
	Endothelial growth factor (ECGF)
Adhesive proteins	Fibrinogen
	von Willebrand factor
	Fibronectin
	Thrombospondin
Bactericidal	β-lysin

surface of the activated platelet or diffuse into the clot milieu where they promote or protect the developing clot. By contrast, other α granule factors have no known coagulant effects, but instead modulate inflammation and wound repair by acting locally on leukocytes and endothelial cells. For example, transforming growth factor-β is well known to influence wound healing, tissue remodeling, and fibrosis.[28] Thrombin-stimulated platelets release two neutrophil-activating peptide-2 (NAP-2) variants that are capable of stimulating polymorphonuclear (PMN) neutrophils, thereby producing an inflammatory response.[29]

Conversely, other hematopoietic cells are capable of modulating platelet reactivity by soluble factors. In addition to the tonic inhibitory effects described above by healthy endothelial cells, unstimulated neutrophils inhibit activation and recruitment of thrombin-stimulated or collagen-stimulated platelets by a modulation of the platelet lipoxygenase pathway enhanced by aspirin.[30] Erythrocytes, by contrast, promote platelet reactivity, increasing platelet ADP and thromboxane A_2 release in response to collagen.[31] This procoagulant property is not inhibited by aspirin treatment and actually obviates the effects of low-dose aspirin.[32] Thus, overall platelet responsiveness is a complex integration of many factors, and circulating erythrocytes and PMN may contribute to setting the tone of platelet reactivity.

Leukocyte-Platelet Adhesion

The discovery of receptors mediating activated platelet-leukocyte binding suggested a novel mechanism for communication that, in addition to soluble factor release, promotes cross-talk between coagulant and inflammatory pathways. Indeed, a growing body of evidence suggests that activated platelets exert significant proinflammatory effects by binding to the leukocyte surface simultaneously with leukocyte stimulation by soluble factors. This adhesion/cytokine co-stimulation has been referred to as a "tethering and signaling" sequence and is critical for leukocyte-endothelial cell interactions as well.[33,34] Leukocyte-platelet adhesion may take one of two forms in vivo. The first is caused by freely circulating activated platelets binding to monocytes or PMN, which produces circulating leukocyte-platelet conjugates. The second form of adhesion occurs at the surface of vessel wall-*adherent* platelets, which permits monocytes or PMN to bind to a developing thrombus. The remainder of this chapter will first discuss the receptor-ligand pairs involved in leukocyte-platelet interactions, followed by a discussion of the consequences of these two forms of adhesion.

Inside the resting platelet, a glycoprotein known as P-selectin, (also known as CD62P, GMP-140, and PADGEM) resides on the inner lumen of the α granule membrane.[35,36] Activation-induced fusion of the α granule with the platelet surface membrane exposes P-selectin to the extracellular milieu. Following its initial discovery, the percentage of platelets expressing P-selectin was used as a measure of in vitro platelet activation. One of the first in vivo demonstrations of circulating P-selectin–positive platelets was in cardiopulmonary bypass (CPB), where the percentage of circulating platelets expressing P-selectin increased progressively over the course of bypass.[37] Patients exhibited wide variability in their activation response, but in some patients, as many as 50% of circulating platelets expressed P-selectin by the end of CPB (Figure 5–3). In subsequent work, transfusion of Indium-labeled platelets demonstrated that P-selectin–positive platelets had a relatively short circulatory half-life,[38] which suggests that any increase in P-selectin–positive platelets in the circulation was evidence of *recent* platelet activation. This finding was supported by the steady decline in circulating P-selectin–positive platelets af-

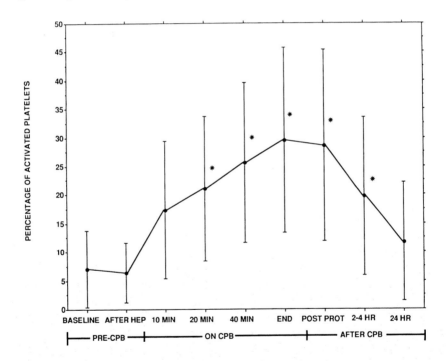

FIGURE 5–3.   Platelet activation during cardiopulmonary bypass (CPB). The percentage of circulating platelets expressing P-selectin was measured in whole blood taken before surgery (BASELINE), 5 minutes after heparinization (AFTER HEP), during CPB at 10 minutes (10MIN), 20 minutes (20 MIN), 40 minutes (40 MIN), before separation from CPB (END), and after CPB at 5 minutes after protamine (POST PROT), 2 to 4 hours (2–4H), and 24 hours (24H). All values are mean ± SD. Reprinted with permission.[37]

ter CPB, such that by the first postoperative day, levels had returned to baseline. Increased circulating P-selectin–positive platelets have also been demonstrated in other clinical settings characterized by acute platelet activation; in a recent study, acute coronary syndrome patients had higher circulating P-selectin–positive platelets than normal volunteers or patients admitted for noncoronary events.[39]

Circulating leukocyte-platelet conjugates

P-selectin was subsequently identified as an adhesion receptor that enabled activated platelets to bind to monocytes, PMN, and some T-cell subsets[40,41] through leukocyte constitutive expression of P-selectin glycoprotein ligand-1 (PSGL-1).[42] It was unclear whether this novel heterotypic adhesion occurred in vivo or whether it was largely an in vitro phenomenon with minimal clinical consequences. Following development of a whole-blood assay for the measurement of leukocytes with bound platelets,[43] CPB was again the clinical setting in which platelet adhesion to circulating leukocytes was first demonstrated.[44] In parallel with increasing numbers of circulating P-selectin-positive platelets, circulating monocytes and, to a lesser extent, PMN were shown to have platelets bound to their surface (Figure 5–4). The platelet-monocyte conjugates in particular persisted in the circulation for hours even after the numbers of circulating P-selectin–positive platelets had returned to baseline. It was not known at the time whether these leukocyte-platelet conjugates had any clinical consequences or whether the adhesion was simply an epiphenomenon, perhaps serving to clear the circulation of activated platelets. Since that initial demonstration, increased leukocyte-platelet conjugates have also been demonstrated in patients with unstable angina[45] and in septic patients with multiple organ failure.[46] In vitro, activated platelets induce superoxide anion release by monocytes and PMN through P-selectin–mediated binding to their surfaces[47]; during hemodialysis, PMN with bound activated platelets produced greater amounts of reactive oxygen species, again via a P-selectin–dependent pathway.[48]

In vitro, P-selectin–dependent adhesion has been identified as the adhesive half of the tethering and signaling mechanism described above. The list of cytokines whose signaling effects are enhanced by P-selectin–dependent tethering is growing at a rapid rate. Proinflammatory consequences of this type of costimulation include lysozyme production by stimulated PMN, whereby coincubation with activated platelets markedly amplifies lysozyme levels released after exposure to activated platelet supernatant.[49] In monocytes, activated platelet adhesion via P-selectin induces nuclear translocation of nuclear factor-κB,[50]

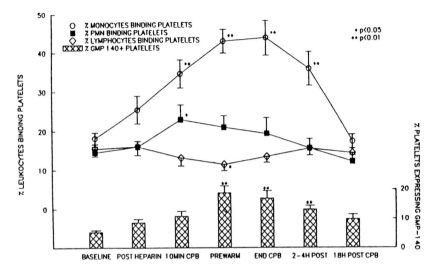

FIGURE 5–4. Platelet activation and leukocyte-platelet conjugates during cardiopulmonary bypass (CPB). The percentage of leukocyte-platelet conjugates (line graphs) were measured in whole blood taken before surgery (BASELINE), 5 minutes after heparinization (POST HEPARIN), 10 minutes after the start of CPB (10MIN CPB), before rewarming (PREWARM), before separation from CPB (END CPB), 2 to 4 hours after termination of CPB (2–4H POST), and 18 hours after CPB (18H POST CPB). The percentage of circulating platelets expressing P-selectin (here termed GMP-140, right axis) is displayed in the bar graphs for the same time points. All values represent mean ± SD for the 17 patients. Reprinted with permission.[44]

a transcription factor required for expression of monocyte immediate-early response genes.[33] The product ultimately released by these platelet-bound monocytes is determined by the cytokine costimulus. The potent proinflammatory chemokines IL-8 and monocyte chemotactic peptide-1 are released from platelet-bound monocytes costimulated by a platelet-activation by-product currently referred to as RANTES (regulated upon activation normal T cell expressed presumed secreted).[51] By contrast, platelet adhesion and costimulation by platelet activating factor causes monocytes to secrete tumor necrosis factor-α and monocyte chemotactic peptide-1.[50] Thus, platelet adhesion to PMN and monocytes in the circulation may augment leukocyte recruitment by enhanced release of chemotactic peptides, as well as increasing the levels of proinflammatory cytokines produced by those leukocytes. Under situations of localized platelet activation, such tethering-signaling events would be more likely to occur in the vicinity of the growing thrombus, helping to constrain inflammatory activity to the hemorrhagic site. However, the finding of significant numbers of circulating monocyte-platelet conjugates many hours after termination of CPB[44] raises the possibility that such leukocytes are primed and ready for this costimulus, potentially disseminating their inflammatory response throughout the circulation. Such a possibility was given support by the recent study of CPB,[52] in which IL-1β and IL-6 levels correlated with platelet P-selectin expression.

Growing evidence demonstrates that platelets facilitate localization of PMN to sites of thrombosis and inflammation. A study of clotting on the surface of a femoral DacronR graft in baboons demonstrated that PMN and platelets together produce enhanced fibrin deposition on the graft surface, a cooperativity that was dependent on P-selectin–dependent PMN adhesion.[53] A recent study looking at ischemia/reperfusion injury in rat myocardium[54] found that PMN infiltration and the corresponding myocardial injury were exacerbated when the ischemic tissue was reperfused with PMN plus platelets compared with platelets alone. This enhancement in PMN egress by platelets was inhibited by P-selectin blockade (Figure 5–5).

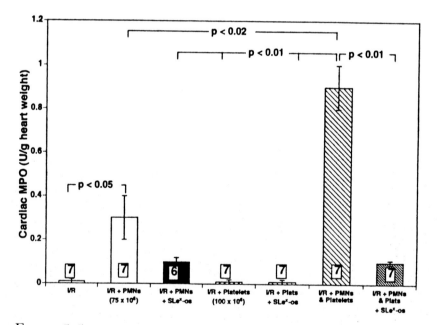

FIGURE 5–5. Cardiac myeloperoxidase (MPO) activity in cardiac tissue samples obtained from ischemia/reperfusion (I/R) rat hearts, with polymorphonuclear (PMN) neutrophils and/or platelets (Plats). All values are mean ± SEM of 7 hearts. Addition of a sialyl Lewis^x-oligosaccharide (SLe^x-os), an inhibitor of P-selectin–dependent adhesion, inhibited MPO activity in hearts perfused with platelets and PMN. Reprinted with permission.[54]

Leukocyte Binding to Immobilized P-Selectin

In addition to forming circulating leukocyte-platelet conjugates, immobilized P-selectin can facilitate leukocyte egress from the circulation, particularly under arterial flow conditions. The selectin family of adhesion receptors mediates heterotypic interactions between platelets, leukocytes, and endothelial cells.[55] P-selectin is also expressed by activated endothelial cells after mobilization from the Wiebel-Palade bodies.[56] Much of the research examining the effects of leukocyte binding to an adherent source of P-selectin under flow has been performed using purified protein layers or activated endothelial cells, but these data are pertinent to adherent activated platelets as well. On activated endothelial cells, P-selectin expression permits rapid attachment-detachment between the endothelial cell P-selectin and PSGL-1 on circulating PMN and monocytes.[57] This transient interaction causes the leukocytes to roll along the vessel wall in a manner analogous to the rolling described for platelets along adherent vWF. Such rolling slows the overall velocity of the leukocytes, thus enabling formation of higher-affinity and more stable adhesion mediated by β_2-integrins, which then allow the leukocyte to migrate through the endothelial cells into the perivascular tissue and cause inflammation.[58] P-selectin knockout mice therefore exhibit a relative immunologic impairment that is characterized by diminished leukocyte marginating ability.[59]

Similarly, adherent platelets expressing P-selectin on the surface of a clot, on a thrombosed atherosclerotic plaque, or on an extracellular matrix can induce rolling in PMN and monocytes under moderate-to-high shear, potentially recruiting them to the site of bleeding (Figure 5–6).[60,61]

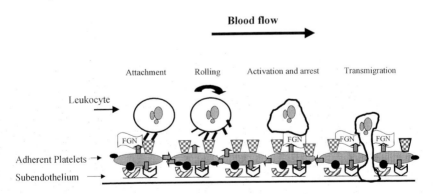

FIGURE 5–6.   Leukocyte attachment to adherent platelets. Leukocytes use PSGL-1(▮▮) to attach to and roll on P-selectin (▧) expressed on the surface of activated adherent platelets. Under certain conditions, these rolling leukocytes then activate and form the higher affinity interaction of CD11b/CD18 with platelet-bound fibrinogen; leukocytes then dissociate from P-selectin and migrate into the surrounding tissue (other platelet symbols defined in Figure 5–1).

For PMN, firm adhesion requires sequential binding by several receptor-ligand pairs on the adherent platelets and flowing PMN.[62,63] First, platelets immobilized to collagen express P-selectin, which then support PMN rolling as described above. The collagen-adherent platelets also produce platelet activating factor, which activates and transforms the rolling PMN into immobilized cells[64] mediated by PMN CD11b/CD18 binding to fibrinogen, which is adherent to both GpIIb-IIIa[65] and ICAM-2[66] on the platelet surface. Transmigration of PMN through the layer of adherent platelets may be facilitated by PMN activation, which down-regulates P-selectin binding[67] through clustering of PSGL-1 and renders it relatively inaccessible for platelet adhesion.[68] Similarly, activation-induced release of neutrophil elastase locally cleaves platelet-fibrinogen bonds, further promoting PMN egress from the circulation.[69]

Monocytes binding to a surface of adherent platelets behave similarly to PMN, using P-selectin–dependent adhesion to slow their velocity and facilitate β_2 integrin–dependent adhesion and migration into the perivascular tissue.[70] Platelet-monocyte interactions may modulate long-term atherogenic and thrombotic events, as well as those of inflammation. P-selectin binding to PSGL-1 on monocytes in one study was shown to induce monocytes to express tissue factor on their surface.[71] This finding has not been duplicated with purified P-selectin,[50] which suggests that isolated platelet adhesion or adhesion coupled with stimulation by a product of platelet activation is necessary to induce a monocyte procoagulant state.[72]

The field of leukocyte-platelet adhesion is rapidly evolving as researchers use a combination of animal models, benchtop flow chambers, and in vivo investigations to discern the complex interactions between these cell types. Many of the effects from heterotypic adhesion are subtle and modulate not the nature of the target cell's response itself, but rather its magnitude. Future therapeutic strategies for safer manipulation of the coagulation and inflammation pathways may take the form of fine tuning strategies through manipulation of these heterotypic cell-cell interactions. The recent recognition that flow and shear themselves modulate both homotypic and heterotypic cell adhesion has generated a greater appreciation for the dynamic state of the interactions between hematopoietic cells in vivo. Our subsequent understanding of the downstream (effector) results of such interactions may lead to more sophisticated therapy of cell-dependent pathologies.

References

1. Marcus AJ: Thrombosis and inflammation as multicellular processes: Pathophysiologic significance of transcellular metabolism. Blood 76:1903–1907, 1990

2. Almony GT, Lefkovits JK, Topol EJ: Antiplatelet and anticoagulant use after myocardial infarction. Clin Cardiol 19:357–365, 1996
3. Ruggeri ZM: Mechanisms initiating platelet thrombus formation. Thromb Haemost 78:611–616, 1997
4. Livio M, Gotti E, Marchesi D, Mecca G, Remuzzi G, De Gaetano G: Uraemic bleeding: role of anaemia and beneficial effect of red cell transfusions. Lancet 2:1013–1015, 1982
5. Ruggeri ZM: von Willebrand factor. J Clin Invest 99:559–564, 1997
6. Kroll MH, Harris TS, Moake HL, Handin TI, Schafer HI: von Willebrand factor binding to platelet GpIb initiates signals for platelet activation. J Clin Invest 88:1568–1573, 1991
7. Ferguson JJ, Waly HM, Wilson JM: Fundamentals of coagulation and glycoprotein IIb/IIIa receptor inhibition. Eur Heart J 19(Suppl D):D3-D9, 1998
8. Saelman EUM, Niewenhuis HK, Hese KM, de Groot PG, Heijnen HFG, Sage EH, McKeown W, Gralnick HR, Sixma JJ: Platelet adhesion to collagen types I through VIII under conditions of stasis and flow is mediated by GpIa/IIa. Blood 83:1244–1250, 1994
9. Kehrel B, Wierwille S, Clemetson KJ, Anders O, Steiner M, Knight CG, Fanrdale RW, Okuma M, Barnes MJ: Glycoprotein VI is a major collagen receptor for platelet activation: It recognizes the platelet-activating quaternary structure of collagen, whereas CD36, glycoprotein IIb/IIIa, and von Willebrand factor do not. Blood 91:491–499, 1998
10. Dunlop LC, Andrews RK, Lopez JA, Berndt MC: Congenital Disorders of Platelet Function. In: Loscalzo J, Shafer A, eds. Thrombosis and Hemorrhage. Baltimore: Williams & Wilkins, 1998: 685–689
11. Moroi M, Jung SM, Okuma M, Shinmyozu K: A patient with platelets deficient in glycoprotein VI that lack both collagen-induced aggregation and adhesion. J Clin Invest 84:1440–1445, 1989
12. Nieuwenhuis HK, Akkerman JW, Houdijk WP, Sixma JJ: Human blood platelets showing no response to collagen fail to express surface glycoprotein Ia. Nature 318:470–472, 1985
13. Nichols WC, Coone KA, Ginsburg, Ruggeri ZM. von Willebrand Disease. In: Loscalzo J, Shafer A, eds. Thrombosis and Hemorrhage. Baltimore: Williams & Wilkins, 1998:729–756
14. Lefkovits J, Plow EF, Topol EJ: Platelet glycoprotein IIb/IIIa receptors in cardiovascular medicine. N Engl J Med 332:1553–1559, 1995
15. Vorchheimer DA, Badimon JJ, Fuster V: Platelet glycoprotein IIb/IIIa receptor antagonists in cardiovascular disease. JAMA 281:1407–1414, 1999

16. Zucker MB, Nachmias VT: Platelet activation. Arteriosclerosis 5:2–18,1985

17. Anderson GM, Hall LM, Yang JX, Cohen DJ: Platelet dense granule release reaction monitored by HPLC-fluorometric determination of endogenous serotonin. Anal Biochem 206:64, 1992

18. Dephino RA, Kaplan K: The Hermansky-Pudlak syndrome: report of three cases and review of pathophysiologic and management considerations. Medicine 64:192–202, 1985

19. Scandura JM, Walsh PN: Factor X bound to the surface of activated human platelets is preferentially activated by platelet-bound factor IXa. Biochem 35:8890–8901, 1996

20. Swords NA, Mann KG: The assembly of the prothrombinase complex on adherent platelets. Arterioscler Thromb 13:1602–1612, 1993

21. Banner EW: The factor VIIa/tissue factor complex. Thromb Haemost 78:512–515, 1997

22. Weiss HJ, Turitto VT, Baumgartner HR, Nemerson Y, Hoffman T: Evidence for the presence of tissue factor activity on subendothelium. Blood 73:968, 1989

23. Ofosu FA, Longbin L, Freedman J: Control mechanisms in thrombin generation. Semin Thromb Haemost 22:303–308, 1996

24. Muszbek L, Pogar J, Boda Z: Platelet factor XIII becomes active without the release of activation peptide during platelet activation. Thromb Haemost 69:282–285, 1993

25. Braaten JV, Jerome WG, Hantgan RR: Uncoupling fibrin from integrin receptors hastens fibrinolysis at the platelet-fibrin interface. Blood 83:982–993, 1994

26. Marcus AJ, Safier SV, Hajjar KA, Ullman HL, Islam N, Broekman MJ, Eiroa SM: Inhibition of platelet function by an aspirin-insensitive endothelial cell ADPase: Thromboregulation by endothelial cells. J Clin Invest 88:1690, 1991

27. Marcus AJ, Broekman MJ, Drosopuolos JH, Islam N, Alonycheva TN, Safier LB, Hajjar KA, Posntee DN, Schoenborm MA, Schooley KA, Gayle RB, Maliszewski CR: The endothelial cell ecto-ADPase responsible for inhibition of platelet function is CD39. J Clin Invest 99:1351–1360, 1997

28. Letterio JJ, Roberts AB: Regulation of immune responses by TGF-β. Ann Rev Immunol 16:137–161, 1998

29. Piccardoni P, Evangelista V, Piccoli A, de Daetano G, Walz A, Cerletti C: Thrombin-activated human platelets release two NAP-2 variants that stimulate polymorphonuclear leukocytes. Thromb Haemost 76:780–785, 1996

30. Valles J, Santo MT, Marcus AJ, Safier LB, Broekman MJ, Islam N, Ullman HL, Aznar J: Downregulation of human platelet reactivity

by neutrophils: Participation of lipoxygenase derivatives and adhesive proteins. J Clin Invest 92:1357–1365, 1993

31. Valles J, Santos MT, Azner J, Marcus AJ, Martinez-Sales V, Portoles M, Broekman MJ, Safier LB: Erythrocytes metabolically enhance collagen-induced platelet responsiveness via increased thromboxane production, adenosine diphosphate release, and recruitment. Blood 78:154–162, 1991

32. Valles J, Santos MT, Azner J, Osa A, Lago A, Cosin J, Sanchez E, Broekman MJ, Marcus AJ: Erythrocyte promotion of platelet reactivity decreases the effectiveness of aspirin as an antithrombotic therapeutic modality: The effect of low-dose aspirin is less than optimal in patients with vascular disease due to prothrombotic effects of erythrocytes on platelet reactivity. Circulation 97:350–355, 1998

33. Zimmerman GA, Prescott S, McIntyre T: Endothelial cell interactions with granulocytes: Tethering and signaling molecules. Immunol Today 13:93–100, 1992

34. McEver RP, Moore KL, Cummings RD: Leukocyte trafficking mediated by selectin-carbohydrate interactions. J Biol Chem 270: 11025-11028, 1995

35. McEver RP, Martin MN: A monoclonal antibody to a membrane glycoprotein binds only to activated platelets. J Biol Chem 259: 9799–9804, 1984

36. Berman CL, Yeo EL, Wencel-Drake JD, Furie BC, Ginsberg MH, Furie B: A platelet α-granule membrane protein that is associated with the plasma membrane after activation: Characterization and subcellular localization of platelet activation-dependent granule-external membrane protein. J Clin Invest 78:130–137, 1986

37. Rinder CS, Bohnert J, Rinder HM, Mitchell J, Ault KA, Hillman RS: Platelet activation and aggregation during cardiopulmonary bypass. Anesthesiology 75:388–393, 1991

38. Rinder HM, Murphy M, Mitchell JG, Stocks J, Ault KA, Hillman RS: Progressive platelet activation with storage: evidence for shortened survival of activated platelets after transfusion. Transfusion 31:409–414, 1991

39. Ault KA, Cannon CP, Mitchell J, McCahan J, Tracy RP, Novotny WF, Reimann JD, Braunwald E: Platelet activation in patients after an acute coronary syndrome: Results from the TIMI-12 trial. Thrombolysis in myocardial infarction. J Am Coll Cardiol 33: 634–639, 1999

40. Larsen E, Celi A, Gilbert GE, Erban JK, Bonfanti R, Wagner DD, Furie B: PADGEM protein: A receptor that mediates the interaction of activated platelets with neutrophils and monocytes. Cell 59:305–312, 1989

41. Vachino G, Chang XJ, Veldman GM, Kumar R, Sako D, Fouser LA, Berndt M, Cummings DA: P-selectin glycoprotein ligand 1 is the major counter-receptor for P-selectin on stimulated T-cells and is widely distributed in non-functional form on many lymphocytic cells. J Biol Chem 270:21966-21974, 1995

42. Moore KL, Eaton SF, Lyons DE, Lichenstein HS, Cummings RD, McEver RP: The P-selectin glycoprotein ligand from human neutrophils displays sialylated, fucosylated, O-linked poly-N-acetyl-lactosamine. J Biol Chem 269:23318-23327, 1994

43. Rinder HM, Bonan J, Rinder CS, Ault KA, Smith BR: Dynamics of leukocyte-platelet adhesion in whole blood. Blood 78:1730–1734, 1991

44. Rinder CS, Bonan JL, Rinder HM, Mathew J, Hines R, Smith BR: Cardiopulmonary bypass induces leukocyte-platelet adhesion. Blood 79:1201–1205, 1992

45. Ott I, Neumann F-J, Gawaz M, Schmitt M, Schomig A.: Increased neutrophil-platelet adhesion in patients with unstable angina. Circulation 94:1239–1246, 1996

46. Gawaz M, Fateh-Mighadam S, Pilz G, Gurland H-J, Werdan K.: Platelet activation and interaction with leukocytes in patients with sepsis or multiple organ failure. Eur J Clin Invest 25:843–851, 1995

47. Nagata K, Tsuji T, Todoroki N, Katagiri Y, Tanoue K, Yamazaki H, Hanai N, Irimura T: Activated platelet induce superoxide anion release by monocytes and neutrophils through P-selectin (CD62). J Immunol 151:3267, 1993

48. Bonomini M, Stuard S, Carreno M-P, Settefrati N, Snatrelli P, Haeffner-Cavaillon N, Albertazzi A.: Neutrophil reactive oxygen species production during hemodialysis: Role of activated platelet adhesion to neutrophils through P-selectin. Nephron 75:402–411, 1997

49. Del Maschio A, Corvazior E, Maillt F, Kazatchkine M, Maclouf J: Platelet-dependent induction and amplifications of PMN lysosomal enzyme release. Br J Hematol 72:329–335, 1989

50. Weyrich A, McIntyre T, McEver R, Prescott S, Zimmerman G: Monocyte tethering by P-selectin regulates monocyte chemotactic protein-1 and tumor necrosis factor-α secretion. Signal integration and NF-κB translocation. J Clin Invest 95:2297–2303, 1995

51. Weyrich A, Elstad M, McEver R, McIntyre T , Moore K, Morrissey J, Prescott S, Zimmerman G:. Activated platelet signal chemokine synthesis by human monocytes. J Clin Invest 97:1525–1534, 1996

52. Ferroni P, Speziale G, Ruvolo G, Giovannelli A, Pulcineeli FM, Lenti L, Pangatelli P, Criniti A, Tonelli E, Marino B, Gazzaniga PP: Platelet activation and cytokine production during hypothermic cardiopulmonary bypass: A possible correlation? Thromb Haemost 80:58–64, 1998

53. Palabricca T, Lobb T, Furie BC, Aronovitz M Benjamin C, Hsu YM, Sajer SA, Furie B: Leukocyte accumulation which promotes fibrin deposition is mediated in vivo by P-selectin (CD62) on adherent platelets. Nature 359:848–851, 1992

54. Lefer A, Campbell B, Scalia T, Lefer DJ: Synergism between platelets and neutrophils in provoking cardiac dysfunction after ischemia and reperfusion. Circulation 98:1322–1328, 1998

55. Bevilacqua MP, Nelson RM: Selectins. J Clin Invest 91:379–387, 1993

56. McEver RP, Beckstead JH, Moore KL, Marshall-Carlson L, Bainton DF: GMP-140, a platelet α-granule membrane protein, is also synthesized by vascular endothelial cells and is localized in Weibel-Palade bodies. J Clin Invest 84:92–99, 1989

57. Lawrence MB, Springer TA: Leukocytes roll on a selectin at physiologic flow rates: Distinction from and prerequisite for adhesion through integrins. Cell 65:859–873, 1991

58. Springer TS: Traffic signals for lymphocyte recirculation and leukocyte emigration: The multistep paradigm. Cell 76:301–314, 1994

59. Frenette PS, Mayadas TN, Hynes HR, Wagner DD: Susceptibility to infection and altered hematopoiesis in mice deficient in both P- and E-selectins. Cell 84:563–574, 1996

60. Kirchhofer D, Riederer MA, Baumgartner HR: Specific accumulation of circulating monocytes and polymorphonuclear leukocytes on platelet thrombi in a vascular injury model. Blood 89:1270–1278, 1997

61. Hagberg A, Roald H, Torstein L: Adhesion of leukocytes to growing arterial thrombi. Thromb Haemost 80:852–858, 1998

62. Diacovo TG, Roth SM, Bucola JM, Bainton DF, Springer TA: Neutrophil rolling, arrest, and transmigration across activated, surface adherent platelets via sequential action of P-selectin and the β2-integrin CD11b/CD18. Blood 88:146–157, 1996

63. Kuijper PMN, Torres G, Lammers J-W, Sixma JJ, Koenderman L, Zwaginga J: Platelet and fibrin deposition at the damaged vessel wall: Cooperative substrates for neutrophil adhesion under flow conditions. Blood 89:166–175, 1997

64. Ostrovsky L, King A, Bond S, Mitchell D, Lorant DE, Zimmerman G, Larsen R, Niu XF, Kubes P: A juxtacrine mechanism for neutrophil adhesion on platelets involves platelet-activating factor and a selectin-dependent activation process. Blood 91:3028–3036, 1998

65. Weber C, Springer TA: Neutrophil accumulation on activated, surface-adherent platelets in flow is mediated by interaction of Mac-1 with fibrinogen bound to αIIbβ3 and stimulated by platelet activating factor. J Clin Invest 100:2085–2093, 1997

66. Kuijper PHM, Torres HIG, Lammers J-W, Sixma JJ, Koenderman L, Zwaginga JJ: Platelet associated fibrinogen and ICAM-2 induce firm adhesion of neutrophils under flow conditions. Thromb Haemost 80:443–448, 1998
67. Rinder HM, Tracey JL, Rinder CS, Leitenberg D, Smith BR: Neutrophil but not monocyte activatio inhibits P-selectin-mediated platelet adhesion. Thromb Haemost 72:750–756, 1994
68. Lorant DE, McEver TP, McIntyre TM, Moore KL, Prescott SM, Zimmerman GA. Activation of PMN reduces their adhesion to P-selectin and causes redistribution of P-selectin ligands. J Clin Invest 96:171–176, 1995
69. Plow EF: The major fibrinolytic proteases of human leukocytes. Biochim Biophys Acta 630:47–56, 1980
70. Kuijper PMN, Torres G, Lammers J-W, Houben LAM, Zwaginga J, Koenderman L: P-selectin and MAC-1 mediate monocyte rolling and adhesion under flow conditions. J Leukoc Biol 64:647–673, 1998
71. Celi A, Pellegrini G, Lorenzet R, De Blasi A, Ready N, Furie BC, Furie B: P-selectin induces the expression of tissue factor on monocytes. Proc Natl Acad Sci USA 91:8767–8771, 1994
72. Amirkhosravi A, Alexander M, May K, Francis DA, Warnes G, Biggerstaff J, Francis JL: The importance of platelets in the expression of monocyte tissue factor antigen measured by a new whole blood flow cytometric assay. Thromb Haemost 75:87–95, 1996

Mark H. Ereth, M.D.

6 A Contemporary View of Coagulation

contemporary: *adj* 1: happening, existing, living, or coming into being during the same period of time. 2: a: simultaneous b: marked by characteristics of the present period: modern, current

coagulation: *n* 1: to cause to become viscous or thickened into a coherent mass: curdle, clot. 2: to gather together or form into a mass or group

A modern and comprehensive survey or discussion of the characteristics of blood that causes it to become thickened in a coherent mass is not possible. The old concept of the bricks (platelets) being held together by the mortar (fibrin) to form a solid structure against the hole in the wall (vascular defect) is at best a poor analogy in our modern understanding of thrombotic and hemostatic processes. In this chapter, I will review what is known about these complex and interrelated events that are actively being studied in hundreds of laboratories and thousands of operating rooms around the world.

Coagulation is a complex, interrelated, and dynamic (patho)physiologic process involving enzymatic and cellular mechanisms, vascular and inflammatory processes, and humoral responses. In this survey of coagulation factors and platelet function, I will place special emphasis on platelet procoagulant activities and the importance of the platelet surface in coagulation.

The Relationship Between Coagulation, Inflammation, and Endothelium, edited by Bruce Spiess, Lippincott Williams & Wilkins, Baltimore © 2000.

ENDOTHELIUM AND VASCULAR INTEGRITY

Cell-dependent processes provide the framework, and as I will discuss here, the actual surface or milieu for plasmatic and other factors involved in coagulation and inflammatory activities (Figure 6–1). This pyramid of endothelium, white cells, and platelets provides a simplified yet critical visualization of the close interrelationships between hemostasis and inflammation and the central theme of this monograph. The endothelium and endothelial function are the subject of detailed discussions in other chapters of this text. However, a brief discussion is appropriate as we begin to review coagulation, platelets, and platelet procoagulant functions.

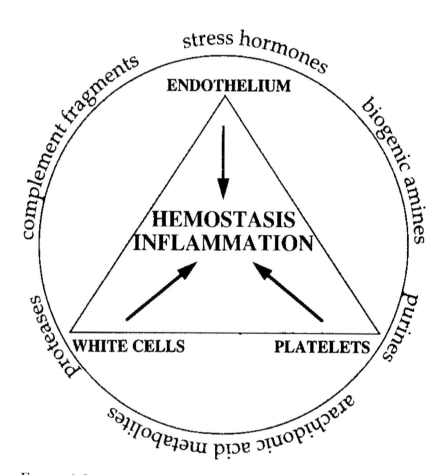

FIGURE 6–1. Interaction of various cell and humoral processes. Reprinted with permission from BD Spiess: J Cardiovasc Pharm 27:VI, 1996.

The intimal surface of the entire vascular system is lined by a mono-layer of endothelial cells. In concert, these endothelial cells comprise a large-body organ weighing only 1.5 kg that is close to 600 miles in length and has a surface area that is nearly that of a soccer field (4,260 m²). The endothelium provides for coagulation and anticoagulation activities, vasoconstrictive and vasorelaxing functions, synthesis and degradation of various proteins and mediators, and actively participates in inflammation in addition to providing a blood-tissue barrier. The endothelial cells maintain blood fluidity by physically acting as a barrier to prevent exposure of circulating blood elements to the thrombogenic subendothelial components of the vessel (von Willebrand factor [vWF] and collagen). These cells also synthesize and secrete a variety of regulatory compounds that have anticoagulant properties (Figure 6–2).[1–3] Endothelial cells continuously secrete a coating of proteoglycan containing heparin.

The surface of the endothelial cell is covered with a hyaluronic acid and branches of linked proteins that electrostatically repel circulating coagulation factor precursors. These protein complexes are covered with heparin chains and are continually built up and consumed. The interaction of heparin with antithrombin III (ATIII) accelerates the anti-coagulant activity of ATIII, inhibiting the formation of procoagulants

Vascular Integrity and Endothelium

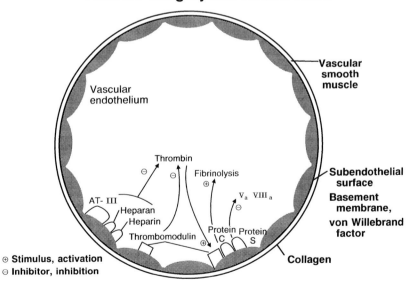

FIGURE 6–2. Endothelial function contributes to vascular integrity by providing a number of pathways by which thrombin generation or activity is limited (localized antithrombotic and profibrinolytic processes). AT-III, antithrombin III; Va, factor Va; VIIIa, factor VIIIa.

such as thrombin (factor IIa), factor IXa, and factor Xa.[4] The endothelial cell also inhibits thrombin through protein S, protein C, and thrombomodulin (Figure 6–2). Endothelial cells synthesize and release prostacyclin and nitric oxide. Both prostacyclin and nitric oxide are labile molecules that act as autocoids to inhibit platelet activity in the immediate vicinity of their sites of production (Figure 6–3).[5,6]

Platelets in motion and in proximity to endothelial cells are unresponsive to agonists.[7] This platelet unresponsiveness may be because of an ecto-ADPase on the surface of endothelial cells, which metabolizes ADP released from activated platelets (Figure 6–3). This endothelial cell ecto-ADPase, which causes a blockade of the platelet aggregation response, has been described as CD39.[8] Platelets do not adhere to normal vascular endothelial cells but only to those areas of endothelial disruption that provide bonding sites for adhesive proteins such as vWF, through the platelet glycoprotein Ib (GpIb) complex, and fibrinogen, as well as fibronectin through the integrin receptors.[9]

The response of the vessel to injury and hemorrhage is vasoconstriction and endothelial cellular release of vWF.[10] vWF then binds to

Ecto ADPase and Nitric Oxide

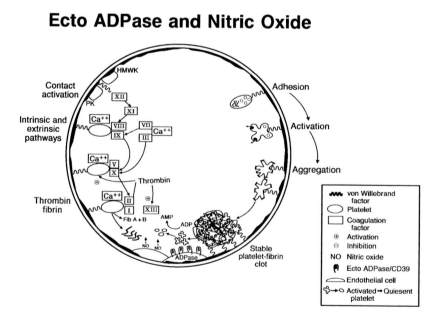

FIGURE 6–3. Ecto-ADPase and nitric oxide (NO) cause localized inhibition of clot formation. Ecto-ADPase can convert activated platelets to quiescent platelets.

the collagen in the vascular basement membrane and acts as an adhesive site for platelets. This is the first step in the capture of circulating platelets and the initiation of the platelet plug. After initial adherence to subendothelial surfaces, platelets spread out on the surface and recruit additional platelets in an accelerating fashion, which rapidly forms a coagulum of aggregated platelets.

COAGULATION PROTEINS

The coagulation system has traditionally be divided (for conceptual and in vitro laboratory testing purposes) into the intrinsic and extrinsic pathways ending in a final common pathway, which results in the formation of an insoluble fibrin clot.[11]

Although this monograph examines the crosstalk between endothelial, inflammatory, and thrombotic processes, there is much interaction between the intrinsic and extrinsic pathways, as well as the final common pathway, contact activation, fibrinolysis, and platelets. A simplified schematic overview of thrombosis and fibrinolysis is presented in Figure 6–4. Coagulation factors, with a few exceptions, are glycoproteins that are synthesized in the liver; most coagulation factors circulate as inactive proteins called "zymogens."

The molecular assembly of cofactor, enzyme, and substrate is a clear and recurrent theme in blood coagulation and provides for the maximal efficiency and speed of molecular reactions. In each of these four interrelated groups of coagulation factor cascades—contact activation, intrinsic, extrinsic, and common pathways—there are critical operant cofactors (Figure 6–4D). In the extrinsic system, tissue factor (TF) is a membrane protein that is analogous to high-molecular-weight kininogen in the contact system, factor VIII in the intrinsic system, and factor V in the final common pathway.

Factor activation proceeds in a sequential fashion, with each factor acting as a substrate in an enzymatic reaction catalyzed by the previous factor in the sequence. Enzymatic cleavage of a protein fragment changes the inactive zymogen to an active enzyme. This enzyme is termed a "serine protease" because the active site for its protease activity is a serine amino acid residue.

Extrinsic Activation

The principle initiating pathway of in vivo blood coagulation is the extrinsic system, which uses components from both blood and vascular elements. TF is synthesized in macrophages and endothelial cells and is

Thrombosis and Fibrinolysis

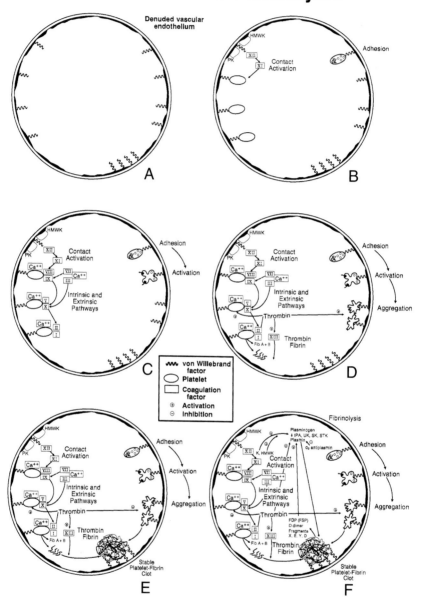

FIGURE 6–4. Serial cross sections of precapillary arterials after vascular endothelium has been disrupted, (A) exposing von Willebrand factor. (B) Unactivated platelets become adherent to von Willebrand factor via glycoprotein Ib, and contact activation of the coagulation cascade is also initiated. (C) Platelets become activated, releasing their intracellular vacuole contents and shedding procoagulant-containing microparticles accompanied by intrinsic and extrinsic coagulation pathway activation.

localized mostly in the adventitia of blood vessels. The major plasmic component of the extrinsic pathway is factor VII, which, after vascular or endothelial cell injury, works in concert with TF factor VIIIa and phospholipid to convert factor IX to the activated form (protenase complex) and resulting in the generation of activated factor X. The interaction between these four coagulation factor cascades is observed early in that factor XIIa of the contact system greatly increases the coagulant activity of factor VII. Factor Xa also displays both positive and negative feedback effects within these systems. The factor VII-TF enzyme complex operates on two principle substrates, factor IX and factor X (both vitamin K–dependent proteins). Factor VIII, which exists primarily in plasma in an activated form, forms a noncovalent complex with vWF, and functions to accelerate factor IXa conversion of factor X to Xa. Also of interest is the fact that the direct conversion of factor X to Xa by the factor VIIa-TF complex bypasses the need for factor VIII or IX.

Intrinsic System

Running parallel to and yet closely interacting with the extrinsic system is the intrinsic system, which is defined as coagulation initiated by components contained entirely within the vascular system. Here the contact system provides for activation of factor XI, which then promotes the intrinsic system with activation of factor IX to IXa and leads to protenase complex generation and a factor VII–independent pathway for generation of tenase. In the intrinsic system, the activation of factor IX requires only the presence of ionized calcium, whereas the activation of factor IX by VIIa requires calcium and TF embedded in a cell membrane lipid bilayer. The conversion of factor XI to XIa occurs in the absence of calcium by exposure to anionic polymers. The relative importance of contact activation in the intrinsic system is a subject of current debate.

Contact System

The contact system proteins participate in the initiation of the inflammatory response, complement activation, fibrinolysis, and kinin formation (Figure 6–4C).[12] This system is also critical and operant when blood contacts foreign surfaces, such as during cardiopulmonary bypass. The

FIGURE 6–4.—Continued. (D) Activated platelets recruit and can aggregate with other platelets via glycoprotein IIb/IIIa receptors as the final common coagulation pathway generates fibrin monomers. (E) Activated and aggregated platelets surrounded by prelimarized fibrin form a stable clot. (F) Early on, fibrinolysis is initiated by inflammatory processes that result in the generation of plasmin, which initiates clot breakdown.

zymogen factor XII (Hageman factor) binds to negatively charged surfaces and initiates the sequence of reactions (autoactivation), which causes generation of activated factor XII (XIIa). This exposes of a catalytic site, increases its local concentration, and provides for the generation of kallikrein and activated factor XI. A negatively charged surface is necessary for the contact system; however, later reactions in the clotting cascade require the presence of phospholipids or cell membrane surfaces. The exact nature of the contact system has never been fully clarified in vivo. Some even suggest that this would most appropriately be renamed "procoagulant initiation" and that this really only occurs in extreme inflammation and during cardiopulmonary bypass (Owen WG: Contact activation, does it exist in vivo? Personal communication, 1999). Profound inherited defects of the contact system are very rare, usually have little or no clinical effect, and are thus not studied.

Final Common Pathway

The combined or independent activities of the extrinsic, intrinsic, or contact pathways results in formation of factor Xa, which provides for the conversion of prothrombin to thrombin (IIa). In this reaction, the prothrombinase complex is formed by factor Xa, factor V, phospholipid, and calcium. The prothrombinase complex provides for a markedly increased rate of prothrombin activation, more than 300,000-fold over that which is achievable with only the enzyme factor Xa and the substrate prothrombin. Many of the procoagulant properties of platelets begin to come into play at this point. Factor V, which participates in this prothrombinase complex, is located on the platelet membrane, is supplied after platelet activation occurs, and is secreted from the platelet α granules.

Modulators of Coagulation Factor Pathways

At the site of injury there is active enzymatic control exerted to slow the coagulation reaction and prevent excessive spread. Thrombin is the most important coagulation pathway modulator. It activates cofactors V and VIII and factors I and XIII and stimulates platelet recruitment (Figure 6–4). To prevent excessive clot spread, it induces the release of tissue plasminogen activator (tPA) and urokinase-type plasminogen activator (uPA) from endothelial cells, and with thrombomodulin, it activates protein C (Figure 6–2 and 6–4F).

Additional inhibitors, commonly called "serpins" (a contraction of serine protease inhibitor), include ATIII, heparin cofactor II, α_2-antiplasmin (α_2-PI), and C1-inhibitor function in a variety of ways.[14] ATIII is the most important inhibitor of coagulation, and it serves as a protease scavenger by forming complexes with many of the coagulation factors that have moved away from the growing clot. ATIII blocks the action of thrombin (IIa) by covalently binding to its active serine site. ATIII also blocks the action of other coagulation factors (XIIa, XIa, IXa, and Xa), kallikrein, and plasmin. Protein C, along with cofactors protein S, calcium, and phospholipid, degrades factors VIIIa and Va.[15] α_2-PI reacts very rapidly with plasmin and is considered a primary regulator of fibrinolysis (Figure 6–4F).

PLATELETS

Platelets are the smallest (2–3 μm) of all hematologic cells. They have RNA but are devoid of DNA and, therefore, are unable to synthesize new proteins. They are formed in the bone marrow from megakaryocytes, which fragment to produce platelets. The platelets have a plasma half-life of 9 to 10 days. Platelets contain microtubules, α granules, and dense granules. Both types of granules contain a number of compounds, factors, and cofactors that enhance coagulation.

The formation of a platelet plug is the initial response to vascular injury. A good hemostatic response is highly dependent on proper platelet adhesion, activation, and aggregation.[16] Blood flow in the capillaries is laminar, which causes margination of platelets along the vessel wall and produces maximal physical contact and interaction. With injury and denudation of the vessel endothelium, platelets attach to the vWF bound to the exposed collagen of the subendothelium (Figure 6–5A). GpIb is a platelet membrane component that attaches to vWF, thus anchoring the platelet to the vessel wall.[17] GpIb is thought to be the receptor most responsible for platelet adhesion to the subendothelial matrix. Platelets also have membrane GpIa and GpIIa, which may attach directly to exposed collagen.[16]

Upon contact with collagen, platelets release the contents of their α and dense granules. The α granules contain platelet factor 4 and 4a, beta thromboglobulin, and integrin proteins (fibronectin, fibrinogen, vitronectin, and vWF). Dense granules contain ADP, serotonin, epinephrine, norepinephrine, and calcium. The released ADP acts to recruit additional platelets to the injury site and stimulates platelet G proteins. The G protein activates membrane phospholipase, which causes the formation of arachidonate and eventually thromboxane A_2 via platelet cyclooxygenase. Thromboxane and serotonin are both potent vasoconstrictors. Simultaneous with platelet granule release, the platelets undergo a change in shape from discoid to a spiculated sphere (Figure 6–5A). The normal equatorial band of microtubules, which maintain the discoid shape of platelets, disappears, the α and dense storage granules

Platelet Adhesion, Activation, and Aggregation: Glycoprotein Receptors

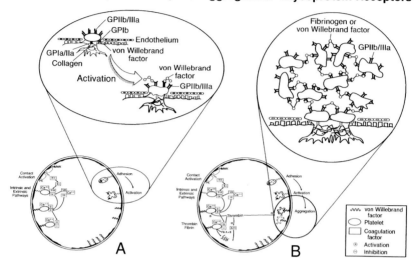

FIGURE 6–5. Platelet glycoprotein receptors (GPIb, GPIIb/IIIa) are intimately involved in the adhesion, activation, and aggregation process. During activation, the receptors are exposed and provide for cross-linking with receptors on other platelets via fibrinogen or plasmatic von Willebrand factor.

decentralize, and formation of pseudopodia occurs. This exposes the platelet integrin protein membrane GPIIb-IIIa receptors. Aggregation occurs when molecular bridges form between adjacent platelet GPIIb-IIIa receptors via binding to the RGD (arginine-glycine-aspartic acid) sequences of fibrinogen (Figure 6–5B).[11] Once platelet aggregation has occurred, fibrin cross-linking via the coagulation factor cascade is required to cement the platelets into an aggregate tough enough to withstand pressure and shear forces (Figure 6–4E). As the network of fibrin is formed, platelets extend cytoplasmic projections out along fibrin strands. Late in the process of platelet plug formation, platelets retract these fibrin adherent pseudopodia, which reduces the clot volume and concentrates the fibrin matrix directly over the site of injury.

Under normal circumstances, quiescent and unactivated platelets survey the inner lining of the blood vessel walls without significant interaction. However, they respond very rapidly to alterations of vessel wall surfaces by attaching firmly at the site of the vascular defect where exposure of subendothelial structures provide an initial site for adhesion. A single layer of platelets initially adheres to the reactive surface, binding vWF or other subendothelial structures via the GPIb receptor. Accrual of additional platelets then occurs, which provides for enhanced aggregation. Both of these processes depend on the binding of membrane receptors to mobilized or soluble ligands and are modulated by stimulus-coupled biochemical and cytoskeletal responses.[18] Activated platelets, as opposed to quiescent platelets, are required to become irreversibly attached at sites of vascular injury even under high shear conditions. vWF is synthesized in endothelial cells and megakaryocytes, and upon cleavage of a single peptide, complex intercellular processing leads to dimerization of a pro-vWF, which then undergoes covalent polymerization. Multimeric forms are stored in the Weibel-Palade bodies in endothelial cells as well as α granules in megakaryocytes and eventually platelets. The degree of vWF polymerization directly correlates with platelet prothrombotic activity. The largest multimeric forms are found in the subendothelial and platelet α granules, whereas the plasmatic forms of soluble vWF tend to be smaller multimeric size.[10] vWF promotes thrombus formation by mediating the adhesion of platelets to the injured vessel wall and to one another. Circulating plasmatic vWF provides an important initiating platelet adhesion function, whereas the subendothelial vWF provides for initial tethered adhesion, translocation, and rolling of the platelet along the vessel surface, which eventually leads to firm adhesion and recruitment of additional platelets.[10] Platelet α granule vWF is not released until platelets are fully activated and, accordingly, is not available in the initial phases of platelet contribution to thrombus formation.

Shortly, but not immediately, after platelets are activated, expel the contents of their α and dense granules, and undergo the shape change, platelet microparticles are externalized and shed. Platelet microparticles originating from the plasma membrane contain membrane GpIb and GpIIb-IIIa, as well as membrane skeletal proteins. Microparticles are shed during platelet activation but at a rate slightly slower than that of activation processes. These unilamellar vesicles have an average diameter of about 0.2 μm, and the extent of microvesicle formation is thought to parallel the timecourse of generation of procoagulant activity, which is likely a measure of platelet procoagulant activity. Greater than 25% of the procoagulant activity and factor Va binding sites are associated with microvesicles, with the remainder present on the remnant cells. Platelet shedding of microvesicles is closely associated with surface exposure of phosphatidylserine (PS). This shedding of vesicular material is certainly not unique to platelets and is another indication of the interrelated relationships between areas of cellular and humoral systems.[19] Erythrocytes, endothelial cells, and tumor cells all exhibit a similar shedding phenomenon, which is also accompanied by a loss of phospholipid asymmetry and the surface exposure of the procoagulant phosphatidylserine.[20] Platelet microvesicle production is likely to be the result of a number of cellular mechanisms that are as yet fully undescribed and, notably, seem to have an absolute requirement for extracellular calcium.

PLATELET PROCOAGULANT FUNCTIONS

An important contribution of platelets to coagulation is the surface exposure of a specific phospholipid, which provides a catalytic surface for the assembly of enzyme complexes of coagulation cascade.[21] This platelet procoagulant response leads to a dramatic increase in the rate of thrombin formation, which accelerates fibrin generation and the consolidation of a primary hemostatic plug. In addition, the catalytic surface also provides negative feedback control of the coagulation cascade via activated protein C. Platelets and their microvesicles are the primary source of procoagulant lipid surfaces. Membrane proteins serve to transport specific phospholipids from the outer to the inner leaflet of the platelet plasma membrane, and the shedding of microvesicles from platelets provides for important platelet procoagulant functions.

PS provides for much greater procoagulant activity than the other common anionic phospholipid phosphatidylinositol. Some authors have even suggested that PS might be considered as the exclusive molecule responsible for platelet procoagulant activity.[22] In the quiescent platelet, PS is almost exclusively located in the cytoplasmic leaflet of the plasma membrane. Upon activation, the phospholipid asymmetric distribution is lost, which causes a tremendous increase in procoagulant activity and the formation of factors Va and VIIIa.[23] Procoagulant factor properties of the platelet surface are most strongly promoted by collagen exposure and less so by thrombin. Weak platelet agonists such as ADP, epinephrine, or platelet activating factor provide very minimal initiation of procoagulant properties. Of interest is the fact that the combined action of collagen and thrombin, and the complement membrane attack complex C5b-9 along with calcium, provide the most intense platelet procoagulant response.[24] This is not directly related to shape change, platelet aggregation, or secretion. It is, however, a somewhat delayed response that occurs after initial adhesion, activation, and aggregation. The full expression of platelet procoagulant membrane surface function usually requires at least 5 minutes compared with only 2 minutes for the completion of platelet aggregation.[25] PS and other amino phospholipids are preferentially located in the cytoplasmic side of the platelet membrane bilayer. Under normal conditions, an asymmetrical distribution of phospholipids is maintained until cells are perturbed, which prevents unwanted coagulation.[26] The expression of procoagulant activity occurs when this phospholipid membrane asymmetry is lost. The relative increase of surface-exposed PS is closely related to the cell's ability to stimulate protenase and prothrombinase activity. During the process of platelet activation, phospholipids migrate and membrane fusion events take place, which releases derived microparticles. Of interest is the finding that GPIIb-IIIa receptor antagonists inhibit the development of some platelet procoagulant activities.[27] Intact platelet membranes may have greater procoagulant activity than platelet-released microvesicles.[28]

PLATELET AND COAGULATION FACTORS: SURFACE BINDING

Negatively charged phospholipid surfaces are the site of assembly for enzyme complexes of two important and consecutive reactions in the coagulation cascade.[29] These two important actions are the production of the tenase complex and the prothrombinase complex. A complex of factors IXa and VIIIa activate factor X (tenase complex). An enzyme complex composed of factors Xa and Va provides for the prothrombinase reaction, which converts prothrombin to thrombin.[30,31] It is the binding of factor IX, factor X, and prothrombin through calcium-mediated bridging that causes an increase in the local concentration and provides for favorable spatial relationship between the coagulation factors. This significantly increases the rate of conversion reaction. The presence of this catalytic phospholipid surface can increase the rate of thrombin formation by several orders of magnitude. PS is the major negatively charged phospholipid that is responsible for these catalytic properties.[32] Of interest is the fact that, irrespective of the actual surface charge, those membranes containing PS retain full procoagulant activity. As part of the tissue thromboplastin complex, PS also provides a major catalytic function in the extrinsic coagulation pathway.

It seems that the expression of platelet procoagulant activity is regulated by an amino phospholipid translocase.[25] This as yet to be described active membrane lipid pump serves to regulate membrane lipid asymmetry and is likely important in the procoagulant properties of platelets and a variety of other cells.

The gradual increase in the surface exposure of PS enables an efficient assembly of tenase and prothrombinase enzyme complexes. Once again the balance or cross reactivity of various protein components is illustrated by the fact that surface-exposed PS provides binding sites for tenase and prothrombinase, yet at the same time promotes the assembly of a complex composed of activated protein C and protein S, which allows for the proteolytic inactivation of factors Va and VIIIa.[33] As previously mentioned, procoagulant surfaces are exposed on platelets as well as endothelial cells and erythrocytes. These normally thromboresistant surfaces can exhibit procoagulant properties associated with microvesicle formation when agonists that increase cytosolic calcium (histamine, thrombin, and complement C5b-9) provide a challenge. It has also been observed that virally infected endothelial cells and tumor cells demonstrate procoagulant exposure of PS, release procoagulant microvesicles, and increase prothrombinase activity.[34]

FIBRINOLYSIS

Fibrinolysis is a normal physiologic activity that occurs in the vicinity of a clot and serves to remodel the formed clot and remove the thrombus when the endothelium heals. Cleavage of plasminogen (a serine protease synthesized by the liver that circulates as a zymogen) by the proper serine protease forms plasmin. As fibrinogen is being converted to fibrin, plasmin may be incorporated into the fibrin clot. Fibrinolysis may also be initiated by intrinsic or extrinsic pathways (Figure 6–5F). Both pathways activate plasminogen conversion to plasmin. The intrinsic fibrinolytic pathway occurs when factor XIIa, formed by contact activation, cleaves plasminogen to plasmin. The extrinsic fibrinolytic pathway occurs when the endothelial cells release uPA and tPA. uPA and tPA are serine proteases that split plasminogen to plasmin. The binding of tPA with fibrin concentrates its activity to the thrombus site and accelerates activity. Plasmin splits fibrinogen and fibrin into smaller and smaller fragments. The final breakdown product, D-dimer fragments, are not able to polymerize. They also act as potent serine protease inhibitors. Inhibition of fibrinolysis occurs at the level of the activators (by plasminogen activator inhibitors) or the level of plasmin (mainly by α_2-PI). Plasmin associated with the fibrin surface is protected from rapid inhibition by α_2-PI and may therefore efficiently degrade the fibrin of a thrombus. Plasma normally does not contain any plasmin because the scavenging protein, α_2-PI, consumes any plasmin formed from localized fibrinolysis. A full discussion of fibrinolysis occurs in Chapter 7.

SUMMARY

The field of platelet procoagulant function is rapidly evolving as investigators and clinicians attempt to apply in vitro results to the in vivo setting. Management of platelet and coagulation function (and dysfunction) in the future will rely on a greater understanding of the interaction between cellular and noncellular components of thrombosis and hemostasis.

Acknowledgments

The authors wish to thank Ms. Malinda Woodward for her assistance with manuscript preparation and Ms. Christine Welch for computer graphics.

References

1. Mason RG, Sharp D, Chuang HY, Mohammad SF: The endothelium: Roles in thrombosis and hemostasis. Arch Pathol Lab Med 101:61–64, 1977
2. Furlong B, Henderson AH, Lewis MJ, Smith JA: Endothelium-derived relaxing factor inhibits in vitro platelet aggregation. Br J Pharmacol 90:687–692, 1987
3. Griffith TM, Edwards DH, Lewis MJ, Newby AC, Henderson AH: The nature of endothelium-derived vascular relaxant factor. Nature 308:645–647, 1984
4. Hirsh J: Heparin. N Engl J Med 324:1565–1574, 1991
5. Azuma H, Ishikawa M, Sekizaki S: Endothelium-dependent inhibition of platelet aggregation. Br J Pharmacol 88:411–415, 1986
6. Mollace V, Salvemini D, Sessa WC, Vane JR: Inhibition of human platelet aggregation by endothelium-derived relaxing factor, sodium nitroprusside or iloprost is potentiated by captopril and reduced thiols. J Pharmacol Exp Ther 258:820–823, 1991
7. Marcus AJ, Safier LB, Hajjar KA, Ullman HL, Islam N, Broekman MJ, Eiroa AM: Inhibition of platelet function by an aspirin-insensitive endothelial cell ADPase: Thromboregulation by endothelial cells. J Clin Invest 88:1690–1696, 1991
8. Marcus AJ, Broekman MJ, Drospoulous JH, Islam N, Alyonycheva TN, Safier LB, Hajjar KA, Posnett DN, Schoenborn MA, Schooley KA, Gayle RB, Maliszewski CR: The endothelial cell Ecto-ADPase responsible for inhibition of platelet function in CD39. J Clin Invest 99:1351–1360, 1997
9. Kunicki TJ, Newman PJ, Amrani DL, Mosesson MW: Human platelet fibrinogen: Purification and hemostatic properties. Blood 66:808–815, 1985
10. Ruggeri ZM: Perspectives series: Cell adhesion in vascular biology. J Clin Invest 99:559–564, 1997
11. Furie B, Furie BC: Molecular and cellular biology of blood coagulation. New Engl J Med 326:800–806, 1992
12. Colman RW: Surface-mediated defense reactions: The plasma contact activation system. J Clin Invest 73:1249–1253, 1984
13. Deleted in proof
14. Salvesen G, Pizzo SV: Proteinase Inhibitors: α-Macroglobulins, Serpins, and Kunins. In: Colman RW, Hirsh J, Marder VJ, Salzman EW, eds. Basic Principles and Clinical Practice. 3rd ed. Philadelphia: JB Lippincott, 1994:241–258
15. Broze GJ, Miletich JP: Biochemistry and Physiology of Protein C, Protein S, and Thrombomodulin. In: Colman RW, Hirsh J, Marder VJ, Salzman EW, eds. Basic Principles and Clinical Practice. 3rd ed. Philadelphia: JB Lippincott, 1994:259–276

16. Colman RW, Cook JJ, Niewiarowski S: Mechanisms of Platelet Aggregation. In: Colman RW, Hirsh J, Marder VJ, Salzman EW, eds. Basic Principles and Clinical Practice. 3rd ed. Philadelphia: JB Lippincott, 1994:508–523

17. Kunicki TJ: Platelet membrane glycoproteins and their function: An overview. Blut 59:30–34, 1989

18. Savage B, Shattil SJ, Ruggeri ZM: Modulation of platelet function through adhesion receptors. J Biol Chem 267:11300–11306, 1992

19. Smeets EF, Comfurius P, Bevers EM, Zwaal RFA: Calcium-induced transbilayer scrambling of fluorescent phospholipid analogs in platelets and erythrocytes. Biochim Biophys Acta 1195:281–286, 1994

20. Hamilton KK, Hattori R, Esmon CT, Sims PJ: Complement proteins C5b-9 induce vesiculation of the endothelial plasma membrane and expose catalytic surface for the assembly of the prothrombinase complex. J Biol Chem 265:3809–3814, 1990

21. Bevers EM, Comfurius P, Zwaal RFA: Mechanisms Involved in Platelet Procoagulant Response. In: Authi KS, Watson SP, Kakkar VV, eds. Mechanisms of Platelet Activation and Control. New York: Plenum Press, 1993:195–207

22. Thiagarajan P, Tait JF: Binding of annexin V/placental anticoagulant protein I to platelets. J Biol Chem 265:17420–17423, 1990

23. Bevers EM, Comfurius P, Zwaal RFA: Changes in membrane phospholipid distribution during platelet activation. Biochim Biophys Acta 736:57–66, 1983

24. Ahmad SS, Rawala-Sheikh R, Ashby B, Walsh PN: Platelet receptor-mediated factor X activation by factor IXa: High-affinity IXa receptors induced by factor VIII are deficient on platelets in Scott syndrome. J Clin Invest 84:824–828, 1989

25. Schroit AJ, Zwaal RFA: Transbilayer movement of phospholipids in red cell and platelet membranes. Biochim Biophys Acta 1071:313–329, 1991

26. Larson PJ, Camire RM, Wong D, Fasano NC, Monroe DM, Tracy PB, High KA: Structure/function analyses of recombinant variants of human factor Xa: Factor Xa incorporation into prothrombinase on the thrombin-activated platelet surface is not mimicked by synthetic phospholipid vesicles. Biochemistry 37:5029–5038, 1998

27. Pedicord DL, Thomas BE, Nousa SA, Dicker IB: Glycoprotein IIb/IIIa receptor antagonists inhibit the development of platelet procoagulant activity. Thromb Res 90:247–258, 1998

28. Swords NA, Tracy PB, Mann KG: Intact platelet membranes, not platelet-released microvesicles, support the procoagulant activity of adherent platelets. Arterioscler Thromb 13:1613–1622, 1993

29. Mann KG, Nesheim ME, Church WR, Haley P, Krishnaswamy S:

Surface-dependent reactions of the vitamin K-dependent enzyme complexes. Blood 76:1–16, 1990

30. Bouchard BA, Catcher CS, Thrash BR, Adida C, Tracy PB: Effector cell protease receptor-1, a platelet activation-dependent membrane protein, regulates prothrombinase-catalyzes thrombin generation. J Biol Chem 272:9244–9251, 1997

31. Swords NA, Mann KG: The assembly of the prothrombinase complex on adherent platelets. Arterioscler Thromb 13:1602–1612, 1993

32. Rosing J, Speijer H, Zwaal RFA: Prothrombin activation on phospholipid membranes with positive electrostatic potential. Biochemistry 27:8–11, 1988

33. Esmon CT: The protein-C anticoagulant pathway. Arterioscler Thromb 12:135–145, 1992

34. van Dam-Mieras MC, Bruggeman CA, Muller AD, Debie WH, Zwaal RF: Induction of endothelial cell procoagulant activity by cytomegalovirus infection. Thromb Res 47:69–75, 1987

Wayne L. Chandler, M.D.

The Fibrinolytic Response During Cardiopulmonary Bypass: Pro or Anticoagulant?

7

Cardiopulmonary bypass (CPB) has profound effects on the body including activation of the complement, kallikrein/kinin, coagulation, fibrinolytic and platelet systems to name just a few.[1-5] Activation and dysregulation of these systems can lead to a number of deleterious effects, which include increased bleeding, thrombosis, and respiratory distress. To prevent or mitigate these problems, we need to understand how CPB affects various hemostatic and inflammatory systems, how the different systems interact once activated, and the clinical consequences of activation. These effects are not the same in all patients. Variations in the genetic make-up of individual patients may also play a role in how they respond to CPB. This review will concentrate on the fibrinolytic system, including enhanced fibrinolysis during surgery, reduced fibrinolysis postoperatively, individual variations in the fibrinolytic response to CPB, and possible clinical effects of these alterations in the fibrinolytic system. We will begin with a short review of how the fibrinolytic system is regulated.

THE FIBRINOLYTIC SYSTEM: A BRIEF REVIEW

The function of the fibrinolytic system is the proteolytic degradation of fibrin and other structural proteins by the active enzyme plasmin.[6] In the vascular system, fibrinolysis controls the size and location of thrombus formation. Fibrinolysis is regulated by controlling the rate of plasminogen activation (Figure 7-1). Tissue plasminogen activator

The Relationship Between Coagulation, Inflammation, and Endothelium, edited by
Bruce Spiess, Lippincott Williams & Wilkins, Baltimore © 2000.

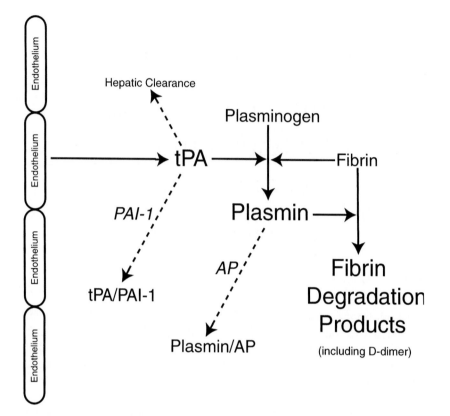

FIGURE 7–1. Diagram of the fibrinolytic system. tPA, tissue plasminogen activator; PAI-1, plasminogen activator inhibitor 1; AP, antiplasmin.

(tPA) is released from vascular endothelial cells. tPA and plasminogen bind to fibrin and tPA converts plasminogen into plasmin. Plasmin, in turn, degrades the fibrin, which releases tPA and prevents further plasminogen activation. Although tPA can activate plasminogen in the absence of fibrin, the rate of plasminogen activation by tPA is approximately 500 times faster when fibrin is present.

The rate of intravascular plasminogen activation is directly related to the concentration of active plasminogen activator in blood. Two types of plasminogen activator are found in humans, tPA and urokinase plasminogen activator (uPA). tPA is the primary intravascular plasminogen activator. Its principle source is the vascular endothelial cell. uPA is the primary extravascular plasminogen activator. It is released from a variety of cell types and is thought to be involved in cell migration and tissue remodeling. uPA plays a small role in fibrinolysis during CPB.[7,8]

tPA, however, is very important during CPB. The level of active tPA is controlled by three processes: (1) secretion of tPA from endothelium; (2) inhibition of active tPA; and (3) clearance of tPA by the liver.[9] tPA is constantly secreted from endothelial cells at an average rate of about 0.1 to 0.2 pmol/L/sec. A variety of factors, including β-adrenergic agonists like epinephrine,[10–12] vasoactive peptides like bradykinin,[13,14] and active serine proteases like thrombin,[15] can stimulate the endothelium to secrete tPA at rates that are 2- to 10-fold above their basal rate, which produces rapid increases in the active tPA concentration in plasma and therefore increases the rate of fibrinolysis. After tPA is secreted, its activity is removed from the circulation in two ways: reaction with inhibitors and hepatic clearance.

The most important inhibitor of tPA is plasminogen activator inhibitor 1 (PAI-1), a protein produced by the liver, adipose tissue, and endothelial cells. PAI-1 is also stored in platelets, which release PAI-1 at the site of a thrombus to block fibrinolysis. tPA reacts with PAI-1 to form an inactive tPA/PAI-1 complex that is removed by the liver. The level of PAI-1 in the blood determines the fraction of tPA that circulates in an active form (Figure 7–2).[9,16] As the level of PAI-1 rises in the blood, the level of active tPA falls while the level of tPA/PAI-1 rises. For example, an active PAI-1 level of 90 pmol/L will inhibit approximately 60% of circulating tPA, leaving 40% in an active form. When PAI-1 levels rise to 400 pmol/L, approximately 12% of the tPA will be active and 88% will be inhibited. When PAI-1 levels rise above 1,000 pmol/L, only a few percent of the tPA circulates in an active form, and the patient is at risk of thrombosis.

Three factors are known to regulate the level of PAI-1 in blood: (1) genetic polymorphisms in the promoter region of the PAI-1 gene that affect basal PAI-1 levels; (2) circadian variations in the secretion rate of PAI-1; and (3) acute-phase increases in PAI-1 secretion. Several polymorphisms have been reported in the promoter region of the PAI-1 gene, but only one seems to be consistently associated with changes in the level of PAI-1 in plasma (recently reviewed by Juhan-Vague et al[17]). This polymorphism consists of an insertion (5G)/deletion (4G) polymorphism at position −675 of the PAI-1 promoter.[18] The 4G allele has been associated with higher plasma PAI-1 activity in patients with coronary artery disease, non–insulin-dependent diabetics, and healthy controls. In addition, individuals who are homozygous for the 4G allele show stronger associations between fibrinogen, triglycerides, and plasma PAI-1 levels. In a small Swedish study, the 4G allele was associated with an increased risk of myocardial infarction at young age.[19] However no relationship was seen between the 4G/5G polymorphism and myocardial infarction in a large study of myocardial infarction patients aged 25 to 64 years.[20]

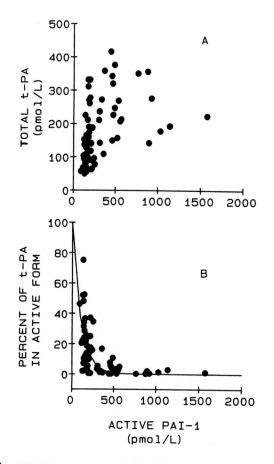

FIGURE 7–2.   (A) Concentration of active PAI-1 versus the total tPA concentration, n = 68. (B) Concentration of active PAI-1 versus the fraction of total tPA that was active (ie, active tPA divided by total tPA), n = 68. The solid line represents the best exponential fit. t-PA, tissue plasminogen activator; PAI-1, plasminogen activator inhibitor 1. Reprinted with permission.[16]

PAI-1 levels follow a prominent circadian rhythm, with peak levels in the morning around 6:00 AM.[21–23] On average, PAI-1 levels are twice as high in the morning as in the evening, but some patients show up to a 10-fold variation in PAI-1 over a 24-hour period. This morning elevation in PAI-1 leads to a reduction in the level of active tPA and fibrinolytic activity.[9] Reduced fibrinolytic activity in the morning may contribute to the increased risk of myocardial infarction, sudden death, and stroke in the morning hours.[24]

PAI-1 is a strong acute-phase reactant that rises 2- to 50-fold in response to acute-phase stimuli such as infection, inflammation, trauma, or surgery.[25] PAI-1 levels are correlated with other acute-phase reactants such as C-reactive protein, fibrinogen, and factor VIII. The rise in PAI-1 is usually transient and lasts hours to days. In some chronic conditions such as cancer, the acute-phase rise in PAI-1 may last for months to years.

In addition to PAI-1, tPA can also be inhibited by α_2-antiplasmin and C_1-inhibitor.[26,27] These proteins react with tPA at a slower rate than PAI-1 and account for only a few percent of the tPA inhibited in most situations.[11,28] By themselves, they are not sufficient to control tPA activity in blood. Patients with PAI-1 deficiency are unable to control fibrinolysis, which causes a delayed bleeding tendency.[29]

Another important regulator of fibrinolysis is hepatic clearance of tPA. Both active tPA and tPA/PAI-1 complex are rapidly cleared from the blood by the liver. Approximately 60% to 90% of active tPA and 30% to 50% of the tPA/PAI-1 complex are removed by the liver in a single pass.[30,31] tPA clearance is directly proportional to hepatic blood flow.[32] When hepatic blood flow decreases, tPA levels rise. This can be seen transiently during sustained submaximal exercise when blood flow is shunted away from the liver to muscle or chronically in patients with cirrhosis.[33] The rise in tPA in patients with cirrhosis can lead to an increased risk of bleeding, particularly during surgery.

In patients with normal liver function, the half-life of active tPA is 2 to 4 minutes, while the half-life of the tPA/PAI-1 complex is 5 to 7 minutes.[30,31] Although this difference in half-lives is small, it has an important effect on the interpretation of different fibrinolytic assays. The two most common assays for tPA measure (1) tPA activity and (2) total tPA antigen. The total tPA antigen assay measures both active tPA and tPA/PAI-1 complex. When PAI-1 activity is low in blood, most of the tPA is in an active form, which is cleared faster by the liver. When PAI-1 levels are high in the blood, most of the tPA is converted to tPA/PAI-1 complex, which is cleared more slowly by the liver and causes total tPA levels to rise in the blood. Thus, under basal conditions, high PAI-1 levels are associated with low tPA activity but high total tPA antigen (Figure 7–2). This phenotype has been associated with an increased risk of arterial thrombosis in a number of studies.[34–39] When tPA secretion increases rapidly, both active and total tPA rise together.[10,12] In this case total tPA levels follow active tPA not PAI-1. Interpretation of total tPA antigen levels requires information on the clinical or experimental conditions at the time the samples were drawn.

Changes in the level of active tPA in blood directly affect the rate of plasmin generation. Because plasminogen activation is accelerated by fibrin, the overall rate of plasmin formation is also dependent on the amount of fibrin present. Fibrinolysis is most rapid when high levels of tPA and fibrin are present in blood. When plasmin is formed, it is rapidly inhibited by α_2-antiplasmin, similar to tPA inhibition by PAI-1. Plasmin reacts with α_2-antiplasmin to form an inactive plasmin/antiplasmin (PAP) complex in blood. Plasmin/antiplasmin complex levels can be used as an indication of the rate of plasmin formation.

Plasmin lyses fibrin, which forms a variety of fibrin degradation products. One of the most commonly measured forms of degraded fibrin is D-dimer, which consists of the D domain ends of two adjacent fibrin molecules that have been cross-linked in the clot by factor XIII and then released by plasmin.

In summary, the level of active tPA in blood controls the rate of fibrinolysis. Active tPA levels, in turn, are controlled by the rate of tPA secretion, the rate of tPA inhibition by PAI-1, and the rate of hepatic clearance. tPA regulation is a very dynamic process; secretion rates for active tPA can change 10-fold in minutes, whereas inhibition of tPA by PAI-1 can change 50-fold in a matter of hours. In the next sections, we will see how these different regulatory factors are affected by CPB and the postoperative state.

THE EFFECTS OF CPB ON FIBRINOLYSIS

Hunt et al[3] compared changes in the hemostatic and fibrinolytic systems in patients undergoing CPB with those undergoing other types of thoracic surgery not involving extracorporeal circulation. They found that the major activation of coagulation and fibrinolysis was the result of CPB and not the surgery itself. Figure 7–3 shows the typical response

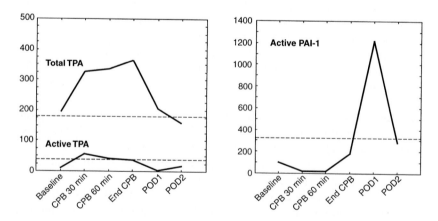

FIGURE 7–3.   Typical response of the fibrinolytic system to cardiopulmonary bypass. TPA, tissue plasminogen activator; PAI-1, plasminogen activator inhibitor 1; CPB, cardiopulmonary bypass; POD, postoperative day.

of the fibrinolytic system to CPB.[4] Soon after going on CPB, most patients show a rise in tPA secretion, which causes an elevation in active and total tPA in the blood and a fall in PAI-1 activity as it is consumed by the increased tPA that is released. The rise in active tPA levels is followed by a rise in plasmin/antiplasmin complexes as the increased tPA generates increased plasmin and a rise in D-dimer fibrin degradation fragments as the plasmin begins to degrade the fibrin that is being formed during the surgery.[2,40–42] Active tPA levels are typically highest during the first 30 minutes of CPB, then fall slowly while still remaining elevated above baseline. On average, active tPA levels rise 4-fold above baseline during CPB, but may rise up to 100-fold in some patients. Once CPB has ended, active tPA levels fall rapidly to normal or reduced levels. Liver blood flow is well preserved during CPB, which causes little change in tPA clearance compared to baseline.[43] In contrast to tPA, which rises rapidly during CPB, there is little or no change in uPA during CPB.[7,8]

There are several theories for the cause of the increased tPA release (Figure 7–4). Circulation of blood over the artificial surface of the bypass circuit causes activation of the kallikrein/kinin (contact phase), complement, and coagulation systems. Changes in each of these systems have been implicated in stimulating the rise in tPA. In vitro, the kallikrein/kinin system can be activated by "contact" between plasma and a negatively charged surface such as kaolin, cellite, or ground glass. This causes an increase in formation of kallikrein from prekallikrein, bradykinin from high-molecular-weight kininogen (HMWK) and activation of factor XII. Contact activation occurs in the activated clotting time assay and the activated partial thromboplastin time. In vivo under normal conditions, this type of contact activation does not occur because there is no known equivalent in the body of the negatively charged surface used in these assays. It is now thought that contact activation occurs on the endothelial surface, where cell metalloproteinases activate prekallikrein to kallikrein independent of factor XII.[44] Contact activation under normal conditions is a misnomer; it does not activate coagulation and is more likely a initiator of fibrinolysis, as will be discussed below. It should be noted that deficiencies of prekallikrein, HMWK, and factor XII are associated with an increased risk of thrombosis, not bleeding.

The kallikrein/kinin system is activated by CPB. There is increased generation of kallikrein (as indicated by a rise in kallikrein/C_1-inhibitor complexes) and activated factor XII.[2,40] The rise in both of these factors occurs within minutes of starting CPB, which suggests that contact activation is associated with exposure of blood to the artificial surface of the bypass circuit.[40] During CPB, it is possible that the bypass circuit is acting as a true contact activator, but the precise mechanism has not

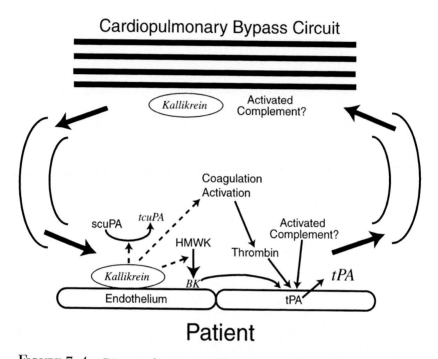

FIGURE 7–4. Diagram showing possible pathways of fibrinolytic activation during cardiopulmonary bypass (CPB). Kallikrein and activated complement fragments may be generated in the CPB circuit. Kallikrein can bind to vascular endothelial cells where it can stimulate fibrinolysis by three pathways: (1) conversion of high-molecular-weight kininogen into bradykinin, which in turn stimulates tPA release; (2) activation of the coagulation system, which generates thrombin followed by tPA release; and (3) direct conversion of inactive single-chain urokinase plasminogen activator into the active two-chain form (tcuPA). In addition, it is possible that the activated complement fragments may also be able to stimulate tPA release or accelerate fibrinolysis in other ways. tPA, tissue plasminogen activator; HMWK, high-molecular-weight kininogen; BK, bradykinin; scuPA, single-chain urokinase plasminogen activator; tcuPA, two-chain urokinase plasminogen activator.

been determined. The plastic used in bypass circuits does not present a strong negatively charged surface like that used for in vitro assays.

Kallikrein generated during CPB is now thought to bind to endothelial cells where it stimulates fibrinolysis in two ways (Figure 7–4).[44] First, kallikrein produces bradykinin from HMWK. Bradykinin has several important effects including vasodilatation, increased vascular permeability, and increased fibrinolytic activity. Bradykinin is a powerful stimulator of tPA release from endothelium.[13,14] In addition to bradykinin generation, kallikrein on the endothelial surface can directly activate single-chain urokinase plasminogen activator to the functional two-chain form, urokinase. Thus, kallikrein on the endothelial surface leads to tPA release and single-chain urokinase plasminogen activator activation. While active tPA levels may increase 100-fold during CPB, only minor changes in uPA activity have been reported, so most of the increase in fibrinolytic activity during CPB is thought to be caused by changes in tPA.[7,8]

Another possible mechanism for enhancing fibrinolysis during CPB is complement activation. Deposition of C5b-9 complex on endothelial cells has been reported to accelerate activation of plasminogen by tPA in the absence of fibrin.[45] Patients with hereditary angioedema because of deficiency of C_1-inhibitor show increased complement and fibrinolytic activation with elevated levels of plasmin/antiplasmin complexes.[46] The complement system is strongly activated by CPB.[47] There is increased generation of C3a, C3b/c, C5a, and C5b-9 membrane attack complex but not C4b/c during CPB.[1] C4b/c is generated as part of the classical pathway of complement activation involving immune complexes. Lack of C4b/c generation during CPB suggests that the classical pathway is not involved and that activation of complement during CPB involves the alternate pathway. Complement activation starts within minutes after CPB is initiated, which suggests that exposure of blood to the artificial surface in the bypass circuit is responsible for the complement activation.[48] Peak levels of C3a and C3b/c occur at the end of CPB, followed by a rapid declined once CPB is stopped. It is possible that complement activation, either through acceleration of plasminogen activation on the endothelial surface or direct release of tPA, may contribute to the acceleration of fibrinolysis.

Finally, increased thrombin generation has been proposed as a direct cause of tPA release during CPB.[49] It has been shown that thrombin stimulates human endothelial cells to release tPA.[15] CPB activates both the coagulation system and platelets.[2,50,51] The mechanism may be a combination of contact-phase activation, increased exposure of tissue factor, and plasmin-induced activation of platelets. CPB increases (1) *thrombin generation,* as shown by elevated levels of prothrombin activation peptide (F1.2); (2) *thrombin activity,* which produces increased fibrin and fibrinopeptide A; and (3) *thrombin inhibition,* as measured by thrombin/antithrombin complex (TAT) levels. Platelets are activated by CPB, as indicated by falling platelet counts and release of β-thromboglobulin and platelet factor 4. Activation of the hemostatic system occurs immediately after going on CPB, which indicates that the artificial surface of the bypass circuit is involved. Thrombin can also be formed on the surface of activated endothelial cells. In turn, thrombin stimulates the rapid release of tPA from the endothelial cells, which initiates fibrinolysis.[15]

While CPB may initially increase fibrinolytic activity by stimulating tPA release, the systemic inflammatory state caused by a combination of CPB and surgery produces an acute-phase response that results in increased PAI-1 production. Because PAI-1 production requires up-regulation of transcriptional/translational pathways rather than release of stored protein, it takes several hours to start. PAI-1 levels begin to rise about 2 hours after the start of surgery. This often coincides with the end of CPB. Once CPB is over, PAI-1 levels continue to rise and peak during the first 12 to 36 hours postoperatively. Typically active PAI-1 levels increase about 12-fold from baseline levels and return to normal by the second postoperative day.[4] This rise in PAI-1 causes faster inhibition of tPA and a fall in the level of active tPA and fibrinolysis postoperatively.

D-dimer levels rise soon after surgery begins, after fibrin begins to form. D-dimer levels rise rapidly during CPB when tPA is released, which increases plasmin generation; D-dimer levels again rise after protamine is given and the coagulation system is released from inhibition by heparin.[52] D-dimer levels fall during the early postoperative period when increased PAI-1 suppresses fibrinolysis, and fibrin formation decreases along with wound healing and reduced blood loss.

Thus, within the first 6 hours after starting open-heart surgery, there are massive alterations in the normal regulation of the fibrinolytic system. This process begins with a rapid rise in tPA and an associated increase in fibrinolytic activity during CPB. This is followed in the immediate postoperative period by a rise in PAI-1 secretion and an associated fall in active tPA levels, which leads to decreased fibrinolytic activity.

INTERINDIVIDUAL RESPONSES TO CPB

While Figure 7–3 shows the typical fibrinolytic response seen in most patients undergoing CPB, this pattern is not seen in all subjects. We found that only 40% of patients undergoing CPB showed this "typical" response.[4] Approximately 10% of patients had no change in tPA or PAI-1, 24% had no change in tPA but had a rise in PAI-1 postoperatively, while the remaining 26% had no change PAI-1 but had an intraoperative rise in active tPA.

The cause of these different fibrinolytic response patterns to CPB is currently unknown. Evidence is accumulating to support the hypothesis that patients may show different responses to CPB based on polymorphisms in the promoter region of the genes that regulate production of these proteins. As described above, patients with the 4G/5G deletion/insertion polymorphism in the PAI-1 gene produce higher levels of PAI-1, particularly in response to elevated plasma triglyceride levels. Another example is the promoter region of the β-fibrinogen gene where polymorphisms are associated with higher basal fibrinogen levels and an increased response to acute-phase stimuli.[53] A recent study suggested that patients with the factor V Leiden mutation may have an increased risk of thrombosis if aprotinin therapy is used because aprotinin can inhibit activated protein C.[54] Thus, some individuals may be genetically programmed to respond differently to CPB. If further studies support this theory, it may be possible to predict which patients are at a greater risk of untoward responses based on preoperative genetic analysis.

CLINICAL CORRELATIONS

Elevated fibrinolytic activity is associated with an increase in risk of bleeding. Increased fibrinolytic activity can be because of increased tPA secretion, reduced inhibition of fibrinolysis, or reduced clearance of tPA. As described above, the most common cause of increased fibrinolysis and associated bleeding in CPB is increased tPA secretion. The extent of fibrinolytic activation correlates positively with the degree of blood loss.[52,55,56] Much of this blood loss is thought to be caused by direct lysis of hemostatic fibrin clots by excess plasmin generated during CPB. Other studies have suggested that an increase in plasmin levels may also have a detrimental effect on platelets.[5] Plasmin formed during CPB may both partially activate and degrade platelet protein receptors, which makes platelets less responsive to normal hemostatic activation pathways. Partial activation of platelets may enhance nonspecific thrombin generation, while platelet degradation reduces normal hemostasis.

Reduced inhibition of fibrinolysis is usually because of reduced levels of PAI-1 or α_2-antiplasmin. Several families with PAI-1 deficiency have been described.[29] In all cases, PAI-1 activity in blood was low, and the patients had multiple episodes of serious bleeding primarily after surgery or trauma. The bleeding was often delayed and was associated with wound hematomas. Homozygous deficiency of α_2-antiplasmin causes an even more severe bleeding disorder, with a lifelong history of easy bruising, epistaxis, hematuria, menorrhagia, hemarthrosis, and bleeding after trauma or surgery, which is again typically delayed.[29] During CPB, PAI-1 activity falls because of hemodilution and the rise in tPA release, which consumes active PAI-1.[4] Many patients have no detectable PAI-1 activity after 30 minutes on CPB. Antiplasmin is also reduced during CPB by hemodilution; however, in all but the worst cases, it is not reduced to a major extent by fibrinolytic activation. Patients with either PAI-1 or antiplasmin deficiencies would be risk for increased bleeding during and after CPB.

tPA levels can rise and the risk of bleeding can increase when tPA clearance by the liver is decreased. The worst form of this risk is in orthotopic liver transplantation, where hepatic clearance is essentially eliminated during the anhepatic phase of surgery.[57] tPA levels may rise substantially, increasing the risk of hemorrhage. A more common cause of reduced tPA clearance is cirrhosis.[33] tPA clearance is directly proportional to effective liver blood flow past functioning hepatocytes. As liver function and blood flow worsen in cirrhosis, tPA levels rise and the risk of bleeding increases. In addition, liver production of PAI-1 and α_2-antiplasmin are decreased in cirrhosis, further worsening the hyperfibrinolytic state. In patients with normal liver function, hepatic clearance is well maintained during CPB.[43] In patients with reduced hepatic function, the hyperfibrinolytic state normally seen during CPB could be accentuated.

Reduced fibrinolytic activity is associated with an increased risk of thrombosis. Reduced fibrinolytic activity is usually caused by reductions in the level of active tPA in plasma, which in turn is caused by elevated PAI-1 levels. Elevated PAI-1 can occur in three situations, chronic increases in basal PAI-1 secretion, elevated PAI-1 secretion in the morning versus the evening, and transient acute-phase increases in PAI-1. Prior studies have shown that chronically reduced blood fibrinolytic activity,[58] elevated plasma PAI-1 activity,[38,39] PAI-1 antigen,[38] and tPA antigen[34–38] are associated with an increased risk of myocardial infarction. One consistent finding in many studies has been a strong association between elevated PAI-1 activity or antigen and elevated levels of total tPA antigen.[16,59–61] As described above, plasma clearance of active tPA is faster than clearance of the tPA/PAI-1 complex. High levels of active PAI-1 convert more tPA into tPA/PAI-1 complex, effectively slowing the clearance of total tPA antigen and explaining in part why high levels of PAI-1 activity are associated with increases in total tPA antigen.

The most common cause of increased basal PAI-1 secretion is the insulin resistance syndrome.[62] This syndrome corresponds to a prediabetic state of decreased insulin sensitivity associated with increased central obesity and elevated plasma insulin, triglycerides, and PAI-1. Other causes of increased basal PAI-1 activity included polymorphisms in the promoter region of the PAI-1 gene that lead to increased production of PAI-1. Both groups of patients have a long-term increased risk of myocardial infarction, and may have an increased risk of myocardial ischemia or infarction after CPB. In addition to increases in the basal secretion of PAI-1, most patients show a transient elevation of PAI-1 secretion after CPB. Preoperative and postoperative increases in PAI-1 are associated with an increased risk of postoperative venous thrombosis.[63]

E-AMINOCAPROIC ACID AND TRANEXAMIC ACID

ε-amino-caproic acid and tranexamic acid are specific inhibitors of the fibrinolytic system.[64] They block binding of plasminogen, tPA, and plasmin to lysine sites on fibrin, which slows plasmin formation and plasmin lysis of fibrin. ϵ-amino-caproic acid reduces D-dimer formation during and after CPB but has no effect on thrombin generation.[41,65]

THE EFFECT OF HEPARIN-COATED BYPASS CIRCUITS

Heparin coating of bypass circuits reduces the activation of the kallikrein/kinin and complement systems and seems to reduce the release of active tPA but has no effect on thrombin or plasmin generation. te Velthuis et al[66] reported a 58% reduction in kallikrein/C_1-inhibitor complexes during CPB when a heparin-coated CPB circuit was used, which suggests that the heparin coating reduced activation of the kallikrein/kinin system. The heparin coating was not associated with a reduction in either thrombin generation, as measured by F1.2 levels, or plasmin generation, as measured by PAP levels. They concluded that heparin coating reduced contact activation but not activation of coagulation or fibrinolysis.

Several groups have reported that heparin coating reduces complement activation 30% to 50% at the end of CPB or after heparin reversal with protamine but not during CPB.[50,67,68] There was no evidence of reduced complement activation early in CPB. Again, there was no evidence that heparin coating reduced thrombin generation, plasmin generation or F1.2, PAP, or D-dimer levels.

Spiess et al[69] reported that heparin-coated CPB circuits reduced tPA release compared with standard circuits. Both active and total tPA levels were lower 30 minutes after starting CPB in the heparin-coated group. There were no differences in active or total tPA levels between groups at the end of CPB or the next day. Furthermore, there were no differences in PAI-1 activity or thrombin generation between groups. Again, this suggests that systemic thrombin generation is not the primary stimulus for tPA release. Using the same type of heparin-coated surface, Gorman et al[50] reported no difference in total tPA antigen in patients undergoing CPB using heparin-coated versus standard CPB circuits. They did not measure active tPA, though, which is a more sensitive indicator of tPA changes during CPB.[4] Using different types of heparin-bonded circuits, several groups have reported no difference in PAP complexes using heparin-coated versus standard CPB circuits.[50,66,70] Thus, plasmin generation does not seem to be affected by the heparin coating.

In summary, heparin coating causes modest reductions in kallikrein/kinin activation and possibly complement activation, but no change in thrombin generation. The reduction in active tPA release reported in one study of heparin-coated circuits suggests that kallikrein/kinin or complement activation may be more important in stimulating tPA release than thrombin. This possible reduction in active tPA release was not associated with a corresponding reduction in plasmin generation. The rate of plasmin generation is a function of both active tPA levels and mass of fibrin available to accelerate plasminogen activation. The lack of difference in plasmin generation rates between heparin-coated and standard circuits indicates either that the reduction in tPA release is not consistent or that variations in fibrin mass between subject groups was sufficient to eliminate any small differences in plasmin generation. Most studies of heparin-coated versus standard circuits are small and often use different heparin coating methods. Further work is needed to determine whether heparin-coated circuits have any real effect on the fibrinolytic system.

APROTININ THERAPY

Aprotinin is a serine protease inhibitor that rapidly neutralizes plasmin and, to a lesser extent, kallikrein.[64] Aprotinin has been reported to reduce the release of tPA during CPB and to decrease the levels of plasmin/antiplasmin complex and D-dimers.[2,41,42,71] The interaction of aprotinin with the fibrinolytic system is complex. In two studies, aprotinin therapy was reported to reduce tPA release during CPB but had no apparent affect on thrombin generation as measured by F1.2 and TAT complex levels.[2,42] As with heparin-coated bypass circuits, thrombin generation did not seem to be related to tPA release. Aprotinin also had no significant effect on complement activation during CPB.[67,72,73] In contrast, aprotinin reduces kallikrein activity and kallikrein/C_1-inhibitor complex levels.[2] Thus, it is possible that reduced tPA release, both using heparin-coated bypass circuits and aprotinin therapy, is related to reduced kallikrein activity.

The effects of aprotinin on plasmin and fibrin-degradation product levels are more complicated. Plasmin formation is related both to the concentration of active tPA in the blood and the mass of fibrin available to accelerate plasminogen activation. In the absence of aprotinin, the average rate of plasmin generation can be estimated from the level of plasmin/antiplasmin complexes in plasma. When aprotinin is present, it competes with antiplasmin to inhibit plasmin. Thus, even if the rates of plasmin formation were similar, the level of plasmin/antiplasmin complex would be reduced when aprotinin was present because it replaces antiplasmin as the inhibitor for part of the plasmin generated. Reduced PAP levels during aprotinin therapy may be caused by a combination of reduced active tPA release from kallikrein inhibition and increased plasmin inhibition by aprotinin. So far, no one has actually measured the level of plasmin/aprotinin complexes in plasma to see if reduced PAP levels are because of reduced plasmin formation in addition to increased plasmin inhibition.

As with plasmin formation, D-dimer levels are related both to the activity of the fibrinolytic system and to the mass of fibrin present in the vasculature. Studies showing a reduction in D-dimer formation during aprotinin therapy have also found reduced tPA and/or plasmin levels.[2,41,42] Whether aprotinin reduces thrombin generation and fibrin formation is still a matter of controversy. Some studies,[71,74–76] but not others,[2,41,42,51,77] have indicated that aprotinin reduces thrombin formation as measured by F1.2 and TAT levels. Similarly, there is no agreement on the effect of aprotinin on the postoperative rise in PAI-1 levels. Studies have reported that postoperative PAI-1 levels were lower,[76] higher,[77] and essentially unchanged[42] in aprotinin treated patients versus controls. In part, the differences in the these studies may relate to dose of aprotinin used, heparin levels maintained,[78] adults versus children,[75] variations in the response of individual patients in small studies, and other factors. The reduction in D-dimer levels even in studies where F1.2 and TAT were not decreased indicates that reduced plasmin activity is the principle mechanism that is responsible for lowering D-dimer levels during CPB.[2,42]

Aprotinin therapy is associated with a reduction in blood loss after CPB.[79] The mechanism of reduced blood loss with aprotinin therapy is still controversial. It may include a combination of direct inhibition of kallikrein activity leading to reduced tPA secretion,[2] direct inhibition plasmin leading to reduced lysis of hemostatic fibrin clots,[42,80] reduced activation of the coagulation system,[74] and preservation of platelet function by reducing plasmin-mediated degradation and partial activation of platelet receptors.[5,81,82]

FUTURE DIRECTIONS

CPB causes an increase in fibrinolytic activity during CBP because of increased tPA release followed by plasmin formation. Hyperfibrinolysis during CPB is followed by hypofibrinolysis in the postoperative period because of increased PAI-1 and reduced active tPA. Thus, CPB produces both an anticoagulant and procoagulant fibrinolytic response. Future work will be directed toward developing therapies or new circuit materials and coatings that can reduce activation of the hemostatic and inflammatory systems. This should result in better hemostasis and less blood loss. One possibility is increasing levels of natural inhibitors, such as antithrombin III, during CPB to suppress activation and return the hemostatic system to a state of homeostasis.

Further work is also needed to understand the specific cytokines or other factors that are involved in the postoperative acute-phase response. When the acute-phase response can be controlled, the risk of postoperative ischemia and infarction may be reduced. Finally, genetic analysis will identify risk factors associated with an increased risk of bleeding and thrombosis during and after surgery. This information can then be used to determine which patients will most benefit from new and potentially expensive therapies.

References

1. Bruins P, te Velthuis H, Yazdanbakhsh AP, Jansen PGM, van Hardevelt FWJ, de Beaumont EMFH, Wildevuur CRH, Eijsman L, Trouwborst A, Hack E: Activation of the complement system during and after CPB surgery, postsurgery activation involves C-reactive protein and is associated with postoperative arrhythmia. Circulation 96:3542–3548, 1997
2. Marx G, Pokar H, Reuter H, Doering V, Tilsner V: The effects of aprotinin on hemostatic function during cardiac surgery. J Cardiothorac Vasc Anesth 5:467–474, 1991
3. Hunt BJ, Parratt RN, Segal HC, Sheikh S, Kallis P, Yacoub M: Activation of coagulation and fibrinolysis during cardiothoracic operations. Ann Thorac Surg 65:712–718, 1998
4. Chandler WL, Fitch JCK, Wall MH, Verrier ED, Cochran RP, Soltow LO, Spiess BD: Individual variations in the fibrinolytic response during and after cardiopulmonary bypass. Thromb Haemost 74:1293–1297, 1995
5. Shigeta O, Kojima H, Jikuya T, Terada Y, Atsumi N, Sakakibara Y, Nagasawa T, Mitsui T: Aprotinin inhibits plasmin-induced platelet activation during cardiopulmonary bypass. Circulation 96:569–574, 1997
6. Chandler WL: The human fibrinolytic system. Crit Rev Oncol Hematol 24:27–45, 1996
7. Spannagle M, Dooijewaard G, Dietrich W, Kluft C: Protection of single-chain urokinase-type plasminogen activator (scu-PA) in aprotinin treated cardiac surgical patients undergoing cardiopulmonary bypass. Thromb Haemost 73:825–828, 1995
8. Valen G, Eriksson E, Risberg B, Vaage J: Fibrinolysis during cardiac surgery: Release of tissue plasminogen activator in arterial and coronary sinus blood. Eur J Cardiothorac Surg 8:324–330, 1994
9. Chandler WL: A kinetic model of the circulatory regulation of tissue plasminogen activator. Thromb Haemost 66:321–322, 1991

10. Chandler WL, Veith RC, Fellingham GW, Levy WC, Schwartz RS, Cerqueira MD, Kahn SE, Larson VG, Cain KC, Beard JC, Abrass IB, Stratton JS: Fibrinolytic response during exercise and epinephrine infusion in the same subjects. J Am Coll Cardiol 19:1412–1420, 1992

11. Chandler WL, Levy WC, Stratton JR: The circulatory regulation of t-PA and u-PA secretion, clearance and inhibition during exercise and during the infusion of isoproterenol and phenylephrine. Circulation 92:2984–2994, 1995

12. Chandler WL, Levy WC, Veith RC, Stratton JR: A kinetic model of the circulatory regulation of tissue plasminogen activator during exercise, epinephrine infusion, and endurance training. Blood 81: 3293–3302, 1993

13. Emeis JJ: Regulation of the acute release of tissue-type plasminogen activator from the endothelium by coagulation activation products. Ann NY Acad Sci 667:249–258, 1992

14. Brown NJ, Nadeau JH, Vaughan DE: Selective stimulation of tissue-type plasminogen activator (t-PA) in vivo by infusion of bradykinin. Thromb Haemost 77:522–525, 1997

15. Booyse FM, Bruce R, Dolenak D, Grover M, Casey LC: Rapid release and deactivation of plasminogen activators in human endothelial cell cultures in the presence of thrombin and ionophore A23187. Semin Thromb Hemost 12:228–230, 1986

16. Chandler WL, Trimble SL, Loo SC, Mornin D: Effect of PAI-1 levels on the molar concentrations of active tissue plasminogen activator (t-PA) and t-PA/PAI-1 complex in plasma. Blood 76:930–937, 1990

17. Juhan-Vague I, Alessi MC: Fibrinolysis and risk of coronary artery disease. Fibrinolysis 10:127–136, 1996

18. Dawson S, Wiman B, Hamsten A, Green F, Humphries S, Henney AM: The two allele sequences of a common polymorphism in the promoter of the plasminogen activator inhibitor-1 (PAI-1) gene respond differently to Interleukin-1 in HepG2 cells. J Biol Chem 268:10739–10745, 1993

19. Eriksson P, Kallin B, van 't Hooft FM, Bavenholm P, Hamsten A: Allele-specific increase in basal transcription of the plasminogen-activator inhibitor 1 gene is associated with myocardial infarction. Proc Natl Acad Sci USA 92:1851–1855, 1995

20. Ye S, Green F, Scarabin PY, Nicaud V, Bara L, Dawson SJ, Humphries SE, Evans A, Luc G, Cambon JP, Arveiler D, Henney AM, Cambien F: The 4G/5G genetic polymorphism in the promoter region of the plasminogen activator inhibitor-1 (PAI-1) associated with differences in plasma PAI-1 activity but not with risk of myocardial infarction in the ECTIM study. Thromb Haemost 74:837–841, 1995

21. Andreotti F, Davies GJ, Hackett DR, Khan MI, De Bart ACW, Aber VR, Maseri A, Kluft C: Major circadian fluctuations in fibrinolytic factors and possible relevance to time of onset of myocardial infarction, sudden cardiac death and stroke. Am J Cardiol 62:635–637, 1988

22. Angleton P, Chandler WL, Schmer G: Diurnal variation of tissue-type plasminogen activator and its rapid inhibitor (PAI-1). Circulation 79:101–106, 1989

23. Chandler WL, Mornin D, Whitten RO, Angleton P, Farin FM, Fritsche TR, Veith RC, Stratton JR: Insulin, cortisol and catecholamines do not regulate circadian variations in fibrinolytic activity. Thromb Res 58:1–12, 1990

24. Muller JE, Tofler GH, Stone PH: Circadian variation and triggers of onset of acute cardiovascular disease. Circulation 79:733–743, 1989

25. Chandler WL, Stratton JR: Laboratory evaluation of fibrinolysis in patients with a history of myocardial infarction. Am J Clin Pathol 102:248–252, 1994

26. Huisman LGM, van Griensven JMT, Kluft C: On the role of C_1-inhibitor as inhibitor of tissue-type plasminogen activator in human plasma. Thromb Haemost 73:466–471, 1995

27. Nordenhem A, Wiman B: Tissue plasminogen activator (tPA) antigen in plasma: Correlation with different tPA/inhibitor complexes. Scand J Clin Lab Invest 58:475–484, 1998

28. Rånby M, Bergsdorf N, Nilsson T: Enzymatic properties of the one- and two-chain form of tissue plasminogen activator. Thromb Res 27:175–183, 1982

29. Francis CW, Marder VJ: Physiologic Regulation and Pathologic Disorders of Fibrinolysis. In: Colman RW, Hirsh J, Marder VJ, eds. Hemostasis and Thrombosis. Basic Principles and Clinical Practice. Philadelphia: JB Lippincott, 1994:1076–1103

30. Brommer EJ, Derkx FH, Schalekamp MA, Dooijewaard G, v d Klaauw MM: Renal and hepatic handling of endogenous tissue-type plasminogen activator (t-PA) and its inhibitor in man. Thromb Haemost 59:404–411, 1988

31. Chandler WL, Alessi MC, Aillaud MF, Henderson P, Vague P, Juhan-Vague I: Clearance of TPA and TPA/PAI-1 complex: Relationship to elevated TPA antigen in patients with high PAI-1 activity levels. Circulation 96:761–768, 1997

32. de Boer A, Kluft C, Kroon JM, Kasper FJ, Schoemaker HC, Pruis J, Breimer DD, Soons PA, Emeis JJ, Cohen AF: Liver blood flow as a major determinant of the clearance of recombinant human tissue-type plasminogen activator. Thromb Haemost 67:83–87, 1992

33. Joist HJ: Hemostatic Abnormalities in Liver Disease. In: Colman RW, Hirsh J, Marder VJ, eds. Hemostasis and Thrombosis. Basic

Principles and Clinical Practice. Philadelphia: JB Lippincott, 1994:906–920

34. Jansson JH, Nilsson TK, Olofsson BO: Tissue plasminogen activator and other risk factors as predictors of cardiovascular events in patients with severe angina pectoris. Eur Heart J 12:157–161, 1991

35. Jansson JH, Olofsson BO, Nilsson TK: Predictive value of tissue plasminogen activator mass concentration on long-term mortality in patients with coronary artery disease. Circulation 88:2030–2034, 1993

36. Thompson SG, Kienast J, Pyke SD, Haverkate F, van de Loo JC: Hemostatic factors and the risk of myocardial infarction and death. European Concerted Action on Thrombosis and Disabilities Angina Pectoris Study Group. N Engl J Med 332:635–641, 1995

37. Ridker PM, Vaughan DE, Stampfer MJ, Manson JE, Hennekens CH: Endogenous tissue-type plasminogen activator and risk of myocardial infarction. Lancet 341:1165–1168, 1993

38. Juhan-Vague I, Pyke SDM, Alessi MC, Jespersen J, Haverkate F, Thompson SG: Fibrinolytic factors and risk of myocardial infarction or sudden death in patients with angina pectoris. Circulation 94:2057–2063, 1996

39. Hamsten A, Walldius G, Szamosi A, Blomback M, De Faire U, Dahlen G, Landou C, Wiman B: Plasminogen activator inhibitor in plasma: Risk factor for recurrent myocardial infarction. Lancet 2:3–9, 1987

40. Grossmann R, Babin-Ebell J, Misoph M, Schwender S, Neukam K, Hickethier T, Elert O, Keller F: Changes in coagulation and fibrinolytic parameters caused by extracorporeal circulation. Heart Vessels 11:310–317, 1996

41. Eberle B, Mayer E, Hafner G, Heinermann J, Dahm M, Prellwitz W, Dick W, Oelert H: High-dose e-aminocaproic acid versus aprotinin: Antifibrinolytic efficacy in first-time coronary operations. Ann Thorac Surg 65:667–673, 1998

42. Ray MJ, Marsh NA: Aprotinin reduces blood loss after cardiopulmonary bypass by direct inhibition of plasmin. Thromb Haemost 78:1021–1026, 1997

43. Hampton WW, Townsend MC, Schirmer WJ, Haybron DM, Fry DE: Effective hepatic blood flow during cardiopulmonary bypass. Arch Surg 124:458–459, 1989

44. Schmaier AH: Contact activation: A revision. Thromb Haemost 78:101–107, 1997

45. Christiansen VJ, Sims PJ, Hamilton KK: Complement C5b-9 increases plasminogen binding and activation on human endothelial cells. Arterioscler Thromb Vasc Biol 17:164–167, 1997

46. Nielsen EW, Johansen HT, Hogasen K, Wuillemin W, Hack CE, Mollnes TE: Activation of the complement, coagulation, fibrinolytic

and kallikrein-kinin systems during attacks of hereditary angioedema. Scand J Immunol 44:185–192, 1996

47. Mollnes TE: Complement and biocompatibility. Vox Sang 74 (Suppl 2):303–307, 1998

48. Plotz FB, van Oeveren W, Bartlett RH, Wildevuur CR: Blood activation during neonatal extracorporeal life support. J Thorac Cardiovasc Surg 105:823–832, 1993

49. Teufelsbauer H, Proidl S, Havel M, Vukovich T: Early activation of hemostasis during cardiopulmonary bypass: evidence of thrombin mediated hyperfibrinolysis. Thromb Haemost 68:250–252, 1992

50. Gorman RC, Ziats NP, Rao AK, Gikakis N, Sun L, Khan MMH, Stenach N, Sapatnekar S, Chouhan V, Gorman JH, Niewiarowski S, Colman RW, Anderson JM, Edmunds LH: Surface-bound heparin fails to reduce thrombin formation during clinical cardiopulmonary bypass. J Thorac Cardiovasc Surg 111:1–12, 1996

51. Dietrich W, Schopf K, Spannagl M, Jochum M, Braun SL, Meisner H: Influence of high- and low-dose aprotinin on activation of hemostasis in open heart operations. Ann Thorac Surg 65:70–78, 1998

52. Gram J, Janetzko T, Jespersen J, Bruhn H: Enhanced effective fibrinolysis following the neutralization of heparin in open heart surgery increases the risk of post-surgical bleeding. Thromb Haemost 63:241–245, 1990

53. Humphries SE, Thomas A, Montgomery HE, Green F, Winder A, Miller G: Gene-environment interactions in the determination of plasma levels of fibrinogen. Fibrinolysis Proteolysis 11(Suppl 1):3–7, 1997

54. Sweeney JD, Blair AJ, Dupuis MP, King TC, Moulton AL: Aprotinin, cardiac surgery, and factor V Leiden. Transfusion 37:1173–1178, 1997

55. Ray MJ, Marsh NA, Hawson GAT: Relationship of fibrinolysis and platelet function to bleeding after cardiopulmonary bypass. Blood Coag Fibrinol 5:679–685, 1994

56. Khuri S, Wolfe J, Josa M, Axford TC, Szymanski I, Assousa S, Ragno G, Patel M, Silverman A, Park M, Valeri CR: Hematologic changes during and after cardiopulmonary bypass and their relationship to the bleeding time and nonsurgical blood loss. J Thorac Cardiovasc Surg 104:94–107, 1992

57. Dzik WH, Arkin CF, Jenkins RL, Stump DC: Fibrinolysis during liver transplantation in humans: Role of tissue-type plasminogen activator. Blood 71:1090–1095, 1988

58. Meade TW, Ruddock V, Stirling Y, Chakrabarti T, Miller GJ: Fibrinolytic activity, clotting factors and long-term incidence of ischaemic heart disease in the Northwick Park Heart Study. Lancet 342:1076–1079, 1993

59. Juhan-Vague I, Alessi MC, Joly P, Thirion X, Vague P, Declerck PJ,

Serradimigni A: Plasma plasminogen activator inhibitor-1 in angina pectoris, influence of plasma insulin and acute-phase response. Arteriosclerosis 9:362–367, 1989

60. Nicoloso G, Hauert J, Kruithof EKO, Melle GV, Bachmann F: Fibrinolysis in normal subjects, comparison between plasminogen activator inhibitor and other components of the fibrinolytic system. Thromb Haemost 59:299–303, 1988

61. Haverkate F, Thompson SG, Duckert F: Haemostasis factors in angina pectoris: Relation to gender, age and acute-phase reaction. Thromb Haemost 73:561–567, 1995

62. Juhan-Vague I, Alessi MC, Vague P: Increased plasma plasminogen activator inhibitor 1 levels, a possible link between insulin resistance and atherothrombosis. Diabetologia 34:457–462, 1991

63. Prins MH, Hirsh J: A critical review of the evidence supporting a relationship between impaired fibrinolytic activity and venous thromboembolism. Arch Intern Med 151:1721–1731, 1991

64. Verstraete M: Clinical application of inhibitor of fibrinolysis. Drugs 29:236–261, 1985

65. Slaughter TF, Faghih F, Greenberg CS, Leslie JB, Sladen RN: The effects of e-aminocaproic acid on fibrinolysis and thrombin generation during cardiac surgery. Anest Analg 85:1221–1226, 1997

66. te Velthuis H, Baufreton C, Jansen PG, Thijs CM, Hack CE, Sturk A, Wildevuur CR, Loisance DY: Heparin coating of extracorporeal circuits inhibits contact activation during cardiac operations. J Thorac Cardiovasc Surg 114:117–122, 1997

67. Baufreton C, Velthuis HT, Jansen PG, Besnerais PL, Wildevuur CH, Loisance DY: Reduction of blood activation in patients receiving aprotinin during cardiopulmonary bypass for coronary artery surgery. ASAIO J 42:M417-M423, 1996

68. Gu YJ, van Oeveren W, Akkerman C, Boonstra PW, Huyzen RJ, Wildevuur CR: Heparin-coated circuits reduce the inflammatory response to cardiopulmonary bypass. Ann Thorac Surg 55:917–922, 1993

69. Spiess BD, Vocelka C, Cochran RP, Soltow L, Chandler WL: Heparin coated bypass circuits, Carmeda®, suppresses the release of tissue plasminogen activator during coronary artery bypass graft surgery. J Cardiothorac Vasc Anesth 12:299–304, 1998

70. Øvrum E, Brosstad F, Holen EÅ, Tangen G, Abdelnoor M: Effects on coagulation and fibrinolysis with reduced versus full systemic heparinization and heparin-coated cardiopulmonary bypass. Circulation 92:2579–2584, 1995

71. Rossi M, Storti S, Martinelli L, Varano C, Marra R, Zamparelli R, Possati G, Schiavello R: A pump-prime aprotinin dose in cardiac surgery: appraisal of its effects on the hemostatic system. J Cardiothorac Vasc Anesth 11:835–839, 1997

72. Gott JP, Cooper WA, Schmidt FEJ, Brown WM, Wright CE, Merlino JD, Fortenberry JD, Clark WS, Guyton RA: Modifying risk for extracorporeal circulation: Trial of four antiinflammatory strategies. Ann Thorac Surg 66:747–753, 1998

73. Segal H, Sheikh S, Kallis P, Cottam S, Beard C, Potter D, Townsend E, Bidstrup BP, Yacoub M, Hunt BJ: Complement activation during major surgery: the effect of extracorporeal circuits and high-dose aprotinin therapy. J Cardiothorac Vasc Anesth 12:542–547, 1998

74. Dietrich W, Spannagl M, Jochum M, Wendt P, Schramm W, Barankay A, Sebening F, Richter JA: Influence of high-dose aprotinin treatment on blood loss and coagulation patterns in patients undergoing myocardial revascularization. Anesthesiology 73: 1119–1126, 1990

75. Dietrich W, Mossinger H, Spannagl M, Jochum M, Wendt P, Barankay A, Meisner H, Richter JA: Hemostatic activation during cardiopulmonary bypass with different aprotinin dosages in pediatric patients having cardiac operations. J Thorac Cardiovasc Surg 105:712–720, 1993

76. Lu H, Du Buit C, Soria J, Touchot B, Chollet B, Commin PL, Conseiller C, Echter E, Soria C: Postoperative hemostasis and fibrinolysis in patients undergoing cardiopulmonary bypass with and without aprotinin therapy. Thromb Haemost 72:438–443, 1994

77. Hayashida N, Isomura T, Sato T, Maruyama H, Kosuga K, Aoyagi S: Effects of minimal-dose aprotinin on coronary artery bypass grafting. J Thorac Cardiovasc Surg 114:261–269, 1997

78. Okita Y, Takamoto S, Ando M, Morota T, Yamaki F, Matsukawa R, Kawashima Y: Coagulation and fibrinolytic system in aortc sugery under deep hypothermic circulatory arrest with aprotinin: The importance of adequate heparinization. Circulation 96(Suppl II): II-376-II-381, 1997

79. Royston D, Bidstrup B, Taylor K, Sapsford R: Effect of aprotinin on need for blood transfusion after repeat open-heart surgery. Lancet 2:1289–1291, 1987

80. Wahba A, Black G, Koksch M, Rothe G, Preuner J, Schmitz G, Birnbaum DE: Aprotinin has no effect on platelet activation and adhesion during cardiopulmonary bypass. Thromb Haemost 75:844–848, 1996

81. van Oeveren W, Jansen N, Bidstrup B, Royston D, Westaby S, Neuhof H, Wildevuur C: Effects of aprotinin on hemostatic mechanisms during cardiopulmonary bypass. Ann Thorac Surg 44:640–645, 1987

82. van Oeveren W, Harder MP, Roozendaal KJ, Eijsman L, Wildevuur CRH: Aprotinin protects platelets against the initial effect of cardiopulmonary bypass. J Thorac Cardiovasc Surg 99:788–789, 1990

Bruce D. Spiess, M.D.

Heparin: Beyond
8 an Anticoagulant

This chapter will present supporting evidence for a hypothesis and a largely uninvestigated hole in research on the linkage between cardiopulmonary bypass (CPB), coagulation, inflammation, and endothelial function. Since the late 1950s when CPB was first used in humans, heparin has been administered routinely as the pharmacological agent to prevent the CPB machine, particularly the reservoir and the oxygenator, from clotting. A massive amount of research has been done to examine the "coagulopathy of CPB," and we are still working to characterize the exact mechanisms of dysfunction. Because heparin has been used in almost every one of the published studies and the majority of clinical cases, it has become synonymous with CPB. Today, other pharmacologic alternatives are being tested, or in some cases have recently reached approval for use as anticoagulants in CPB. Only now is it possible to consider that heparin may in some way actually be part of the cause of a number of problems that we had previously attributed to the CPB machine or the overall process of bypass. Heparin is not an innocuous drug.

The hypothesis outlined in this chapter is that: (1) heparin possesses a number of deleterious effects; (2) by its use in very high dose, reactions are set up in the coagulation, inflammation, and endothelial systems; and (3) these secondary effects of the bypass heparin interact with physiologic defects previously considered to be caused directly by CPB. Therefore, heparin use primes a number of deleterious reactions.

The Relationship Between Coagulation, Inflammation, and Endothelium, edited by
Bruce Spiess, Lippincott Williams & Wilkins, Baltimore © 2000.

The evidence is present in the literature for the far-reaching effects of heparin but no one has systematically isolated heparin as a causative agent. Previously, there has not been a way to conduct CPB routinely in the absence of heparin.

Cardiac anesthesiologists are familiar with how heparin works; however, a short review may be helpful. Unfractionated heparin is isolated from animal tissues containing large concentrations of mast cells and is supplied to us in an aqueous solution. As unfractionated heparin, it may be relatively impure, which means that only a small fraction of the mucopolysaccharides present within a vial of heparin may possess the properties necessary to bind antithrombin III (ATIII). There are several unique saccharide sequences in heparin that bind ATIII and thrombin. A particular pentasaccharide sequence on heparin is necessary to bind ATIII.[1] However, many of the mucopolysaccharides contain other active sites for other effects of heparin, not just those related to ATIII. It has been estimated that 30% or less of the heparin-like molecules in a vial are active in the anticoagulant role.[2,3] By itself, heparin has little, if any, anticoagulant effect; therefore, it is not an anticoagulant per se. Antithrombin effects only occur when it is in its coenzyme functional binding to the zymogen ATIII.

In CPB, a loading dose of heparin is given that is designed to massively overwhelm the amounts of circulating ATIII and thrombin, thereby creating a biochemical sink for thrombin. It is hoped that, every time a thrombin molecule is created somewhere within the circulation, an ATIII/heparin complex will be immediately adjacent and will provide an avid binding site for that thrombin molecule. By creating a sea of hungry, activated, and scavenging ATIII/heparin complexes, it is intended that thrombin will never see its other active sites (platelets, fibrin, endothelium, and white cells). If thrombin is rapidly bound to heparin/ATIII complexes then thrombin would be unable to create the secondary coagulation and inflammatory amplification reactions. A number of other chapters in this monograph discuss the effects of thrombin. Heparin is used because it works, CPB machines do not clot off routinely, and it is easily reversible (not without problems). However, it is very naive to assume that every thrombin molecule created immediately binds to an available ATIII/heparin complex.

Heparin is a naturally occurring substance that is found in mast cells and elsewhere. It probably has a function in those mast cells to assist in the local inflammatory reactions at sites of tissue injury. By creating local anticoagulation when it is released from mast cells, heparin may well assist white cells in transmigrating across the endothelium, as well as allowing them to move into the interstitium. Massive doses of heparin circulating in the bloodstream are not a natural phenomenon. Not even in pathophysiologic states do we see the level of free heparin in the bloodstream that is intentionally administered in CPB. Therefore, there is no natural disease that allows us to compare with heparinization for CPB.

Heparin (unfractionated and pharmacological) is often confused with heparan. Heparan is a very similar substance to heparin in that varying chain length mucopolysaccharides are created and these are capable of stimulating ATIII to change conformation. Heparan is tethered to the surface of the endothelium by a protein skeleton, and, therefore, heparans are considered glycosaminoglycans. They are continuously being created and sheared off in the bloodstream. Vascular shear stress not only activates platelets and produces changes in endothelial cells, but it also probably increases the turnover rate or destruction of heparan, thereby making the endothelial surface particularly susceptible to attack by other inflammatory events. The circulating ATIII interacts with the endothelial-bound heparan and can bind to it, thereby becoming activated. That combination leads to the normal physiologic effect, which is to create a vascular surface that has profound anticoagulant properties. If heparan fragments are released from their endothelial tethers, they can float free in the bloodstream. A scavenging mechanism exists to deal with these free fragments, and platelets bind them to platelet factor 4 (PF4).[4] That particular membrane glycoprotein is expressed in low levels in all platelets but can be very highly expressed in activated platelets (Chapter 5).

Vascular homeostasis, therefore, is dependent upon having a circulating element, ATIII, which interacts with a bound coenzyme, heparan, and also has a mechanism for dealing with low levels of released ATIII/heparan complexes. As a homeostatic mechanism, this lovely system has a certain buffering capacity. There are local and systemic limits beyond which the capacity to handle a stimulus is exceeded. This is true for any buffering system (eg, acid–base buffering by bicarbonate). One can think of the native anticoagulation and thrombin generation system as being buffered with ATIII, heparan, heparin cofactor I, proteins C/S, tissue plasminogen activator (tPA), and PF4. Although heparin interacts with ATIII to increase the affinity for thrombin by up to 1,000-fold, ATIII may interact with other serine proteases as well.[5–7] ATIII may have actions against the activation of factors IXa, Xa, XIa, and XIIa as well as plasmin and potentially the kallikreins. ATIII is a 58-kDa single-chain α_2-glycoprotein. It belongs to the serpin group of serine protease inhibitors (as does aprotinin). It has an arginine-active site that, when exposed by heparin, finds and binds in a 1:1 interaction with a serine site on thrombin.[6–9] Heparin binds to a lysine site on ATIII and causes a conformational change of ATIII, which exposes the binding site for thrombin. Once the heparin/ATIII complex is formed, the affinity for thrombin is increased; however, ATIII inhibition of other serine proteases may not be increased as greatly as that seen for thrombin. The inhibitory effects of ATIII on plasmin, kallikrein, and activated factors IX, X, XI, and XII are not necessarily heparin dependent.

The administration of large doses of heparin overwhelms the buffering capacity that was just outlined. The liver produces ATIII at a relatively constant rate; ATIII has a biologic half-life of 2.8 to 4.8 days.[10] As such, it is a nonconstitutive protein; its production does not change rapidly in response to stress or other inducements. ATIII levels are considered normal at between 85% and 120% activity. One unit of ATIII is that amount found in a normal (100%) activity of 1cc of human plasma. Low levels of ATIII can occur congenitally or with acquired deficiencies.

Congenital ATIII deficiency is inherited in an autosomal dominant fashion, and therefore those persons with heterozygous deficiency are the ones that we see as ATIII-deficient.[11,12] The incidence of ATIII deficiency is 1 in 2,000 to 5,000.[13] Levels less than 20% to 30% activity (homozygous for the defect) are not usually compatible with life, and any fetus conceived with such low levels or with severely dysfunctional protein will undergo spontaneous abortion.[14–16] However, several case reports do exist in the literature of severe deficiency wherein infants have been born to heterozygous ATIII-deficient mothers.[11,16–19] Some of these infants have survived with exogenous ATIII administration, and others have died with severe arterial thrombosis.[18,19] Patients with congenital ATIII deficiency in the range of 30% to 70% may present with any number of thrombotic complications, although the tendency seems to be for venous thrombotic and embolic events to occur.[15] Arterial thrombosis is extremely rare (less than 1%), and cerebral venous sinus thrombosis has been described in infants.[17] ATIII concentrates have been used to treat mild to moderate congenital deficiencies of ATIII. Although one study of 171 patients with congenital ATIII deficiency notes no difference in mortality from the general population, a second study points towards a reduction in the embolic events if ATIII concentrates are employed.[16]

The acquired deficiencies of ATIII have provided a fertile ground for research. Acquired ATIII deficiency is seen in a number of states including certain chemotherapeutic regimens (L-asparaginase treatment), hepatic failure, nephrotic syndrome, severe preeclampsia, shock, disseminated intravascular coagulation (DIC), and after certain surgeries such as CPB. As well, ATIII deficiency is seen in chronic heparin administration or with acute large doses of heparin. Although these syndromes are not all directly related to CPB, we may well be able to learn about the effects of acute and chronic reductions of ATIII levels from such diverse defects.

Pregnancy is well accepted to be a hypercoagulable state in which fibrinogen concentration and platelet counts rise.[20,21] In preeclampsia, the association of hypercoagulability is complicated by diminishing levels of ATIII, and in its worse situations, preeclampsia progresses from a hypercoagulability to a profound coagulopathy.[22–25] ATIII levels drop during preeclampsia, probably through a consumptive process. Thrombin/antithrombin complexes increase as the ATIII levels drop. The decrease in ATIII levels precedes the clinical expression of a true preeclamptic syndrome by 1 to 2 weeks, and lowered ATIII levels may also be seen in gestational hypertension.[26] There is some evidence that the actual levels of ATIII signal the severity of the preeclampsia because ATIII levels show some correlation with the amount of renal dysfunction in the mother and correlate with fetal and maternal mortality.[24,26] DIC is a hallmark of severe preeclampsia, and one cannot be sure about what role the lowered levels of ATIII play in the production or continuation of that DIC. At least one report on administration of ATIII concentrate to preeclamptic women with DIC did show efficacy of the ATIII and improved coagulation precursor levels.[24] The exact mechanism of preeclampsia still remains under investigation. However, it seems reasonable to say that a diffuse endothelial dysfunction occurs through an as-yet unidentified toxin, which leads to a complex organ dysfunction and coagulopathy. The interactions between endothelial cells, coagulation, and inflammation are perhaps analogous in some way to the dysfunction of CPB.

In a number of septic shock animal models that have been investigated, endotoxemia is a cause of near universally lethal DIC.[27–31] In rats receiving meningococcal endotoxin, severe ATIII deficiency accompanies the onset of the thrombotic organ destruction. In groups of rats who received exogenous ATIII, survival was much improved.[27–30] In humans, the studies have been less than conclusive, yet they remain very encouraging. Studies in children that have been poorly controlled or uncontrolled have claimed significant benefit in stopping the progression of DIC.[32] In an adult-controlled, randomized study of DIC with septic shock patients in an ICU setting, there was a 44% reduction in lethality.[33] Unfortunately, because of the sample size, this study did not reach statistical significance for mortality, but the trend was quite strong ($p = 0.22$ statistical significance). One study in which patients received heparin, heparin and ATIII, or ATIII alone also showed no difference in mortality.[34] There was no placebo group, and the numbers of patients were small; however, they did show a decrease in the coagulopathy in patients that received ATIII. Other studies need to be performed, and the ultimate study on ATIII and septic shock has yet to be performed. One problem with this research is that there are so many different causative agents for septic shock as well as a very wide patient-to-patient variability in response to the insults. The studies that have been published have used different doses of ATIII, and some included heparin, other anticoagulants, and other therapies. When to intervene and at what dose of ATIII, in addition to what end points should be examined for efficacy, are all problems yet to be solved. We do know that patients who have undergone shock and demonstrate levels of ATIII below 50% to 60% of normal activity have an increased morbidity and mortality.[33,35,36] Patients with levels below 20% have near 100% mortality. It is very common for patients undergoing CPB to have levels of ATIII below 40% to 50% at the end of CPB.[37,38]

End-stage hepatic failure will produce mild DIC. The synthetic function of the liver, of course, is important not only for the ATIII production but for a large number of other coagulation proteins and for clearance of tPA and plasma.[39,40] Although ATIII concentrate repletion has been tried in end-stage liver disease, it is hard to conclude from these studies that it is effective in decreasing morbidity or mortality. Some studies do show a benefit in decreasing the level of thrombin production or its effects in creating the low-grade DIC picture.[41] Interestingly, one problem that does occur post–liver transplantation is hepatic artery thrombosis. The cause for this arterial thrombosis is unclear but may again be because of the complex interaction of endothelial cell dysfunction and the circulating procoagulant and inflammatory mediators in the bloodstream. In pediatric liver transplantation, the incidence of hepatic artery thrombosis may be as high as 25%.[42] In one study where ATIII was administered to 25 children undergoing transplantation, there were no hepatic artery thromboses. This study was uncontrolled, did not have a placebo group, and other anticoagulants were used, so it is inconclusive, but again points toward the key axis of endothelial dysfunction and circulating ATIII levels.

In cancer chemotherapy for leukemia, L-asparaginase therapy is used. This therapy can lead to a prothrombotic state that is associated with lowered levels of ATIII, protein C, and protein S.[43–45] Some thought that the L-aspariginase treatment actually is toxic to the endothelial cells, and therefore the natural barrier to coagulation is decreased. That may be unclear, but certainly the parallels to the complex dysfunction seen in CPB is obvious. Treatment of patients undergoing L-aspariginase therapy with ATIII concentrate has been shown to decrease the levels of D-dimer formation and thrombin/antithrombin complexes.[46–48] It is thought that, through the maintenance of ATIII levels at a normal percentage, the risks of fibrinolytic activation and prothrombotic mechanisms can be shutoff. A decrease in the incidence of thrombotic episodes is yet to be proven, but like other ATIII studies, the numbers of patients in the studies to date have been small. Some studies have used fresh frozen plasma as their source of ATIII, and no universal target level of ATIII has been agreed upon.

In CPB, there is some literature supporting the use of or repletion of ATIII levels to normal. In a small series with children and adults undergoing CPB, it was noted that some severely low levels of ATIII are encountered (less than 40%).[37] Routinely, levels as low as 30% to 40% of activity are seen. In those patients with the lowest levels of ATIII, the highest degree of activation of thrombin was noted.[37,38,49] This has been seen in other series with extracorporeal oxygenation support, and in some of this literature it is noted that, when the ATIII levels decrease to critically low levels, oxygenator failure occurs and a new oxygenator must be put into system. That implies that microfibrin deposition is occurring in these systems when the inhibitory effects of ATIII are lost as the levels drop. A patient who required biventricular extracorporeal support has shown heparin resistance as his support became more long term.[49] Repletion of the ATIII levels returned heparin responsiveness and improved coagulation such that consumption of platelets and fibrin was slowed.

One case report notes that a patient with acquired ATIII deficiency was scheduled to undergo coronary artery bypass surgery and received exogenous ATIII to achieve an acceptable level of activated clotting time (ACT) prior to institution of CPB.[51] This patient had an ATIII level of 54% activity on entrance to the operating room after 4 days of continuous heparin therapy for unstable angina. He could not respond to challenges of heparin, and an ACT could not be raised above 347 seconds. The administration of ATIII concentrate raised his ACT to an acceptable 635 seconds, and the circulating ATIII level rose to 120% of normal. The ATIII level still fell during CPB to levels of 73%, which raises the question of how low levels might have been had the exogenous ATIII not been administered. Most likely, the ATIII level would have been in the range of levels as seen with severe DIC, shock, and death in animal studies. Several trials of ATIII are now being completed, and examination of those data shows that a very wide variability exists in the population in response to ATIII. Clearly, some patients achieve very low levels of ATIII in the ranges described for septic shock, DIC, or congenital deficiency states.

White cells release plasma elastase in response to activation. Elastase functions as an inhibitor of ATIII function. In the microenvironment where coagulation occurs if endothelial dysfunction exists, the enhanced white cell activity may worsen the potential for endothelial cell attack by white cells through released elastase.[52] Interestingly, heparin actually stimulates the release of plasma elastase from white cells. Therefore, heparin, which should be acting as an anticoagulant in binding and activating ATIII, may be decreasing its concentration and activity as well.

It is known that variability in response to CPB is the norm and that some patients have profound reactions in fibrinolytic response.[53] It may well be that this same variability of response is present in the level of drop experienced with ATIII. Because ATIII is so important for the maintenance of normal endothelial barrier function to platelet adhesion and leukocyte attack, the precipitous drop of ATIII levels as driven by heparin administration cannot be ignored.[50] The ultimate outcome study is lacking at this point; however, some research studies are underway that examine the exogenous administration of ATIII to the pump or intravenous administration to the patient to replete the ATIII bound by heparin. Questions exist about what is an appropriate dose and whether repletion is necessary, or whether a pharmacological supranormal level is required in the presence of such massive doses of heparin.

Fibrinolysis is stimulated during CPB.[53] It has been described as one of the most common problems of CPB leading to coagulopathy. tPA production is variable and can be extreme, which leads to plasmin activation.[53] It seems that heparin can cause the release of tPA from endothelial cells.[54]

Furthermore, heparin causes activation or release of serum urolcinase-type plasmogen activator (scuPA) from endothelial cells.[55] scuPA acts both as a fibrinolytic and as a secondary trigger of tPA release and activation. A protein stops the production or release of scuPA as well as tPA. Although it would be tempting to attribute a great deal of the tPA production during CPB to heparization, that may be incorrect. In a study of heparin-bound CPB circuits, where routine levels of circulating heparin were administered and the ACT was maintained at greater than 450 seconds, tPA production was greatly reduced. Therefore, although tPA can be demonstrated to be released by heparin in some studies, it does seem that the non–heparin-bound bypass circuit plays a major role in stimulating fibrinolysis.

The ATIII decrease in the circulating milieu of the plasma is one aspect of massive heparin administration. Heparin is supplied as a salt and it is very water soluble. When it is in the bloodstream, it chelates calcium.[56] This can lead to a sudden vasodilatation and blood pressure decrease. It is unclear whether a concomitant myocardial depression occurs as well, secondary to this sudden calcium depletion. We, in anesthesiology, have not focused considerable attention on the effects of massive heparin infusion because when heparin is administered CPB often is imminent. We know that the circulation will be supported within seconds to minutes of the time that we "heparinize." However, if the time after heparinization is long enough, one will note that, in most patients, there is a gradual or sudden decline in the blood pressure and in the filling pressures of the heart.

The drug we accept in a vial as heparin is relatively unpurified. Not only are the mucopolysaccharides supplied as "heparin" of all different sizes and molecular weights, but they possess a wide chemical composition. These polysaccharides clearly have a number of functions in the animal organs from which they have been harvested. We use them only for their anticoagulant activities, but what other functions do they have? The vial probably carries a number of chemically foreign substances that can cause allergic reactions. Persons allergic to pork should not receive porcine insulin, just as patients allergic to beef should not receive bovine lung heparin.[57] Allergic reactions do occur, and although we only remember the worst case scenarios in our clinical experience that demonstrate anaphylactic shock, one has to wonder if other immunologically mediate subclinical events are occurring.[58-60]

One immunologically mediated reaction to heparin is very extensively studied: the Heparin-Induced Thrombocytopenic (HIT) syndrome. Again, as clinicians, we may regard this as a relatively rare phenomenon, but in reality, the creation of antibodies to heparin are quite universal. Its manifestations in our practice may become ever more important and apparent as we see patients on longer heparin therapy. HIT is caused by the manufacture and release of immunoglobulin G (IgG) to the glycoprotein PF4.[61-63] That is, of course, the native glycoprotein that scavenges loose heparan from the plasma. If unfractionated heparin is administered to a patient and then a patient undergoes a second administration, or if a patient has a prolonged administration of heparin (ie, he/she may develop and release these antibodies), the antibody attaches to the surface of platelets and does one of two things: it can either attack the individual platelet, which leads to the early demise of that platelet, or it can cause activation of the platelet, which leads to a prothrombotic event. Platelet-to-platelet bridging by the Immuglobin leads to "white clot" syndrome. The attack on individual platelets leads to a population crash and eventual thrombocytopenia. That is one of the hallmarks of the syndrome: thrombocytopenia after the administration of heparin over a period of time. In the acute situation, a potentially catastrophic and lethal series of events can occur. If the amount of circulating IgG is large enough and a bolus of heparin is infused, the immunoglobulin can crosslink the platelets. This leads to platelet clumping and the formation of diffuse platelet plugs throughout the microcirculation. The immunoglobulins act as independent activators of the platelets, and, secondarily, thrombin may be generated. It is entirely possible for a platelet plug to be formed without any thrombin generation, however (white clot syndrome). The sudden diffuse and massive precipitation of platelets leads to other defects, which include activation of coagulation, organ hypoxemia, and a DIC syndrome. There is no routine way to anticoagulate a patient once this has been triggered; and, as stated earlier, limb ischemia, critical organ ischemia, and death do occur. Therefore the suspicion of HIT syndrome is very important in the prevention of the syndrome (ie, avoidance of heparin administration).

A number of potentially useful new pharmacologies are being tested that could form strategies to avoid the use of heparin as an anticoagulant in situations of a known HIT patient.[62]

It is most likely that the patients described as having the HIT syndrome represent the "tip of the iceberg" in terms of the variability in human immunoglobulin response to exogenous heparin administration.[61] Some recent assays using radioimmunoassay and ELISA techniques have been developed. These assays allow us to find the quantitative amounts of PF4 immunoglobulin circulating in the body. It seems that a very large percentage of the population has low levels of PF4 antibody, perhaps between 5% and 40% on entrance to the operating rooms.[61,64] However, after CPB and the massive heparin administration that we use, the prevalence of detectable antibody may exist in over 50% of the population.[61,64] If antibody is present, being actively coded for, and released we do not know what the effects of low levels of antibody are on the circulating platelet function. We are now all becoming aware of the horrific potential of HIT. It is known that low levels of antibody are present in all patients undergoing CPB and that such antibody activity is at least, in part, responsible for platelet dysfunction. It is also possible that, by decreasing the native scavenging behavior of platelets for released heparan, circulating heparan can have anticoagulant and other effects that it was never biologically intended to manifest. It all traces back to the fact that massive heparin administration is unnatural and upsets a delicate homeostatic buffering balance.

Heparin does activate platelets.[65–67] The mechanism for that activation is unclear to this author, but it may be, in part, because of the immunoglobulin reaction just described in its worse case as HIT. Platelets circulate in an inactivated form with only a relatively small number of glycoprotein membrane interactive sites available on their surfaces. PF4 has been described as it relates to heparan binding and the probable site for IgG binding during HIT. The GPIIb/IIIa site is of key importance for the final stabilization of a clot through binding of fibrinogen. Platelets normally have about 1,000 of these expressed on their surface, but when they are activated, they can increase that number by 50- to 100-fold. The GPIIb/IIIa binding site is the most prolific or ubiquitous cell ligand in the body. It is found on white cells as well as other cells. It is of great importance that, when platelets are exposed to exogenous heparin, they rapidly express their GPIIb/IIIa binding sites and therefore behave like activated platelets.[68,69] There is considerable evidence that the destruction of these binding sites, both the GPIb and GPIIb/IIIa sites, is important in the bleeding diathesis of CPB.[69,70] If a platelet normally hides its active binding sites during normal circulation but is forced to express them (activated) by exogenous heparin, it may well be that our injection of heparin forces the platelets to let down a defense mechanism. In essence, they expose those key binding sites to attack by the chemical agents circulating during CPB. Plasmin is known to downgrade the activity of these binding sites. It is yet a matter of some debate as to whether the sites are actually destroyed, reinternalized, or competitively bound with plasmin or fibrin degradation byproducts. However, if the sites are expressed on platelet surfaces, they are exposed to the noxious environment and setup for dysfunction. The administration of heparin may be the inciting event that leads to the eventual demise of so many key platelet-binding sites. We will not know the answer to that hypothesis until an alternative anticoagulant is available for study side by side with heparin and, therefore, the platelet dysfunction always ascribed to CPB may be initially, at least, partly caused by the large-scale heparin administration.

The use of heparin obligates the use of a reversal agent, which has historically meant the use of protamine. A large literature exists regarding the "evils" of protamine and I would refer the readers to some of the references.[71,72] Although protamine by itself has certain effects, the heparin/protamine complex is particularly offensive. Data exist showing that protamine alone does not cause the much-feared pulmonary hypertensive reaction sometimes referred to as a type III protamine reaction.[73] It is the heparin/protamine complex together that triggers the release of thromboxane and severe pulmonary hypertension. There is a phenomenon that occurs after protamine administration with regards to platelet number. Circulating platelet counts drop immediately after the administration of protamine.[74,75] This drop can be dramatic. It is most often approximately 30% but can be as high as 90%. In animal species with the greatest incidence of pulmonary hypertension (sheep), the drop in platelet count immediately after protamine administration is universally in the 90% range.[76] However, in platelet-depleted animals, the pulmonary hypertension may still occur. Therefore, it is thought that the thromboxane release is from pulmonary macrophages and that platelet drops are secondary to the activation along the endothelial border of pulmonary macrophages by the heparin/protamine complex.[73] That may be so in the sheep, but to what extent that mechanism is active in humans is unknown.

However, we know that heparin will bind to circulating platelets, probably at the GPIb or GPIIb/IIIa binding site. If protamine finds heparin there and creates a heparin/protamine complex at that binding site, it is very likely that such a binding site would then become unavailable for fibrin or von Willebrand factor binding. The acute drop in platelet count may be caused by margination of platelets with large loads of heparin/protamine complexes attached. The decrease in platelet counts last about 45 to 90 minutes, with a slow return to pre-protamine platelet counts. This time period corresponds to the time when the operating room team is actively looking for clot and attempting to "dry-up" the patient. It may be that the heparin/protamine complex, by binding to the important glycoprotein sites, drives some of our erratic transfusion behavior in the operating rooms. One study shows that the platelets lost are those that have been activated.[76] Does heparin play the key role in setting up that activation? The anxiety produced by first seeing clots and then having the appearance of microvascular bleeding certainly drives the ordering of fresh frozen plasma, cryoprecipitate, and platelet concentrates. It is, of course, very hard to anticipate what will happen next or just when the platelet number or function will return to levels that will support acceptable coagulation.

For many years, it was thought that contact activation of the blood with the synthetic surface of the CPB machine drove the coagulopathy of CPB. Therefore, it was natural to say that factor XIIa and factor XIa were stimulated to cause low levels of thrombin activation. However, patients with factor XIIa deficiency undergo CPB and have the same types of coagulopathies as do other "normal" patients. Tissue factor (TF) activates the extrinsic coagulation process through factor VIIa, and it is thought that this is the most potent and most important mechanism for creating localized activation of the coagulation proteins. Interestingly, we now know that the endothelial cells have the ability to increase production of TF as a response to a wide range of insults. Perhaps it is that local release of TF from activated endothelial cells that leads to the thrombin production that so many feel is a common denominator for the coagulopathy of bypass.[77]

TF pathway inhibitor (TFPI) buffers TF, like so many other serine proteases. TFPI is manufactured by the endothelial cell and is held in the proteoglycan coating of the endothelial cell membrane.[78] Its presence in the cellular coating acts as another part of the anticoagulant cell surface and prevents attack of thrombus, platelet, or white cell adhesion. TFPI is normally not found circulating in significant amounts in the plasma. TFPI is rapidly and profoundly released by the administration of heparin.[79–85]

In low-to-moderate level heparin administration, the levels of TFPI may increase in the plasma by up to 300%.[78,80] Levels of TFPI have been seen to rise as much as 30-fold with the injection of low-molecular-weight heparins.[80] Some have suggested that part of the anticoagulant effect of low molecular weight heparins, indeed their anti-Xa activity, may partially be because of the release of TFPI. The release of TF and TFPI are driven by different mechanisms. TF is inducible and can rapidly have its expression increased, whereas TFPI seems to be stored, and its release from cell surface binding sites is caused by some action on the proteoglycan surface of endothelial cells. An increase in one does not therefore translate into a coordinated corresponding increase in the

other. It has been suggested that perhaps one possible cause for the coagulopathy of CPB is that, after CPB, high levels of TFPI remain circulating in the blood. With these high levels, they form a natural anticoagulant that may well be one that we do not test for at the present time.
There may be wide variability in response of TFPI levels, just as it has
been demonstrated that very large variability exists with fibrinolytic
proteins (tPA and PAI-1). The continued use of heparin, such as is common today in CPB patients, prior to coming to the operating rooms
leads to a depletion of the stores of TFPI. Secondary infusion or second
boluses of heparin do not cause the same amount of release of TFPI. The
role such a depletion effect may have upon efficacy of heparinization for
CPB or for the natural defense of the endothelial border is not known.

Heparin not only creates a very large release of TFPI from endothelial surfaces, but it may also effect the binding and hence degradation of TFPI. The heparin/ATIII complex can actually bind Xa as
noted earlier, and it seems that such a complex has a higher affinity for
Xa than does TFPI.[80] If TFPI and Xa are bound and heparin ATIII is
added, the Xa will dissociate from TFPI and bind to heparin/ATIII complexes.[84,85] Heparin-releasable TFPI is actually used as a marker of endothelial cellular viability or dysfunction. In one study that looked at
patients with highly reactive coronary spasm disease, heparin-
releasable TFPI levels were increased, whereas in the aorta or in patients
without coronary spasm disease, TFPI release with heparin was much
less.[84,85] This would suggest that the health or reactivity of a vascular
endothelium might well have a great deal to do with how tightly TFPI
is held or released with the challenge of heparin. A number of studies
have demonstrated that patients with diffuse vascular disease and/or
ischemic coronary artery disease are hypercoagulable. Levels of fibrinogen, PAI-1, and other factors such as GPIIb/IIIa alleles have been
found that make thrombosis or hypercoagulability more likely in this
group. TF levels are increased at baseline over the general population,
and it is thought that acute TF release from atherosclerotic plaque triggers acute coronary thrombosis. TFPI levels are also increased in patients with ischemic heart disease; however, a localized imbalance of
TFPI release to TF activation may exist.[81]

TFPI binds to TF and/or factor Xa. Rebinding to glycosaminoglycans or proteoglycans (heparan) clears TFPI.[84] Indeed, normal heparan
sulfate proteoglycans are required for the normal reuptake of TFPI.[84]
We know that disturbed endothelial cells lose a considerable amount of
their heparan; therefore, with the effects of CPB upon endothelial cells,
it may be that the capacity of the body to control or eliminate a large
load of TFPI is reduced. The story with TFPI is not complete, and at this
point it is not known to what extent circulating or local TFPI plays a role
in bleeding or thrombosis. It is very well known that heparin causes a

profound release of TFPI and dislodges that natural endothelial antico-agulant from its normal site on the endothelial cell surface.

Not only does heparin exogenously administered create the release of TFPI, it also causes the release of heparan. Once again, one has to wonder if the large doses of heparin might be setting up a situation wherein attack can occur on key cellular elements. We have already discussed that heparin causes the platelets to express their glycoprotein binding sites. If heparan is released from endothelial borders, it may be that heparin either displaces it or somehow competitively forces the release of heparan. Heparan is important in not only binding ATIII to the surface of endothelial cells but is also important in anchoring a number of other anticoagulant/antiinflammatory proteins such as TFPI.

Heparin is implicated in a number of areas of cellular growth, regulation, and vascular wound healing. It is unknown whether a short period of very high circulating plasma heparin levels will have any effect on some of these cellular reactions. These are included in this chapter by way of discussion only to demonstrate that we as cardiac anesthesiologists may not fully appreciate the far-reaching effects that heparin can have. Heparin-bound endothelial growth factor is produced in endothelial cells in response to injury and can be induced by thrombin, angiotensin II, platelet-derived growth factor, and by inflammatory reactions through leukocyte-released superoxide radicals.[86] Messenger RNA for this heparin-binding growth factor can be expressed within minutes of the endothelial cells seeing these insults. Vitronectin, is an extracellular protein that may also play a role in cellular signaling for repair and growth. It can exist in a native form or in a form that binds heparin. The heparin-binding form can interact with the thrombin/ATIII complex (which exists in very high amounts in CPB) or the important reactive complement C5b-9.[87] With heparin-dependent activated vitronectin tissue growth factor-β can be rapidly expressed from aortic endothelial cells. Even growth factors for neural cells are dependent on heparin binding growth factors.

Studies examining heparin-dependent growth factors all note that heparin freely moves between the intravascular space and perivascular interstitium. The role that rapid movement of this important group of molecules plays in the CPB patient is unclear. Heparin rebound has long been described as a potential event with different regions of distribution for protamine and heparin. The water-soluble free movement of heparin may indeed form a method for a reservoir of heparin to exist in the interstitium. It would then move back along diffusion gradients and perhaps reenter the circulation. More important, it may well be that, by creating such a large intravascular level of heparin, we drive heparin into the interseptum and, once we have reversed circulating heparin with protamine, a local extravascular interstitial concentration of heparin still exists. Any amount of ACT or other testing of circulating blood would not show that interstitial heparin. However, its effects upon tissue coagulation at wound sites and potentially its effects upon endothelial cells or white cells would be very real. That hypothesis is untested today, but it does make sense if one understands the movements of large doses of heparin in the body.

Other effects of heparin exist as well. The effects of heparin on the release of lipoprotein lipase and its regulation of free fatty acids into tissues has been investigated.[88] This holds implications in diabetes because animals with diabetes have a greatly increased release of lipoprotein lipase compared with nondiabetic animals in response to heparin. In periods of low insulin, increased levels of free fatty acids are presented to the heart, and all this is exaggerated by heparin stimulation. These free fatty acids have been implicated in the chronic diabetic rat model of cardiomyopathy.[89] Once again, we know little of what relevance such research may have to the CPB patient. But one can be sure that, in the diabetic patients that are so often seen in our operating rooms, our load of heparin may well affect these patients differently than nondiabetics.

In summary, it should be obvious that heparin is not a simple drug that is used to enhance anticoagulation for CPB. Although it is routinely used and we have for years found ourselves dependent upon its binding to ATIII for blocking fibrin formation, heparin has very far reaching effects. It is the complex nature of the interactions between coagulation proteins, platelets, endothelial cells, and inflammatory cells that heparin affects. The unique massive dose administration of heparin may set up many other dysfunctions that have historically been associated with CPB alone. Because heparin does not have an alternative at the present time, research has not separated the effects of heparin from those of CPB. So many functions of heparin are just now beginning to be investigated, particularly those with cellular growth factors, that it is difficult to understand all of the effects of a single large bolus making CPB possible.

References

1. Nader HB, Dietrich CP: Natural Occurrence and Possible Biological Role of Heparin. In: Lave DA, Lindah V, eds. Heparin, Chemical and Biological Properties, Clinical Applications. Boca Raton, FL: CRC Press, 1989:81–96
2. Hirsh J: Heparin. N Engl J Med 324:1565–1574, 1998
3. Thomas DP, Barrowcliffe TW, Johnson EA: The influence of tissue source, salt and molecular weight on heparin activity. Scand J Haematol 25:40–48, 1980

4. Levy J, Cormack J, Morales A: Heparin neutralization by recombinant platelet factor 4 and protamine. Anesth Analg 81:35–37, 1995
5. Bueur SZ, Levy JH, Desposis GJ, Spiess BD, Hallyer DC: Use of antithrombin III concentrate in congenital and acquired deficiency states. Transfusion 38:481–498, 1998
6. Rosenberg RD, Bauer KA, Marcum JA: Protease inhibitors of human plasma. Antithrombin III: "The heparin antithrombin III system". J Med 16:351–416, 1985
7. Murano G, Williams L, Miller-Anderson M: Some properties of antithrombin III and its concentration in human plasma. Thromb Res 18:259–262, 1980
8. Rosenberg RD, Oosta GM, Jordan RE, Gardner WT: The interaction of heparin with thrombin and antithrombin. Biochem Biophys Res Conven 96:1200–1208, 1980
9. Kridel SJ, Chan WW, Knaver DJ: Requirement of lysine residues outside the proposed pentasaccharide binding region for high affinity heparin binding and activation of human antithrombin III. J Biol Chem 271:20935–20941, 1996
10. Collen D, Schetz J, de Cock F, Holmer E, Verstraete M: Metabolism of antithrombin III (heparin cofactor) in man: Effects of venous thrombosis and heparin administration. Eur J Clin Invest 7:27–35, 1977
11. Hirsch J, Piorella F, Pini M: Congenital antithrombin III deficiency. Am J Med 87:345–385, 1989
12. Hathaway WE: Clinical aspects of antithrombin III deficiency. Semin Hematol 28:19–23, 1991
13. Odegard OR, Abildgaurd V: Antithrombin III. Critical review of assay methods: Significance of variations in health and disease. Haemostasis 7:127–134, 1978
14. Blajchman MA, Austin RC, Fernandez-Rachubinski F, Sheffield WP: Molecular basis of inherited human antithrombin deficiency. Blood 80:2159–2171, 1992
15. Finazzi G, Caccia R, Baskui T: Different prevalence of thromboembolism in the subtypes of congenital AT-III deficiency: Review of 404 cases (Letter). Thromb Haemost 58:1094, 1987
16. Rosendaal FR, Heijboer H, Briet E, Buller HR, Brandjes DP, de Bruin K, Hommes DW, Vandenbroucke JP: Mortality in hereditary antithrombin-III deficiency: 1830–1989. Lancet 337:260–262, 1991
17. De Stefano V, Leone G, Mastrangeto S, Tripodi A, Rodeghiero F, Castaman G, Barbui T, Finazzi G, Bizzi B, Mannucci PM: Clinical manifestations and management of inherited thrombophilia: Retrospective analysis and follow-up after diagnosis of 238 patients with congenital deficiency of Antithrombin III, protein C, protein S. Thromb Haemost 72:352–358, 1994

18. Shiozaki A, Arai T, Iaum R, Niiya K, Sakuragawa N: Congenital antithrombin III deficient neonate treated with antithrombin III concentrate. Thromb Res 70:211–216, 1993
19. Bjarke B, Hern P, Blouback M: Neonatal aortic thrombosis. Acta Paediat Scand 63:297–301, 1974
20. Hellgren M, Tengborn L, Abilgaard V: Pregnancy in women with congenital antithrombin III deficiency: experience of treatment with heparin and antithrombin. Gynecol Obstet Invest 14:127–141, 1982
21. Nilsson IM, Kullander S: Coagulation and fibrinolytic studies during pregnancy. Acta Obstet Gynecol Scand 46:273–285, 1967
22. Chang CH, Chang FM, Chen CP, Yao BL, Kuo HC, Lin CC: Antithrombin III activity in normal and toxemic pregnancies. J Formos Med Assoc 91:680–684, 1992
23. Kobajaski T, Terao T: Pre-eclampsia as chronic disseminated intravascular coagulation. Study of two parameters: Thrombin-Antithrombin III complex and D-drivers. Gynecol Obstet Invest 24:170–178, 1987
24. Weiner CP, Bonsib SM: Relationship between renal histology and plasma antithrombin III activity in women with early onset pre-eclampsia. Am J Perinatol 7:139–143, 1990
25. Maki M, Terao T, Ikenoue T, Takemura T, Sekiba K, Shirakawa K, Soma H: Clinical evaluation of antithrombin III concentrate (BI 6.013) for disseminated intravascular coagulation in obstetrics: Well-controlled multicenter trial. Gynecol Obstet Invest 23:230–240, 1987
26. Savelieva GM, Efinov VS, Grislin VL, Shalina RI, Kashezheva AZ: Blood coagulation changes in pregnant women at risk of developing preeclampsia. Int J Gynaecol Obstet 48:3–8, 1995
27. Emerson TE, Fauvel MA, Redens TB, Taylor FB: Efficacy of antithrombin III supplementation in animal models of fulminant *Escherichia coli* endotoxemia or bacteremia. Am J Med 87:275–335, 1989
28. Dichneite G, Paques EP: Reduction of mortality with antithrombin III in septicemic rats: A study of Klebsiella pneumoniae induced sepsis. Thromb Haemost 69:98–102, 1993
29. Hauptman JG, Hassouna HI, Bell TG, Penner JA, Emerson TE: Efficacy of antithrombin III in endotoxin-induced disseminated intravascular coagulation. Circ Shock 25:111–122, 1988
30. Redens TB, Emerson TE: Antithrombin-III treatment limits disseminated intravascular coagulation in endotoxemia. Circ Shock 28:49–58, 1989
31. Weiss DJ, Rashid J: The sepsis-coagulant axis: A review. J Vet Intern Med 12:317–324, 1998

32. Fuse S, Tomita H, Yoshida M, Hori T, Igarashi C, Fujita S: High dose of intravenous antithrombin III without heparin in the treatment of disseminated intravascular coagulation and organ failure in four children. Am J Hematol 53:18–21, 1996

33. Fourrier F, Chopin C, Hwart JJ, Runge I, Caron C, Goudemand J: Double blind, placebo-controlled trial of antithrombin III concentrate in septic shock with disseminated intravascular coagulation. Chest 104:882–888, 1993

34. Blanhut B, Kramar H, Vivazzer H, Bergmann H: Substitution of antithrombin III in shock and DIC: A randomized study. Thromb Res 39:81–89, 1985

35. Wilson RF, Mammen EF, Robson MC, Heggers JP, Soullier G, DePoli PA: Antithrombin, prekallikrein, and fibronectin levels in surgical patients. Arch Surg 121:635–640, 1986

36. Massignon D, Lepape A, Bienvenu J, Barbier Y, Boileau C, Coeur P: Coagulation/fibrinolysis balance in septic shock related to cytokines and clinical state. Haemostasis 24:36–48, 1994

37. Hashimoto Y, Yamagishi M, Sasaki T, Nakano M, Kurosawa H: Heparin and antithrombin III levels during cardiopulmonary bypass: Correlation with subclinical plasma coagulation. Ann Thorac Surg 58:799–805, 1994

38. Despotis GJ, Levine V, Joist JH, Joiner-Maier D, Spitznagel E: Antithrombin III during cardiac surgery: Effect on response of activated clotting time to heparin and relationship to markers of hemostatic activation. Anesth Analg 85:498–506, 1997

39. Zurbon KH, Kirch W, Bruhn HD: Immunological and functional determinations of the protease inhibitors, protein C, and antithrombin III in liver cirrhosis and in neoplasia. Thromb Res 52:325–336, 1988

40. De Caterina M, Tarantino G, Farina C, Arena A, di Maro G, Esposito P, Scopacasa F: Haemostasis imbalance in Pugh-scored liver cirrhosis: Characteristic changes of plasma levels of protein C versus protein S. Haemostasis 23:229–235, 1993

41. Schipper HG, Tencate JW: Antithrombin III transfusion in patients with hepatic cirrhosis. Br J Hematol 52:25–33, 1982

42. Hashikura Y, Kawasaki S, Okumura N, Ishikawa S, Matsunami H, Ikegami T, Nakazawa Y, Makuuchi M: Prevention of hepatic artery thrombosis in pediatric liver transplantation. Transplantation 60:1109–1112, 1995

43. Tabbara IA, Ghazal CD, Chazal HH: Early drop in protein C and antithrombin III is a predictor for the development of venoocclusive disease in patients undergoing hematopoietic stem cell transplantation. J Hematother 5:79–84, 1996

44. Gugliotta L, Mazzucconi MG, Leone G, Mattioli-Belmonte M, De-

fazio D, Annino L, Tura S, Mandelli F: Incidence of thrombotic complications in adult patients with acute lymphoblastic leukemia receiving L-aspariginase during induction therapy: A retrospective study. The GIMEMA Group. Eur J Haematol 49:63–66, 1992

45. Liebman HA, Wada K, Patch MJ, McGehee W: Depression of functional and antigenic plasma antithrombin III (ATIII) due to therapy with L-aspariginase. Cancer 50:451–456, 1982

46. Gugliotta L, D'Angelo A, Mattioli Belmonte M, Vigano-D'Angelo S, Colombo G, Catani L, Gianni L, Lauria F, Tura S: Hypercoagulability during L-aspariginase treatment: The effect of antithrombin III supplementation in vivo. Br J Haematol 74:465–470, 1990

47. Zaunschirm A, Muntean W: Correction of hemostatic imbalance induced by L-aspariginase therapy in children with acute lymphoblastic leukemia. Pediatr Hematol Oncol 3:19–25, 1986

48. Mattioli Belmonte M, Gugliotta L, Delvos U, Catani L, Vianelli N, Cascione ML, Belardinelli AR, Mottola L, Tura S: A regimen for antithrombin III substitution in patients with acute lymphoblastic leukemia under treatment with L-aspariginase. Haematologica 76: 209–214, 1991

49. Desposit GJ, Levine V, Joist H, Santoro SA, Mendeloff E: Multiple episodes of thrombosis with biventricular support devices with inadequate anticoagulation and evidence of accelerated intravascular coagulation. J Thorac Cardiovasc Surg 113:419–422, 1997

50. Cohen JR, Tenenbar N, Sarfati I, Tyras D, Graver LM, Weinstein G, Wise L: In vivo inactivation of antithrombin III is promoted by heparin during cardiopulmonary bypass. J Invest Surg 5:45–49, 1992

51. Van Norman GA, Gernsheimer T, Chandler WL, Cochran RP, Spiess BD: Indicators of fibrinolysis during cardiopulmonary bypass after exogenous antithrombin III administration for acquired antithrombin III deficiency. J Cardiothorac Vasc Anesth 11:760–763, 1997

52. Turner-Gomes SO, Andrew M, Coles J, Trusler GA, Williams WG, Rabinovitch M: Abnormalities in von Willebrand factor and antithrombin III after cardiopulmonary bypass operations for congenital heart disease. J Thorac Cardiovasc Surg 103:87–97, 1992

53. Chandler WL, Fitch JC, Wall MH, Verrier ED, Cochran RP, Soltow LO, Spiess D: Individual variations in the fibrinolytic response during and after cardiopulmonary bypass. Thromb Haemost 74:1293–1297, 1995

54. Fareed J, Walenga JM, Hoppensteadt DA, Messmore HL: Studies on the profibrinolytic actions of heparin and its factors. Semin Thromb Hemost 11:199–207, 1985

55. Bertolesi GE, Farias EF, Alonso DF, Bal de Kier Joffe E, Lauria de

Cidre S, Eijan AM: Insight into the profibrinolytic activity of heparin, effects on the activation of plasminogen mediated by urokinase. Blood Coagul Fibrinolysis 8:403–410, 1997

56. Urban P, Scheidegger D, Buchmann B, Skarran K: The hemodynamic effects of heparin and their relation to ionized calcium levels. J Thorac Cardiovasc Surg 91:303–306, 1986

57. Harada A, Tatsuno K, Kikuchi T, Takahashi Y, Sai S, Murakami Y, Takada K: Use of bovine lung heparin to obviate anaphylactic shock caused by porcine gut heparin. Ann Thorac Surg 49:826–827, 1990

58. Hancock BW, Naysmith A: Hypersensitivity to chlorocresol-preserved heparin. Br Med J 3:746–747, 1975

59. Ansell JE, Clark WP Jr, Compton CC: Fatal reactions associated with intravenous heparin. Drug Intell Clin Parm 20:74–75, 1986

60. Bernstein IL: Anaphylaxis to heparin sodium. Report of a case, with immunologic studies. JAMA 161:1379–1380, 1956

61. Pouplard C, May MA, Iochmann S, Amiral J, Vissac AM, Marchand M, Gruel Y: Antibodies to platelet factor 4-heparin after cardiopulmonary bypass in patients anticoagulated with unfractionated heparin or a low-molecular-weight heparin: Clinical manifestations for heparin-induced thrombocytopenia. Circulation 99:2530–2536, 1999

62. Walenga JM, Jeske WP, Wallis DE, Bakhos M, Lewis BE, Leya F, Fareed J: Clinical experience with combined treatment of thrombin inhibitors and GPIIb/IIIa inhibitors in patients with HIT. Semin Thromb Hemost 25(Suppl 1):77–81, 1999

63. Haas S, Walenga JM, Jeske WP, Fareed H: Heparin-induced thrombocytopenia: the role of platelet activation and therapeutic implications. Semin Thromb Hemost 25:67–75, 1999

64. Warkentin TE: Heparin induced thrombocytopenia: A ten year retrospective. Annu Rev Med 50:129–142, 1999

65. Zucker MB: Effect of heparin on platelet function. Thromb Diath Haemorrh 33:63–65, 1975

66. Thomson C, Forkes CD, Prentice CR: Potentiation of platelet aggregation and adhesion by heparin both in vitro and in vivo. Clin Sci Mol Med 45:485–494, 1973

67. Akela M, McAndle B, Qureski M, Pearson DT: Heparin-enhanced ADP-induced platelet aggregation in patients undergoing cardiopulmonary bypass surgery. Perfusion 1:175–178, 1986

68. Schneider DJ, Tracy PB, Mann KG, Sobel BE: Differential effects of anticoagulants on the activation of platelets ex vivo. Circulation 96:2877–2883, 1997

69. Wahba A, Black G, Koksch M, Rothe G, Preuner J, Schmitz G, Birnbaum DE: Cardiopulmonary bypass leads to a preferential loss of

activated platelets: A flow cytometric assay of platelet surface antigens. Eur J Cardiothorac Surg 10:768–773, 1996

70. Rinder CS, Bohnert J, Rinder HM, Mitchell J, Ault K, Hillman R: Platelet activation and aggregation during cardiopulmonary bypass. Anesthesiology 75:388–393, 1991

71. Horrow JC: Protamine: A review of its toxicity. Anesth Analg 64:348–361, 1985

72. Lovestein E, Zapol WM: Protamine reactions, explosive mediator release, and pulmonary vasoconstriction (Editorial). Anesthesiology 73:373–374, 1990

73. Degges RD, Foster ME, Dang AQ, Read RC: Pulmonary hypertensive effect of heparin and protamine interaction evidence of thromboxane B_2 release from the lung. Am J Surg 154:696–699, 1987

74. Harrow J: Thrombocytopenia accompanying a reaction to protamine sulfate. Can Anaesth Soc J 32:49–52, 1985

75. Lindblad B, Wakefield TW, Whitehouse WM Jr, Stanley JC: The effect of profame sulfate on platelet function. Scand J Thorac Cardiovasc Surg 22:55–59, 1988

76. Wahba A, Black G, Koksch M, Rothe G, Preuner J, Schmitz G, Birnbaum DE: Cardiopulmonary bypass leads to a preferential loss of activated platelets: A flow cytometric assay of platelet surface antigens. Eur J Cardiothorac Surg 10:768–773, 1996

77. Boisclair MD, Lane DA, Philippau H, Esnouf MP, Sheikh S, Hunt B, Smith KJ: Mechanisms of thrombin generation during surgery and cardiopulmonary bypass. Blood 82:3350–3357, 1993

78. Sandset PM: Tissue factor pathway inhibitor (TFPI-an update) Haemostasis 26:154–165, 1996

79. Giraux JL, Tapon-Bretaudrere J, Matow S, Fischer AM: Fucoida, as heparin, induces tissue factor pathway inhibitor release from cultured human endothelial cells. Thromb Haemost 80:692–695, 1998

80. Hansen JB, Sarset PM: Differential effects of low molecular weight heparin and unfractionated heparin on circulating levels of antithrombin and tissue factor pathway inhibitor (TFPI): A possible mechanism for difference in therapeutic efficacy. Thromb Res 91:177–181, 1998

81. Soejima H, Ogawa H, Yasue H, Nishiyama K, Kaikita K, Misumi K, Takazoe K, Kugiyama K, Tsuji I, Kumeda K, Nakamura S: Plasma tissue factor pathway inhibitor and tissue factor antigen levels after administration of heparin in patients with angina pectoris. Thromb Res 93:17–25, 1999

82. Ariens RA, Alberio G, Moia M, Mannucci PM: Low levels of heparin-releasable tissue factor pathway inhibitor in young patients with thrombosis. Thromb Haemost 81:203–207, 1999

83. Jeske W, Hoppensteadt D, Callas D, Koza MJ, Fareed J: Pharmacological profiling of recombinant tissue factor pathway inhibitor. Semin Thromb Hemost 22:213–219, 1996
84. Kamikubo Y, Hamuro T, Takemoto S, Nakahara Y, Kamei S, Nakagaki T, Miyamoto S, Funatsu A, Kato H: A kinetic analysis of human recombinant tissue factor pathway inhibitor with factor Xa utilizing an immunoassay and the effect of antithrombin III/heparin on the complex formation. Thromb Res 89:179–186, 1998
85. Nishiyama K, Ogawa H, Yasue H, Soejima H, Misumi K, Kugiyama K, Tsuji I, Kumeda K: Heparin-releasable endothelial cell associated tissue factor pathway inhibitor (TFPI) is increased in the coronary circulation after coronary spasm in patients with coronary spastic angina. Thromb Res 89:137–146, 1998
86. Kayanolci Y, Higashiyama S, Suzuki K, Asahi M, Kawata S, Matsuzawa Y, Taniguchi N: The requirement of both intracellular reactive oxygen species and intracellular calcium elevation for the induction of heparin-binding EGF-like growth factor in vascular endothelial cells and smooth muscle cells. Biochem Biophys Res Commun 259:50–55, 1999
87. Ribeiro SM, Schultz-Cherry S, Murphy-Ulrich JE: Heparin-binding vitronectin up-regulates latent TGF-beta production by bovine aortic endothelial cells. J Cell Sci 108:1553–1561, 1995
88. Olivecrona T, Bengtsson-Olivecrona G: Heparin and lipases In: Lane DA, Lindahl V, eds. Heparin, Chemical and biological properties, clinical applications. Boca Raton, FL: CRC Press, 1989: 335–361
89. Sambandam N, Abrahani MA, St. Pierre E, Al-Atar O, Cam MC, Rodrigues B: Localization of lipoprotein lipase in the diabetic heart: Regulation by acute changes in insulin. Arterioscler Thromb Vasc Biol 19:1526–1534, 1999

Simon C. Body, M.B., Ch.B., F.A.N.Z.C.A.

Coagulation and Inflammation Polymorphism: Impact on Cardiovascular Outcomes

9

Numerous studies have examined the cellular, subcellular, and humoral inflammatory responses to cardiac surgery and cardiopulmonary bypass (CPB). Cardiac surgery and CPB induce a coagulation and inflammatory response associated with significant patient morbidity and mortality primarily by activation of the cellular elements of blood by CPB circuit materials. Similarly, tissue (especially myocardial) ischemia, reperfusion injury, hypothermia, organ hypoperfusion, and drugs used to modify coagulation, eg, heparin and protamine, may also induce a coagulation and inflammatory response. We are progressing in our translation of the clinical importance of the coagulation and inflammatory responses to the patient's advantage. Indeed, one of the single greatest advances in coagulation and coagulopathy management, aprotinin, was the fortuitous byproduct of efforts to manipulate the inflammatory response to CPB.[1]

We have two outstanding challenges. The first is to identify the role of the inflammatory and coagulation responses in adverse clinical outcomes after CPB and cardiac surgery, such as stroke, cerebral dysfunction syndromes, postoperative graft occlusion, renal failure, and coagulopathy. With detailed knowledge of their etiology, we can progress to identifying therapies that reduce the incidence and expense of these adverse events. The second challenge is to identify those patients who will most likely benefit from prophylactic or therapeutic intervention. There is wide interpersonal variation in the frequency and severity of adverse outcome after CPB and cardiac surgery. The sources of this variability can easily be divided into environmental and genetic causes.

The Relationship Between Coagulation, Inflammation, and Endothelium,
edited by Bruce Spiess, Lippincott Williams & Wilkins, Baltimore © 2000

Environmental sources of variability include anesthetic and surgical techniques, duration and severity of insults, infection, and other therapies that we can manipulate. Our genetic makeup is an important variable in a wide variety of cardiovascular inflammatory and coagulation outcomes. For example, factor V Leiden phenotypic patients have a much higher frequency of venous thromboembolic disease.[2] To date there has been little systematic work relating genetic phenotype to outcomes after CPB. It seems logical and important to establish phenotypes that are associated with those adverse outcomes and subsequently target susceptible individuals. Prophylactic inhibition of CPB-associated inflammation, thus far, not been associated with reliably better clinical outcomes, except for the use of antibiotics and antifibrinolytics. It is much more likely that drug or genetic therapies will have better outcomes when directed at individuals at high risk (either by environmental or genetic causes) for those adverse outcomes.

The purpose of this review is to describe some of the genetic sources of adverse inflammatory and coagulation outcomes after CPB, myocardial infarction (MI) and thrombosis. Additionally, I will examine investigational gene-based therapies for these diseases.

EXAMPLES OF RELATIONSHIPS BETWEEN INFLAMMATORY MARKERS AND CLINICAL OUTCOMES

The inflammatory response to CPB produces systemic organ dysfunction. The observation that older, sicker people undergoing more extensive procedures have worse outcomes can be explained in two possible ways. First, older individuals, those with poorer cardiac function, and those undergoing longer, more extensive procedures have biochemical evidence of a greater inflammatory response. Second, these individuals may be more prone to have a worse clinical outcome for the same, or greater, biochemical or cellular response to injury. Just as important are the numerous observations of a wide variability in biochemical response to the same insult. Despite the examples that follow, there is little evidence of a definitive relationship between an inflammatory or coagulation marker and the risk of an adverse event after CPB, even in relatively homogenous populations.

Coagulation and Fibrinolysis

Chandler et al[3] demonstrated wide variation in tissue plasminogen activator (tPA) and plasminogen activator inhibitor (PAI-1) levels to

CPB in a diverse clinical population undergoing coronary artery bypass graft (CABG), valve replacement, or both. After 30 minutes of CPB, active tPA and PAI-1 levels varied from 8 to 3437 pM (median, 63 pM) and 0 to 1201 pM (median, 18 pM), respectively. Similarly, active tPA and PAI-1 levels varied widely on the first postoperative day (1–29 pM and 42–2902 pM, respectively). This variability could only partially be explained by environmental factors such as combined procedures and long ischemic times. The innovative and insightful portion of this work was to examine the pattern of response in these individuals. The overall averaged data showed an increase in intraoperative tPA, with a decline to sub-baseline levels postoperatively, and no PAI-I response intraoperatively, but an increase postoperatively. However, only 40% of individuals exhibited this overall pattern. Approximately 25% of individuals showed no increase in tPA intraoperatively, but a "normal" PAI-1 response, while a similar number showed a "normal" intraoperative tPA response but no increase in PAI-1 postoperatively. Approximately 10% of individuals showed no tPA or PAI-1 response at all. Although this study did not relate genotype or phenotype to tPA and PAI-1 response, the frequency and pattern of responses matches variations in phenotype seen in the general population. The importance of this paper is the demonstration of patterns of variability in response to a stimulus.

Cytokines

Proinflammatory cytokines (IL-1, IL-6, and tumor necrosis factor [TNF-α]) decrease myocardial contractility and are thought to be responsible for ischemic organ injury.[4] The myocardium is probably responsible for a considerable portion of cytokine production after CPB.[5] In ischemic myocardium, cytokines may be in part responsible for myocardial depression.[6] Circulating cytokines bind to endothelial cell surface cytokine receptors, which cause endothelial injury and activation. Subsequent end-organ injury occurs by several direct and indirect mechanisms. One such indirect mechanism is induction of endothelial inducible nitric oxide synthase (NOS), which causes release into the organ of very high concentrations of nitric oxide (NO). NO has been shown to be a direct myocardial depressant and, in organs undergoing rapid oxidative states, causes injury by the production of deleterious free radicals (eg, peroxynitrite).

Cytokines also initiate coagulation.[7] TNF-α, IL-1, -6 and -10 have been shown to activate the coagulation pathway with thrombogenesis and promote fibrinolysis by tPA release. To date, there is little data demonstrating a link between the magnitude of cytokine response and clinical outcomes.

Complement Activation

Several studies have examined relationships between activated complement products and adverse events. Kirklin et al[8] found that increased levels of $C3a$ were associated with cardiac and pulmonary dysfunction. Polymorphism of the $C4$ gene is associated with $C4b$ levels and postoperative arrhythmias after CPB.[9] The human $C4$ gene is coded at two loci on chromosome 6. One of the loci, $C4A$, has significant polymorphism. The presence of a $C4A$ null allele causes increased complement activation during CPB and an increased intrapulmonary shunt.[10] Inhibition of complement activation during CPB using a monoclonal anti-human $C5$ antibody caused a lower frequency of bleeding and cognitive dysfunction.[11] The relationship between complement activation and adverse outcomes after CPB is not well proven.

Serotonin

Serotonin is released from the dense granules of activated platelets. McNulty et al[12] showed that blood that remained in relative stasis in the pulmonary vasculature during CPB had significantly higher serotonin concentrations. There were good correlations between serotonin concentration and both cardiac index ($r^2 = 0.47$) and right ventricular ejection fraction ($r^2 = 0.36$) and an inverse relationship between serotonin concentration and systemic vascular resistance ($r^2 = 0.36$). These observations show a relationship between platelet activation, measured by serotonin concentrations, and postoperative cardiac function. The importance of platelets in ischemic complications has been confirmed in a population of young (< 70 years) men with angiographically-proven coronary artery disease (CAD). The frequency of coronary events over a 3.7-year follow-up period was strongly related to the baseline circulating serotonin level.[13]

Adhesion Molecules

Considerable work has shown extensive activation of endothelium, neutrophils, and platelets with cooperative aggregation and metabolism in CPB and for unstable coronary syndromes.[14] Many studies, principally for patients with acute MI and angioplasty, have shown that blockade of neutrophil and platelet adhesion reduces the frequency and severity of ischemia and MI.[15–17] Similar results have been shown in animal models of CPB.[18]

EXAMPLES OF GENETIC VARIABILITY IN THROMBOSIS AND FIBRINOLYSIS

There is considerable genetic variability in a wide variety of insult-induced inflammatory and coagulation disorders. Consider 1,000 individuals who undergo CABG; a small proportion of those individuals will have deep vein thrombosis (DVT) and a fatal pulmonary embolus (PE). What determined those who developed a DVT after seemingly identical insults? Others in the group of 1,000 individuals will develop respiratory and renal failure, cerebral dysfunction, and stroke. At least a portion of the risk of developing these adverse events is determined by genetic characteristics.

Fibrinogen

Fibrinogen is a key component of coagulation and is an acute-phase re-actant. Fibrinogen levels are raised in chronic inflammatory disease, cancer, and acute inflammation. Fibrinogen levels and genotype have been shown to predict and probably explain some thrombotic outcomes,[19–21] but not in all studies.[22] The three genes that encode the components of fibrinogen lie in a group of 50 kilo base pairs (Kb) on the long arm of chromosome 4. Transcription of fibrinogen mRNA is controlled by a repressor element approximately 450 base pairs (bp) from the Bβ fibrinogen chain region. An allelic variation between guanine (G) and adenine (A) at $^-455$ bp is present, with 20% of the general population having the A$^-$455 allele (Figure 9–1). Individuals with the A$^-$455 allele (either heterozygotes or homozygotes) have higher circulating fibrinogen levels because of loss of activity of the repressor element present with the G$^-$455 allele.[21–30] Several other polymorphisms of the fibrinogen gene and its activation and repressor elements exist; however, most are not associated with circulating fibrinogen levels.[23,27,31]

In addition to being associated with higher baseline circulating fibrinogen levels, the A$^-$455 allele is associated with greater increases in fibrinogen levels in response to stress.[28] In British Army recruits who underwent a 2-day military exercise there was an increase in fibrinogen levels 2 days after the exercise. GG$^-$455 homozygotes had an increase in circulating fibrinogen of 27%. By contrast, GA heterozygotes and AA$^-$455 homozygotes had increases of 37% and 89%, respectively ($p < 0.01$). In

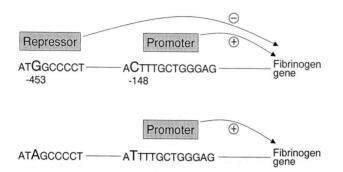

FIGURE 9–1. Diagram of the Bβ-fibrinogen gene promoter showing the binding of the repressor at A⁻455. The G⁻455 allele has a repressor gene that leads to reduced transcription of mRNA for fibrinogen. Modified with permission.[33]

patients with ischemic heart disease (IHD) there are higher fibrinogen levels associated with the A⁻455 allele than in the normal population.[21,22,31] Similar observations have been seen in relation to gender and menopause in women.[22,25,32]

The magnitude of change in circulating fibrinogen level seen with the A⁻455 allele is likely to show a biological effect. A 28 mg/dL change in fibrinogen level seen with the A⁻455 allele will likely impose about a 40% greater risk of IHD.[33] The importance of these observations in relation to CPB and cardiac surgery is unknown.

Tissue Plasminogen Activator

Polymorphism of tPA occurs as a result of a so-called "Alu repeat" insertion in the tPA gene.[34] It is responsible for variation in basal tPA release rates in the normal population and variation in tPA release rates after mental stress.[35] This polymorphism may[36] or may not[37,38] be associated with the risk of MI.

A restriction fragment length polymorphism (RFLP) marker of polymorphism for tPA has also been described.[39] In one study, transplanted donor hearts that were homozygotes for the 2.5 kb mutation RFLP were more likely to suffer coronary artery disease (> 70% at 36 months posttransplantation) than those who were homozygotes or heterozygotes for the 2.9 kb normal RFLP (30% at 36 months posttransplantation), although the study was too small to show significance.[40] In a large study of patients with angina, there was a strong relationship between tPA antigen level and the ongoing risk of developing an MI,[41] although this observation has not been confirmed.[37] Similarly, a relationship between reocclusion after coronary angioplasty and tPA levels has been demonstrated.[42] Because PAI-1 and tPA are antagonists there is considerable opportunity for variability in thrombotic outcomes. Despite the obvious importance of tPA in cardiac surgery, there is little data describing its importance in clinical outcomes and no data relating genotype to clinical outcomes after CPB.

Plasminogen Activator Inhibitor Type I

PAI-1 is a specific serine protease inhibitor of tPA and other plasminogen activators. It is important in local regulation of clot lysis and is the most important regulator of circulating fibrinolytic activity.[43] There are two important mechanisms for variability in circulating PAI-1 levels and its activity. A promoter region for PAI-1 transcription exists 675bp from the PAI-1 gene.[44] The polymorphism is defined by the presence of either four (4G) or five (5G) guanosine residues (Figure 9–2). The two alleles have a roughly equal frequency in the general population. Both the 4G and 5G alleles bind a nuclear factor promoter of the PAI-1 gene. However, the 5G allele is also capable of binding a PAI-1 repressor protein and is associated with lower baseline and stimulated levels of PAI-1: 6% to 10% lower in healthy individuals and an even greater percentage lower when stimulated, compared with non-5G allele individuals.[44-50] The 4G allele produces much more mRNA for PAI-1 than the 5G allele when stimulated by IL-1 and at baseline.

PAI-1 phenotype and circulating levels have been related to the rate of MI and CAD, the development of transplant CAD coronary

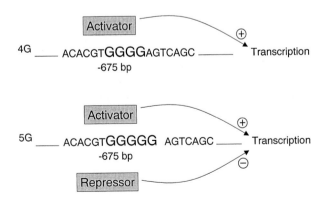

FIGURE 9–2. Diagram of the PAI-1 gene promoter showing the 4G/5G repressor site. The 5G allele has a repressor gene that leads to reduced transcription of mRNA for PAI-1. Modified with permission.[33]

artery bypass graft thrombosis, and venous thromboembolism. In patients having an MI, PAI-1 levels were 20% to 34% higher in 4G homozygotes than heterozygotes or 5G homozygotes.[49] Similarly, 4G homozygotes are more likely (risk ratio = 2.1) to suffer a MI before the age of 45.[45] In patients with type 2 diabetes mellitus, there is a relationship between PAI-1 genotype and the development of CAD.[47] Heart transplant recipients with CAD had higher PAI-1 levels (38 ± 3 pM) than transplant recipients without CAD (26 ± 2 pM) and the severity of allograft CAD was related to PAI-1 level (r^2 = 0.20, $p < 0.001$).[51]

Rifon et al[52] correlated PAI-1 activity with venous and arterial graft occlusion in 82 patients receiving 216 grafts for CABG (136 saphenous vein and 80 internal mammary artery grafts). Twenty-five grafts (22 vein grafts and 3 arterial grafts) were occluded at angiography 10 days postoperatively. Patients with an occluded graft had higher PAI-1 activity (20.9 ± 10.1 U/ml) than those without an occluded graft (10.8 ± 7.6 U/mL, $p < 0.001$). Overall fibrinolytic response (measured by tPA elution with a forearm venous occlusion test) was much lower in patients with a graft occlusion (0.7 ± 0.6 U/mL) than those without a graft occlusion (3.0 ± 4.5 U/mL, $p < 0.003$). PAI-1 polymorphism and circulating levels have also been associated with venous thromboembolic disease.[50] The importance of these data are obvious, but they require a more thorough investigation of the relationships between genotype, PAI-1 levels, and clinical outcomes in order to progress to therapeutic intervention.

THROMBOSIS

Several studies have found an increased risk of nonsurgical thrombotic events in patients with genetic polymorphisms of coagulation factors. Examples are protein C deficiency, protein S deficiency, factor V R506Q (Leiden), and hyperhomocysteinuria. Heterozygotic expression of the above factors is associated with lower rates of thrombosis than homozygotic expression. However, these risks are not the same in people with identical phenotypes, which indicates that other factors are at work. Several inherited disorders have been shown to increase the risk of arterial thromboembolism (ATE) and venous thromboembolism (VTE).

Venous Thromboembolism

An increased risk of VTE is seen in patients with deficiencies of protein C and protein S, heterozygotes for Type I antithrombin III deficiency, and patients with the Leiden allele (R506Q) for factor V. Homozygotes for these deficiencies have a much higher incidence of VTE than heterozygotes. Similarly, individuals with combined deficiencies (eg, factor V R506Q and protein C deficiency) have higher VTE rates than either abnormality alone (Table 9–1).

The molecular basis for some causes of VTE has been well delineated.[53] Protein C is responsible for regulating the activity of activated factors V (FVa) and VIII (FVIIIa) (Figure 9–3). Thrombin binds with high affinity to endothelial thrombomodulin, thereby decreasing its procoagulant properties, but becomes a strong activator of protein C. Activated protein C (PCa) cleaves and inactivates membrane-bound FVa at one of three arginine sites (Arg 306, 506, and 679) and FVIIIa, especially in the presence of its nonenzymatic cofactor protein S.[54] Thus, PCa is an anticoagulant enzyme. The Arg 506 inactivation site is the highest activity site for PCa by a factor of 10-fold. FV R506Q is an infrequently occurring allele whereby an arginine substitution for guanine at nucleotide position 1691 results in the replacement of a glutamine for an arginine at residue 506.[54] This substitution markedly reduces the activity of PCa on FVa but retains the procoagulant activity of FVa and thus increases the risk of FVa-mediated thrombus formation.[55,56] Other reasons for VTE resulting from FV R506Q may be that the substitution causes decreased FV cofactor activity on PCa for inactivated FVIII[57] and increased production of thrombin-activated fibrinolysis inhibitor.[58] Deficiencies of proteins C and S are independent risk factors for VTE and markedly increase the incidence of VTE when concurrently present

TABLE 9–1.   Rate and Odds Ratios of Venous Thromboembolism in the Normal Population and Patients With Deficiencies of Coagulation Factor Proteins by the Age of 65[53,112]

	Sole Defect	Associated With FV-R506Q
Rate*		
Normal population	4 (3/85)	—
FV-R506Q	—	17 (8/46)
Protein C deficiency	35 (12/34)	70 (16/23)
Protein S deficiency	19 (4/21)	72 (13/18)
Antithrombin III deficiency	57 (4/7)	92 (11/23)
Odds ratios†		
Normal population	1	—
FV-R506Q	—	1.6 (0.2–12.0)
Protein C deficiency	7.6 (1.5–38.0)	32.0 (5.9–17.3)
Protein S deficiency	10.0 (1.1–97.0)	112 (12–1044)

*Rate is expressed as percentage with the dataset shown in parentheses.
†The 95% confidence interval is shown in parentheses.

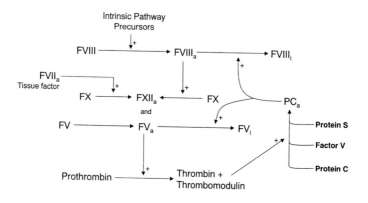

Thrombin has actions on FV, FVII, FXI, fibrinogen and thrombin-activated fibrinolysis inhibitor (TAFI).

FIGURE 9–3. Diagram of the protein C, protein S, factor V pathway. Deficiencies of proteins C and S or the presence of FV 506Q (Leiden) results in higher concentrations of factors Va and VIIIa.

with FV R506Q (Table 9–1). Although we can sometimes establish a post-hoc relationship between VTE and a genetic cause in an individual patient, we do not yet have the ability to predict a likelihood of VTE after cardiac surgery based on a panel of genetic variants.

Arterial Thromboembolic Disease

Arterial thrombotic events such as MI and stroke are associated with abnormally elevated levels of several coagulation factors (Table 9–2). In addition, various factors such as apolipoprotein E (ApoE) and lipoprotein are associated with control of lipoprotein metabolism. The E4 allele of ApoE (APO E4) is associated with a higher risk of ATE. Polymorphisms of lipoprotein a, factor VII, apolipoprotein E,[59] angiotensin converting enzyme, and PAI-1 are important in the pathogenesis of ATE. Other interesting and potentially important polymorphisms are those for tissue factor pathway inhibitor (TFPI)[60–63] and NOS. However, not all initial reports of associations between polymorphisms and outcomes have been supported by larger, more robust studies.[64] One such example is polymorphism of the GpIIa receptor.[65,66]

Prothrombin is synthesized in the liver, and elevated levels are a risk factor for VTE and ATE. In 1996, the first common polymorphism of prothrombin was described.[67] A substitution of adenine for guanine at nucleotide 20210 (FII G20210A) has a prevalence rate of approximately 2.3% in the general population; although, like FV R506G, there

TABLE 9–2.   Genetic Coagulation-Related Risk Factors for
Arterial Thromboembolic Disease

Fibrinogen[20,21,24,27,31,113–116]
Prothrombin[71,72,74,117,118]
Factor V[118,119]
Factor VII[120]
Factor XIII[121]
PAI-1[49,116,122–124]

is a racial predominance in southern Europe and the Middle East and
not in individuals of Asian or African origin. Several studies have confirmed a higher incidence of FII G20210A in patients with VTE and ATE.
For VTE, the odds ratio is approximately 4.[67–69] In women who have suf-
fered a MI, there was an increased incidence of FII G20210A (5.1%) over
controls (1.6%).[70] Other studies have confirmed this observation in
older women[71] and men[72,73] who had an MI and stroke.[74]

Considerable challenges still exist for antithrombotic and antiinflammatory gene therapies. These include identification of appropriate
genes as targets for manipulation, clinical diseases where they have the
greatest utility, patients who are most likely to benefit from their use,
and construction of efficient and benign gene transfer vectors. Some
genes seem to be obvious candidates; principally, they are genes that
encode important anticoagulant and coagulation proteins and enzyme
precursors. Examples of genes that have undergone animal trials are
genes with antiplatelet activity (cyclooxygenase-1, prostacyclin synthase, and NOS),[75–78] genes with anticoagulant activity (thrombomodulin and TFPI),[79] and genes with fibrinolytic activity (tPA and uPA).[80]

CHEMICAL, IMMUNOLOGIC, AND PHYSICAL
METHODS OF REDUCTION OF THE
INFLAMMATORY RESPONSE

Multiple therapeutic strategies have been developed to manipulate the
coagulation and inflammatory responses to CPB. These therapeutic
strategies can be divided into chemical, immunologic, physical, and genetic modifications to the body's response to CPB.

Chemical and Immunologic Methods of Reduction of
the Inflammatory Response

One of the most researched and debated antiinflammatory interventions is the use of corticosteroids during CPB. There is a long history of

contradictory research on the clinical response to corticosteroids for decreasing the adverse consequences to CPB, with many studies failing to find favorable clinical results. Steroids inhibit proinflammatory cytokine production and increase the production of antiinflammatory cytokines, such as IL-10.[6] They also reduce neutrophil activation and leukotriene production. Other favorable noncytokine results have also been reported. This information may provide us with a more selective basis for the use of corticosteroids under some conditions.

The biochemical and antiinflammatory effects of the serine protease inhibitor aprotinin is well established.[81] Aprotinin inhibits kallikrein production, neutrophil elastase release, and complement activation, as well as having a platelet "preserving" effect.[82] It appears to be effective in reducing blood loss and transfusion after a variety of cardiac surgical procedures and reduces biochemical evidence of the inflammatory response.[83,84]

Another antiinflammatory approach involves the production of therapeutic antibodies directed against complement, cytokines, endotoxin, cell membrane proteins, and receptors. Many of these antibodies are approved or undergoing clinical trials, frequently for acute coronary syndromes or sepsis. There are limitations on the use of antibodies to specific proinflammatory molecules. Numerous proinflammatory and antiinflammatory molecules are produced in response to CPB. Knowledge of an individual's inflammatory response will likely increase the success of a targeted therapy. It would be difficult to administer a "cocktail" of antibodies that would provide an appropriate level of inhibition in every patient. In addition, many therapeutic monoclonal antibodies developed from non-human cell lines or hybridomas are immunogenic and develop reactive antibodies, thus limiting repeated therapies. One method to overcome this problem involves the isolation of the Fab portion of the antibody and "humanizing" it by grafting it onto the Fc portion of a human antibody. One such example is the use of a recombinant humanized single-chain monoclonal antibody directed against human C5.[11]

Many other techniques have been tried. Manipulation of the inflammatory response by anesthetic drugs (eg, opioids), reduction in the release of lipopolysaccharide by gut sterilization, and adenosine modulators have all been attempted.

Physical Methods of Reduction of the Inflammatory Response

Surfaced modification of the CPB circuit with heparin or non-heparin coatings has been examined in numerous studies.[85,86] Heparin coating with or without reduced systemic heparinization has been shown to have several biochemical effects; complement, platelet, and leukocyte activation were reduced, and the release of proinflammatory cytokines was reduced in more than 1,100 studies.[87] Despite this, their effect on clinical outcomes is limited. Some studies have seen marginally decreased bleeding, but unchanged transfusion rates. Fewer studies, however, have shown reductions in pulmonary adverse events, duration of ventilation, or other clinical markers of improved outcome.

Leukocyte-mediated endothelial and tissue injury is well described.[83,88–90] Leukocytes have several direct and costimulatory methods of causing organ injury. Leukocyte depletion seems to be an obvious method of reducing organ injury. Alternatively, inhibition of neutrophil adhesion and activation by monoclonal antibodies seems attractive.[18] Physical neutrophil depletion of the CPB circuit blood or blood cardioplegia is reported in many models and in some trials of clinical CPB.[91–95] Most clinical trials have found few improvements in any clinical outcome, but have shown reductions in biochemical markers of inflammation.[84,96] Interestingly, several trials have been unable to reduce leukocyte counts with filters. The only consistent finding in most trials has been an improvement in oxygenation, but this observation has not been translated into clinical benefits such as reduced endotracheal intubation time or reduced frequency of respiratory failure.[97]

Ultrafiltration of plasma and partial or complete replacement with intravenous fluids has been described in pediatric CPB, extra-corporeal membrane oxygenation, and sepsis.[83] Crudely put, it is felt that some "circulating nasty" is removed by ultrafiltration. Levels of IL-1, IL-6, IL-8, TNF-α, and IL-10 have all been reported to be lower after ultrafiltration. The clinical efficacy of ultrafiltration is uncertain, except perhaps in the neonatal/pediatric population, where a beneficial reduction in hemodilution by CPB prime fluids may occur.[98]

GENETIC METHODS OF REDUCTION OF THE INFLAMMATORY RESPONSE

Gene therapy techniques are not simple. They require identification of a gene-related outcome and its biological process, evidence of successful reduction in the adverse outcome when the gene's expression is manipulated, a successful clinical strategy of manipulation of gene expression, and, for some therapies, a methodology of identifying individuals with an abnormal gene prior to the insult. Despite some success at identifying genetic etiologies for a variety of cardiovascular diseases, the majority of diseases and adverse events are the result of a complex interplay of many gene-based processes. Many responses, notably to CPB, are the result of many endogenous mechanisms in a complex interaction that depend on the environmental insult. Thus, they are the result of expression of many genes and will most likely be much more difficult to successfully manipulate. Although this may seem to be a gloomy predication, we have made progress in identifying some molecular targets for gene therapy. Specifically in regards to CPB, these might include tissue factor (TF), PAI-1, complement, proinflammatory cytokines and chemokines, and cellular expression of integrins, vascular adhesion molecules, and selectins.

Three techniques are used for modification of gene expression. Plasmid DNA is the direct incorporation of DNA for the desired gene into the cells of the target tissue. Viral gene therapies use a wide variety of viruses as vehicles for portions of DNA. Antisense oligo (deoxy) nucleotides (ODNs) are essentially the nucleotide base pair opposites of a gene that we wish to inhibit.

Plasmid DNA

Plasmids are synthetic circular DNA molecules that can replicate autonomously in foreign cells. DNA of the desired gene from a donor cell is obtained by restriction endonucleases that cut DNA at specific sites. The DNA segment containing the desirable genetic sequence is isolated and cloned. The isolated DNA is forced into a loop by joining the ends of the DNA with a DNA ligase, thus forming the plasmid. In simplistic terms, they can produce mRNA for the desired protein without incorporation into the genome of the cell. Plasmids can be introduced into target cells by several methods. The most common methodology for plasmid "transfection" is direct application of the plasmid to the cellular target. An example currently undergoing clinical trials is transfection of saphenous vein graft endothelium with plasmid DNA for anti-inflammatory, anticoagulant, and antirecognition genes during CABG or peripheral vascular surgery. Most of the recipient cells maintain the DNA in an extrachromosomal site, which does not allow the donor DNA to become part of the permanent genome. This results in a transient transfection and a temporal decay of effect. Some dividing cells incorporate the donor DNA into the genome and pass the information along to progeny cells. Although this technique appears limited, it may be useful in procedures where good access to the recipient tissue is available. Other means of packaging the plasmid for administration are being used. Advantages of plasmids are their simplicity and short duration. Their disadvantages are low efficiency, short duration, limited stable expression, and possible mutagenicity.

Viral Gene Therapies

Viruses are efficient at delivering their genetic code into recipient cells. Recombinant retroviruses, adenoviruses, and other virsus are useful therapeutic vectors because they can be developed to prevent their own replication or the insertion of the other deleterious genetic code (Table 9–3).

Retroviruses consist of a linear double-stranded RNA genome that is copied into the host DNA genome by a viral RNA-dependent DNA polymerase, which produces a DNA copy. This technique requires the cell to be dividing at the time and therefore limits its utility. Its high transfection rate is aided by envelope proteins and glycoproteins that are recognized by host cell membrane surface proteins and promote fusion of the virus with the cell. To prevent transfection of the native viral genome or replication of the virus those genes are deleted from the viral RNA, thus rendering the retrovirus a relatively safe vector. Because cell division is required to incorporate the DNA into the genome, this technique is of limited efficacy in cardiovascular diseases. By contrast, this may be a very useful technique in the treatment of some cancers. Advantages are high transfection rates and longer gene expression (than plasmid DNA). Disadvantages are that their use is technically challenging and incorporation into the genome requires cell division and possible mutagenicity.

Adenoviruses are a family of nonenveloped viruses containing a linear 36-kb double-stranded DNA genome that infect a broad range of cell types. Gene expression and incorporation of the donor DNA does not require cell division, in contrast to plasmids and retroviruses, although most of the donor DNA remains extrachromosonal. Adeno-viruses can be prevented from replicating by removal of replication genes. This allows space in the 36-kb genome for insertion of large segments of donor DNA (up to 8 kb). Very high concentrations of virus can be delivered

TABLE 9–3. Characteristics of Commonly Used Viral Vectors

Property	Retrovirus	Adeno-Associated Adenovirus	Herpes Virus	Pox Virus	Virus
Insert size	8 kb	8 kb	4 kb	30 kb	>30 kb
Integration into genome	Yes	Rare	Yes	No	No
Cell-division required	Yes	No	Yes	CNS only	Yes
Duration of expression	Good	Brief	Good	Brief	Brief
Tissue specificity	Yes	Yes	No	Yes	No

with high transfection rates. Little or no systemic illness (flu) results from transfection. However, there is commonly a powerful immunologic response to recalled antigens of the viral cost. This limits the efficiency of delivery of the donor DNA. Some synthetic viruses with low immunogenicity are being developed. The advantages of adenoviruses are that large DNA segments can be inserted, they infect a wide variety of cell types, have low toxicity, and have a short duration. Disadvantages are their technical difficulty, strong immunogenicity, and short duration.

Several other human, nonhuman, and synthetic viruses are being developed as high-efficiency vectors. Examples are herpes simplex virus (useful for neural disease because of its neurotropicity), paroviruses (a provirus capable of incorporation of donor DNA into the genome at specific sites without cell division), Sendai virus, and other synthetic virus-like particles.

Inhibitory Gene Therapies

In the above sections, we examined methods of augmentation of gene expression. There are many situations where the inhibition of production of deleterious compounds is desired. One example is inhibition of cell-membrane expression of TF. Unlike other techniques of inhibition, such as corticosteroids, that use pretranscriptional or transcriptional inhibition of TF production (ie, transcription of mRNA for TF is reduced), it is possible to bind mRNA produced by the TF gene to inhibit the production of TF. In other words, the gene is allowed to be active, but its mRNA is prevented form producing the final product (TF, for example). One method is to produce short segments of the synthetic opposite to the mRNA for TF. Remember the A-T and G-C specificity of DNA and RNA. These ODNs mop-up mRNA in a very specific fashion by containing the A-T/G-C opposite of small portions of the mRNA for TF. It is not necessary to have the opposite (antisense) for the entire mRNA transcript. It is often adequate to have small portions (15–20 amino acids in length) of important portions of the mRNA. Several variants of ODNs exist that can bind DNA or RNA in several different ways. They are very easy to prepare and can be delivered by many inexpensive efficient methods, rather similar to plasmid transfection. The major problem with their activity is that they must have a "backbone" to enable physical interaction with the mRNA. The backbone is amenable to degradation by cellular nucleases, thus limiting duration of their efficacy. Another problem is that other genes that we do not wish to target may have very similar or identical sequences that are amenable to attack by an antisense ODN. Not only can the mRNA product be targeted by antisense ODN, the ODN can also target other points in the pathway of gene expression, such as transcription factor binding sites, promoter regions, and intron splice sites on the genomic DNA.

An example of the use of antisense genes is in the production of proinflammatory cytokines or their receptors. Traditionally, antisense ODNs have been used in vitro to examine cytokine production and actions. However, site-specific delivery of antisense ODNs has been shown to reduce cytokine production in vivo. There is also an opportunity for inhibition of expression of intercellular adhesion molecules (ICAM) in circulating leukocytes, platelets, and endothelium (ICAM-1) expression can be inhibited in vivo by antisense ODNs in several cell lines. In a model of cardiac allograft rejection, inhibition of ICAM-1 expression by an antisense ODN was shown to be effective at delaying and/or reducing allograft rejection.[99] In a model of coronary artery endothelial injury that usually produces severe neo-intimal formation, an ODN to the proto-oncogen *c-myb* (usually expressed after vascular injury) markedly reduced the amount of neo-intimal formation and increased the size of the residual lumen (Figure 9–4).[100] Allografted partly-immunosupressed

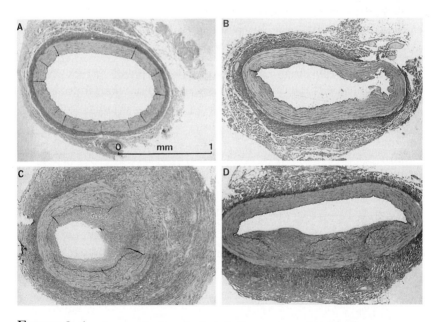

FIGURE 9–4. An oversized angioplasty balloon causes a breach of coronary artery intima and media seen in Panel B. Normal coronary artery is shown in Panel A. Four weeks after the injury there is marked neo-intimal formation and a severe adventitial cellular infiltrate (Panel C). There is marked reduction in luminal area. ODN to the proto-oncogene *c-myb* markedly reduced the amount of neo-intimal formation and increased the size of the residual lumen (Panel D). Reproduced with permission.[100]

mouse hearts normally develop coronary vascular smooth muscle cell (VSMC) and intimal proliferation. When an ODN to Cdk2 kinase was administered, the amount of coronary occlusion and endothelin production normally seen was considerably reduced (Figure 9–5).[101]

The advantages of antisense ODNs are that they can inhibit both proinflammatory and antiinflammatory pathways, are usually very specific, have a short duration, and are relatively easy to prepare and deliver. Their disadvantages are that they are sometimes nonspecific and are prone to degradation.

CLINICAL USES OF GENE THERAPIES UNDER INVESTIGATION

The first successful human gene transfer occurred in 1990. Since that time, more than 3,500 patients have enrolled in gene therapy protocols. Yet very few of these patients have had clinical benefit, primarily because of low incorporation and poor retention of the donor DNA into target cells. Until recently, the lower transfer efficiency has resulted in only short-term expression of transferred genes and, accordingly, no clinically important favorable result. Recently, however, the use of recombinant adeno-associated virus (rAAV) and other viral vectors has increased efficiency without inciting the intense immune response seen with adenovirus vectors that limits the duration of gene expression. It is obvious from the brief description of various types of gene therapy above, that most gene thera-

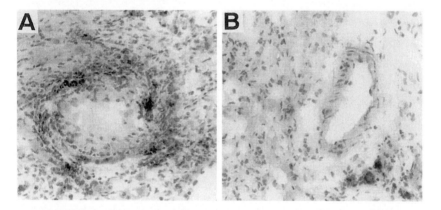

FIGURE 9–5. An ODN to Cdk2 kinase was administered to donor hearts at transplantation. Panel A shows the amount of endothelin-producing cellular infiltrate (dark stain) and intimal hyperplasia in hearts treated with FK506 only. Panel B shows hearts treated with Cdk2 ODN. The amount of endothelin-producing cellular infiltrate and intimal hyperplasia is considerably reduced. Reproduced with permission.[101]

pies are going to be useful for diseases that are of high likelihood for a period of several weeks to months. To give an example, a plasmid therapy to inhibit formation of DVT after orthopedic surgery should be useful. It might be able to be given at the time of surgery and yet not inhibit coagulation during surgery because of the usual lead-up time for gene therapies, but still could be effective for the time of greatest risk of DVT/PE. By contrast, an ODN-based therapy might be effective in reducing the endothelial response to CPB, and to have terminated its action within a few days, to allow normal reparative processes of wound healing.

Although there are numerous potential indications, several lines of investigation are being investigated. These are regression of atherosclerotic lesions, vascular graft thrombosis and stenosis, congestive or hypertrophic cardiomyopathy, lipid disorders, and hemostasis.[102,103]

Angiogenesis

Peripheral and cardiac vascular disease are not always amenable to bypass grafting in certain patients. Induction of angiogensis by gene therapy may provide sufficient revascularization to avoid vessel grafting or provide structural or symptomatic relief in those who cannot undergo conventional grafting.[104] Many animal models of ischemia have shown angiogensis in response to several endothelial growth factors, notably vascular endothelial growth factor (VEGF). The primary difficulties in this approach have been delivering an efficient DNA vector in a site-specific manner. In general, the problem of site-specificity has been approached by delivering the vector via an appropriately placed injection or catheter, or in the case of peripheral vascular disease, by intramuscular injection.

Naked plasmid DNA for human VEGF has been injected directly in to the anterior myocardium of patients with severe maximally treated angina via thoracotomy.[105] Nitroglycerin use decreased markedly and dobutamine-SPECT imaging showed improvement in perfusion in the treated areas (Figure 9–6). Similar results have been seen for peripheral vascular disease.[106,107] By contrast, repeated intracoronary administration of VEGF (not its plasmid) had no effect on anginal symptoms.[108] Adenoviral-based intramyocardial administration of VEGF for IHD, a technique analogous to naked plasmid DNA for VEGF, is under clinical investigation.[109]

Coronary Vein Graft Occlusion

Vein graft occlusion is a recurring problem, with 30% to 50% of saphenous vein-coronary artery grafts occluding within 5 years and a similar percentage of occluded grafts with peripheral vascular lesions. Intimal hyperplasia is responsible for most graft occlusions in the intermediate

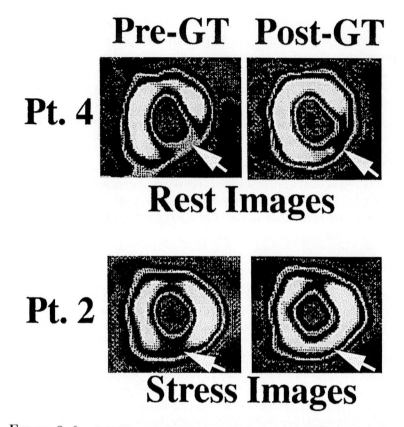

Pre-GT Post-GT

Pt. 4

Rest Images

Pt. 2

Stress Images

FIGURE 9–6. SPECT-sestamibi images of before and after therapy with plasmid DNA encoding VEGF injected directly into the myocardium. Patient 4 (Pt. 4) had a fixed infero-lateral defect (arrow) that resolved after therapy. Patient 2 (Pt. 2) had areas of decreased perfusion inferiorly (arrow) that resolved after therapy, but an anterior defect that was not treated persisted. GT, gene therapy. Reproduced with permission.[105]

term (1–24 months). Vein graft stenosis seems a particularly appropriate target for gene therapy for two reasons. First, several well-recognized genes and cell types are responsible for intimal hyperplasia and VSMC proliferation. Second, the tissue is easily accessed intraoperatively and transfected by several vectors in high concentrations. Endothelial cell transfection is relatively simple and efficient. However, access of viral vectors to VSMCs has been shown to be poor across intact endothelium, such as in vein grafts. By contrast, the use of similar vectors across angioplastied arteries has been shown to be efficient because of de-endothelization of the arterial wall by the angioplasty balloon. Several techniques are being examined to improve transfection of cells remote from the site of application. Several groups have used genes for several biochemical targets (plasmin, urokinase, and endothelial constitutive NOS) in animal models that have been found to reduce intimal hyperplasia by up to 70% over the short term. The targets would be expected to work because of their role in vasodilation, cell-cell recognition, and aggregation.

Coronary Artery Occlusion

Approximately one-third of all stenoses recur after angioplasty. This is a complex process involving many native and circulating cell types. In addition to genetic makeup, there is marked interaction with environmental variables such as smoking.[110] Thus far, several approaches are being investigated: (1) Induction of cell death only in dividing cells. However, there is considerable opportunity for systemic toxicity when distant transfection occurs. (2) Reduction of VSMC migration. The use of a PAI-1 (markedly inhibits VSMC migration) gene has been shown to be effective in some models. (3) Inhibition of VSMC proliferation by delivery of genes that are generally inhibitory to a phase of the VSMC cell replication cycle.

Gene therapy will probably not be a primary therapy for MI because of the need for rapid reperfusion. Expression of the gene usually takes at least 1 day. However, numerous patients have ongoing thrombogenesis after infarction or as a clinical event of unstable angina. Prevention of thrombosis could be achieved by delivery of genes for endothelial NOS, tPA, and other anticoagulant/inflammatory mediators. Similarly, inhibition of procoagulant/inflammatory mediators such as adhesion molecules, cytokines, cytokine receptors, and TF by ODNs may be useful. The latter may be especially useful for short-term prevention of reinfarction after MI.

Ex Vivo Modification and Reimplanation of Vascular Cells

Vascular prosthetic grafts are prone to thrombosis and occlusion. Several groups have modified the expression of vascular proteins in endothelial or other cells ex vivo, and then seeded the cells on to a prosthetic graft, where they proliferated in vivo.[111] Although technically feasible and capable of prolonged expression, the greatest problem with this technique has been the need to obtain suitable cells well in advance of the definitive procedure to enable modification and reseeding on a suitable graft.

SUMMARY

CPB reliably induces a profound inflammatory response. Inflammation was presumably designed to deal with the local injury of a wound or infection, not with the global inflammatory response of CPB. It seems as though the response is excessive and usually able to be controlled by the usual counter-balancing, antiinflammatory processes of the body. We see a failure of the body to control coagulation and inflammation in diseases such as postsurgical DVT, MI, and multisystem organ dysfunction. Many studies have examined methods of modifying inflammatory and coagulation pathways in all of these diseases. Here are just a few illustrative examples: (1) heparin and DVT; (2) thrombolysis after MI; (3) NOS inhibition in ARDS; and (4) aprotinin and reduction of bleeding after CPB. All of these studies have had clearly defined, easily recognizable end points in populations at high risk or suffering from disease. By contrast, modifying the inflammatory response after CPB is a more complicated effort.

Inflammation is a multipathway complex process. It is likely that inhibition of all the pathways of inflammation is not necessary and may even be deleterious. Many studies have shown reduction in some adverse event/outcome with modification of only one pathway, eg, neutrophil depletion and myocardial function. Others have examined the inhibition of several, but not all pathways, upon an outcome, eg, aprotinin and bleeding. Many of the processes we try to inhibit are advantageous for wound healing, fighting infection, and repairing ischemic tissue. Thus, an unknown modicum of therapeutic restraint may be necessary for avoidance or treatment of a CPB-associated adverse event without induction of another adverse event.

The use of various therapeutic strategies requires a thorough understanding of the humoral and cellular mechanisms involved. Because the inflammatory response involves many interactive, cooperative, and inhibitory pathways, we require a thorough understanding of these to examine various therapeutic strategies. For the same reasons, combined and individualized therapies will probably be more effective than single interventions in improving clinical outcomes.

References

1. Royston D, Bidstrup BP, Taylor KM, Sapsford RN: Effect of aprotinin on need for blood transfusion after repeat open-heart surgery. Lancet 2:1289–1291, 1987
2. Rao AK, Sheth S, Kaplan R: Inherited hypercoagulable states. Vasc Med 2:313–320, 1997

3. Chandler WL, Fitch JC, Wall MH, Verrier ED, Cochran RP, Soltow LO, Spiess D: Individual variations in the fibrinolytic response during and after cardiopulmonary bypass. Thromb Haemost 74:1293–1297, 1995

4. Feuerstein GZ, Wang X, Barone FC: Inflammatory gene expression in cerebral ischemia and trauma: Potential new therapeutic targets. Ann NY Acad Sci 825:179–193, 1997

5. Wan S, DeSmet JM, Barvais L, Goldstein M, Vincent JL, LeClerc JL: Myocardium is a major source of proinflammatory cytokines in patients undergoing cardiopulmonary bypass. J Thorac Cardiovasc Surg 112:806–811, 1996

6. Hill GE: Cardiopulmonary bypass-induced inflammation: Is it important? J Cardiothorac Vasc Anesth 12:21–25, 1998

7. ten Cate JW, van der Poll T, Levi M, ten Cate H, van Deventer SJ: Cytokines: Triggers of clinical thrombotic disease. Thromb Haemost 78:415–419, 1997

8. Kirklin JK, Westaby S, Blackstone EH, Kirklin JW, Chenoweth DE, Pacifico AD: Complement and the damaging effects of cardiopulmonary bypass. J Thorac Cardiovasc Surg 86:845–857, 1983

9. Bruins P, te Velthius H, Yazdanbakhsh AP, Jansen PG, van Hardevelt FW, de Beaumont EM, Wildevuur CR, Eijsman L, Trouwborst A, Hack CE: Activation of the complement system during and after cardiopulmonary bypass surgery: postsurgery activation involves C-reactive protein and is associated with postoperative arrhythmia. Circulation 96:3542–3548, 1997

10. Shastri K, Logue G, Stern M, Rehman S, Raza S: Complement activation by heparin-protamine complexes during cardiopulmonary bypass: Effect of C4A null allele. J Thorac Cardiovasc Surg 114:482–488, 1997

11. Rollins S, Fitch J, Shernan S, Rinder C, Rinder H, Smith B, Collard C, Alford B, Li L, Matis L: Anti-C5 single chain antibody therapy blocks complement and leukocyte activation and reduces myocardial tissue damage in CPB patients. Mol Immunol 35:397, 1998

12. McNulty SE, Mannion J, Brennan M, Schieren H: The clinical relevance of hemoglobin, platelet, and serotonin changes in sequestered and circulating blood during cardiopulmonary bypass. J Cardiothorac Vasc Anesth 12:402–407, 1998

13. Vikenes K, Farstad M, Nordrehaug JE: Serotonin is associated with coronary artery disease and cardiac events. Circulation 100:483–489, 1999

14. Kalawski R, Bugajski P, Smielecki J, Wysocki H, Olszewski P, More R, Sheridan DJ, Siminiak T: Soluble adhesion molecules in reperfusion during coronary bypass grafting. Eur J Cardiothorac Surg 14:290–295, 1998

15. Hamm CW, Heeschen C, Goldmann B, Vahanian A, Adgey J, Miguel CM, Rutsch W, Berger J, Kootstra J, Simoons ML: Benefit of abciximab in patients with refractory unstable angina in relation to serum troponin T levels. c7E3 Fab Antiplatelet Therapy in Unstable Refractory Angina (CAPTURE) Study Investigators. N Engl J Med 340:1623–1629, 1999

16. Lincoff AM, Tcheng JE, Califf RM, Kereiakes DJ, Kelly TA, Timmis GC, Kleiman NS, Booth JE, Balog C, Cabot CF, Anderson KM, Weisman HF, Topol EJ: Sustained suppression of ischemic complications of coronary intervention by platelet GP IIb/IIIa blockade with abciximab: one-year outcome in the EPILOG trial. Evaluation in PTCA to Improve Long-term Outcome with abciximab GP IIb/IIIa blockade. Circulation 99:1951–1958, 1999

17. Lincoff AM, Califf RM, Moliterno DJ, Ellis SG, Ducas J, Kramer JH, Kleiman NS, Cohen EA, Booth JE, Sapp SK, Cabot CF, Topol EJ: Complementary clinical benefits of coronary-artery stenting and blockade of platelet glycoprotein IIb/IIIa receptors. Evaluation of Platelet IIb/IIIa Inhibition in Stenting Investigators. N Engl J Med 341:319–327, 1999

18. Byrne JG, Smith WJ, Murphy MP, Couper GS, Appleyard RF, Cohn LH: Complete prevention of myocardial stunning, contracture, low-reflow, and edema after heart transplantation by blocking neutrophil adhesion molecules during reperfusion. J Thorac Cardiovasc Surg 104:1589–1596, 1992

19. Ferlito S, Gallina M, Mangiameli S, Chiaranda G: Thrombotic markers during myocardial infarction. Panminerva Med 37:133–136, 1995

20. Fowkes F, Connor J, Smith F, Wood J, Donnan P, Lowe G: Fibrinogen genotype and risk of peripheral atherosclerosis. Lancet 339:693–696, 1992

21. Green F, Hamsten A, Blomback M, Humphries S: The role of beta-fibrinogen genotype in determining plasma fibrinogen levels in young survivors of myocardial infarction and healthy controls from Sweden. Thromb Haemost 70:915–920, 1993

22. Tybjaerg-Hansen A, Agerholm-Larsen B, Humphries SE, Abildgaard S, Schnohr P, Nordestgaard BG: A common mutation (G-455—>A) in the beta-fibrinogen promoter is an independent predictor of plasma fibrinogen, but not of ischemic heart disease. A study of 9,127 individuals based on the Copenhagen City Heart Study. J Clin Invest 99:3034–3039, 1997

23. Connor JM, Fowkes FG, Wood J, Smith FB, Donnan PT, Lowe GD: Genetic variation at fibrinogen loci and plasma fibrinogen levels. J Med Genet 29:480–482, 1992

24. Scarabin PY, Bara L, Ricard S, Poirier O, Cambou JP, Arveiler D,

Luc G, Evans AE, Samama MM, Cambien F: Genetic variation at the beta-fibrinogen locus in relation to plasma fibrinogen concentration and risk of myocardial infarction. The ECTIM Study. Arterioscler Thromb 13:886–891, 1992

25. Humphries SE, Ye S, Talmud P, Bara L, Wilhelmsen L, Tiret L: European Atherosclerosis Research Study: genotype at the fibrinogen locus (G-455-A beta-gene) is associated with differences in plasma fibrinogen levels in young men and women from different regions in Europe: Evidence for gender-genotype-environment interaction. Arterioscler Thromb Vasc Biol 15:96–104, 1995

26. Iso H, Folsom AR, Winkelmann JC, Koike K, Harada S, Greenberg B, Sato S, Shimamoto T, Iida M, Komachi Y: Polymorphisms of the beta fibrinogen gene and plasma fibrinogen concentration in Caucasian and Japanese population samples. Thromb Haemost 73: 106–111, 1995

27. Heinrich J, Funke H, Rust S, Schulte H, Schonfeld R, Kohler E, Assmann G: Impact of polymorphisms in the alpha- and beta-fibrinogen gene on plasma fibrinogen concentrations of coronary heart disease patients. Thromb Res 77:209–215, 1995

28. Montgomery HE, Clarkson P, Nwose OM, Mikailidis DP, Jagroop IA, Dollery C, Moult J, Benhizia F, Deanfield J, Jubb M, World M, McEwan JR, Winder A, Humphries S: The acute rise in plasma fibrinogen concentration with exercise is influenced by the G-453-A polymorphism of the beta-fibrinogen gene. Arterioscler Thromb Vasc Biol 16:386–391, 1996

29. Margaglione M, Cappucci G, Colaizzo D, Pirro L, Vecchione G, Grandone E, Di Minno G: Fibrinogen plasma levels in an apparently healthy general population: Relation to environmental and genetic determinants. Thromb Haemost 80:805–810, 1998

30. Thomas AE, Green FR, Humphries SE: Association of genetic variation at the beta-fibrinogen gene locus and plasma fibrinogen levels; interaction between allele frequency of the G/A-455 polymorphism, age and smoking. Clin Genet 50:184–190, 1996

31. Behague I, Poirier O, Nicaud V, Evans A, Arveiler D, Luc G, Cambou JP, Scarabin PY, Bara L, Green F, Cambien F: Beta fibrinogen gene polymorphisms are associated with plasma fibrinogen and coronary artery disease in patients with myocardial infarction. The ECTIM Study. Etude Cas-Temoins sur l'Infarctus du Myocarde. Circulation 93:440–449, 1996

32. Henry JA, Bolla M, Osmond C, Fall C, Barker DJ, Humphries SE: The effects of genotype and infant weight on adult plasma levels of fibrinogen, factor VII, and LDL cholesterol are additive. J Med Genet 34:553–558, 1997

33. Humphries SE, Panahloo A, Montgomery HE, Green F, Yudkin J: Gene-environment interaction in the determination of levels of haemostatic variables involved in thrombosis and fibrinolysis. Thromb Haemost 78:457–461, 1997

34. Tishkoff SA, Ruano G, Kidd JR, Kidd KK: Distribution and frequency of a polymorphic Alu insertion at the plasminogen activator locus in humans. Hum Genet 97:759–764, 1996

35. Jern C, Ladenvall P, Wall U, Jern S: Gene polymorphism of t-PA is associated with forearm vascular release rate of t-PA. Arterioscler Thromb Vasc Biol 19:454–459, 1999

36. van der Bom JG, de Knijff P, Haverkate F, Bots ML, Meijer P, de Jong PT, Hofman A, Kluft C, Grobbee DE: Tissue plasminogen activator and risk of myocardial infarction: The Rotterdam Study. Circulation 95:2623–2627, 1997

37. Steeds R, Adams M, Smith P, Channer K, Samani NJ: Distribution of tissue plasminogen activator insertion/deletion polymorphism in myocardial infarction and control subjects. Thromb Haemost 79:980–984, 1998

38. Ridker PM, Baker MT, Hennekens CH, Stampfer MJ, Vaughan DE: Alu-repeat polymorphism in the gene coding for tissue-type plasminogen activator (t-PA) and risks of myocardial infarction among middle-aged men. Arterioscler Thromb Vasc Biol 17: 1687–1690, 1997

39. Degen SJ, Rajput B, Reich E: The human tissue plasminogen activator gene. J Biol Chem 261:6972–6985, 1986

40. Benza RL, Grenett HE, Bourge RC, Kirklin JK, Naftel DC, Castro PF, McGiffin DC, George JF, Booyse FM: Gene polymorphisms for plasminogen activator inhibitor-1/tissue plasminogen activator and development of allograft coronary artery disease. Circulation 98:2248–2254, 1998

41. Juhan-Vague I, Pyke SD, Alessi MC, Jespersen J, Haverkate F, Thompson SG: Fibrinolytic factors and the risk of myocardial infarction or sudden death in patients with angina pectoris. ECAT Study Group. European Concerted Action on Thrombosis and Disabilities. Circulation 94:2057–2063, 1996

42. Terres W, Lund GK, Hubner A, Ehlert A, Reuter H, Hamm CW: Endogenous tissue plasminogen activator and platelet reactivity as risk factors for reocclustion after recanalization of chronic total coronary occlusions. Am Heart J 130:711–716, 1995

43. Zhu Y, Carmeliet P, Fay W: Plasminogen activator inhibitor-1 is a major determinant of arterial thrombolysis resistance. Circulation 99:3050–3055, 1999

44. Dawson SJ, Wiman B, Hamsten A, Green F, Humphries S, Henney AM: The two allele sequences of a common polymorphism in the promoter of the plasminogen activator inhibitor-1 (PAI-1) gene re-

spond differently to interleukin-1 in HepG2 cells. J Biol Chem 268:10739–10745, 1993

45. Eriksson P, Kallin B, van 't Hooft FM, Bavenholm P, Hamsten A: Allele-specific increase in basal transcription of the plasminogen-activator inhibitor 1 gene is associated with myocardial infarction. Proc Natl Acad Sci U S A 92:1851–1855, 1995

46. Ye S, Green FR, Scarabin PY, Nicaud V, Bara L, Dawson SJ, Humphries SE, Evans A, Luc G, Cambou JP, et al.: the 4G/5G genetic polymorphism in the promoter of the plasminogen activator inhibitor-1 (PAI-1) gene is associated with differences in plasma PAI-1 activity but not with risk of myocardial infarction in the EC-TIM study. Etude CasTemoins de I'nfarctus du Mycocarde. Thromb Haemost 74:837–841, 1995

47. Mansfield MW, Stickland MH, Grant PJ: Plasminogen activator inhibitor-1 (PAI-1) promoter polymorphism and coronary artery disease in non-insulin-dependent diabetes. Thromb Haemost 74:1032–1034, 1995

48. Grubic N, Stegnar M, Peternel P, Kaider A, Binder BR: A novel G/A and the 4G/5G polymorphism within the promoter of the plasminogen activator inhibitor-1 gene in patients with deep vein thrombosis. Thromb Res 84:431–443, 1996

49. Ossei-Gerning N, Mansfield MW, Stickland MH, Wilson IJ, Grant PJ: Plasminogen activator inhibitor-1 promoter 4G/5G genotype and plasma levels in relation to a history of myocardial infarction in patients characterized by coronary angiography. Arterioscler Thromb Vasc Biol 17:33–37, 1997

50. Sartori MT, Wiman B, Vettore S, Dazzi F, Girolami A, Patrassi GM: 4G/5G polymorphism of PAI-1 gene promoter and fibrinolytic capacity in patients with deep vein thrombosis. Thromb Haemost 80:956–960, 1998

51. Warshofsky MK, Wasserman HS, Wang W, Teng P, Sciacca R, Apfelbaum, M, Schwartz A, Michler RE, Mancini DM, Cannon PJ, Rabbani LE: Plasma levels of tissue plasminogen activator and plasminogen activator inhibitor-1 are correlated with the presence of transplant coronary artery disease in cardiac transplant recipients. Am J Cardiol 80:145–149, 1997

52. Rifon J, Paramo JA, Panizo C, Montes R, Rocha E. The increase of plasminogen activator inhibitor activity is associated with graft occlusion in patients undergoing aorto-coronary bypass surgery. Br J Haematol 99:262–267, 1997

53. Zoller B, Garcia de Frutos P, Hillarp A, Dahlback B: Thrombophilia as a multigenic disease. Haematologica 84:59–70, 1999.

54. Dahlback B: The protein C anticoagulant system: inherited defects as basis for venous thrombosis. Thromb Res 77:1–43, 1995

55. Dahlback B: Resistance to activated protein C caused by the factor VR506Q mutation is a common risk factor for venous thrombosis. Thromb Haemost 78:483–488, 1997

56. Dahlback B: Procoagulant and anticoagulant properties of coagulation factor V: Factor V Leiden (APC resistance) causes hypercoagulability by dual mechanisms. J Lab Clin Med 133:415–422, 1999

57. Varadi K, Rosing J, Tans G, Pabinger I, Keil B, Schwarz HP: Factor V enhances the cofactor function of protein S in the APC-mediated inactivation of factor VIII: Influence of the factor VR506Q mutation. Thromb Haemost 76:208–214, 1996

58. Bajzar L, Kalafatis M, Simioni P, Tracy PB: An antifibrinolytic mechanism describing the prothrombotic effect associated with factor V Leiden. J Biol Chem 271:22949–22952, 1996

59. Kardia SL, Haviland MB, Ferrell RE, Sing CF: The relationship between risk factor levels and presence of coronary artery calcification is dependent on apolipoprotein E genotype. Arterioscler Thromb Vasc Biol 19:427–435, 1999

60. Moatti D, Seknadji P, Galand C, Poirier O, Fumeron F, Desprez S, Garbarz M, Dhermy D, Arveiler D, Evans A, Luc G, Ruidavets JB, Ollivier V, Hakim J, Aumont MC, de Prost D: Polymorphisms of the tissue factor pathway inhibitor (TFPI) gene in patients with acute coronary syndromes and in healthy subjects : Impact of the V264M substitution on plasma levels of TFPI. Arterioscler Thromb Vasc Biol 19:862–869, 1999

61. Falciani M, Gori AM, Fedi S, Chiarugi L, Simonetti I, Dabizzi RP, Prisco D, Pepe G, Abbate R, Gensini GF, Neri Serneri GG: Elevated tissue factor and tissue factor pathway inhibitor circulating levels in ischaemic heart disease patients. Thromb Haemost 79:495–499, 1998

62. Broze GJ Jr: Tissue factor pathway inhibitor and the revised theory of coagulation. Annu Rev Med 46:103–112, 1995.

63. Broze GJ Jr: Tissue factor pathway inhibitor. Thromb Haemost 74:90–93, 1995

64. Ridker PM, Stampfer MJ: Assessment of genetic markers for coronary thrombosis: Promise and precaution. Lancet 353:687–688, 1999

65. Ridker P, Hennekens C, Schmitz C, Stampfer M, Lindpaintner K; PL[A1/A2] polymorphism of platelet gylcoprotein IIIa and risks of myocardial infarction, stroke, and venous thromboembolism. Lancet 349:385–388, 1997

66. Herrmann S, Poirier O, Marques-Vidal P, Evans A, Arveiler D, Luc G, Emmerich J, Cambien F: The Leu[33]/Pro polymorphism (P1A1/A2) of the glycoprotein IIIa (GP IIIa) receptor is not related to myocardial function in the ECTIM Study. Thromb Haemost 77:1170–1181, 1997

67. Poort SR, Rosendaal FR, Reitsma PH, Bertina RM: A common genetic variation in the 3'-untranslated region of the prothrombin gene is associated with elevated plasma prothrombin levels and an increase in venous thrombosis. Blood 88:3698–3703, 1996

68. Hillarp A, Zoller B, Svensson PJ, Dahlback B: The 20210 A allele of the prothrombin gene is a common risk factor among Swedish outpatients with verified deep venous thrombosis. Thromb Haemost 78:990–992, 1997

69. Bron K, Luddington R, Williamson D, Baker P, Baglin T: Risk of venous thromboembolism associated with a G to A transition at position 20210 in the 3'-untranslated region of the prothrombin gene. Br J Haematol 98:907–909, 1997

70. Rosendaal FR, Doggen CJ, Zivelin A, Arruda VR, Aiach M, Siscovick DS, Hillarp A, Watzke HH, Bernardi F, Cumming AM, Preston FE, Reitsma PH: Geographic distribution of the 20210 G to A prothrombin variant. Thromb Haemost 79:706–708, 1998

71. Watzke HH, Schuttrumpf J, Graf S, Huber K, Panzer S: Increased prevalence of a polymorphism in the gene coding for human prothrombin in patients with coronary heart disease. Thromb Res 87:521–526, 1997

72. Arruda VR, Siquiera LH, Chiaparini LC, Coelho OR, Mansur AP, Ramires A, Annichino-Bizzacchi JM: Prevalence of the prothrombin gene variant 20210 G→ A among patients with myocardial infarction. Cardiovasc Res 37:42–45, 1998

73. Doggen CJ, Cats VM, Bertina RM, Rosendaal FR: Interaction of coagulation of defects and cardiovascular risk factors: Increased risk of myocardial infarction associated with factor V Leiden or prothrombin 20210A. Circulation 97:1037–1041, 1998

74. De Stefano V, Chiusolo P, Paciaroni K, Casorelli I, Rossi E. Molinari M, Servidei S, Tonali PA, Leone G: Prothrombin G20210A mutant genotype is a risk factor for cerebrovascular ischemic disease in young patients. Blood 91:3562–3565, 1998

75. Zoldhelyi P, McNatt J, Xu XM, Loose-Mitchell D, Meidell RS, Clubb FJ Jr, Buja LM, Willerson JT, Wu KK: Prevention of arterial thrombosis by adenovirus-mediated transfer of cycloxygenase gene. Circulation 93:10–17, 1996

76. Yan ZQ, Yokota T, Zhang W, Hansson GK: Expression of inducible nitric oxide synthase inhibits platelet adhesion and restores blood flow in the injured artery. Circ Res 79:38–44, 1996

77. Champion HC, Bivalacqua TJ, D'Souza FM, Ortiz LA, Jeter JR, Toyoda K, Heistad DD, Hyman AL, Kadowitz PJ: Gene transfer of endothelial nitric oxide synthase to the lung of the mouse in vivo: Effect on agonist-induced and flow-mediated vascular responses. Circ Res 84:1422–1432, 1999

78. Qian H, Neplioueva V, Shetty GA, Channon KM, George SE: Nitric oxide synthase gene therapy rapidly reduces adhesion molecule expression and inflammatory cell infiltration in carotid arteries of cholestrol-fed rabbits. Circulation 99:2979–2982, 1999

79. Rade JJ, Schulick AH, Virmani R, Dichek DA: Local adenoviral-mediated expressio of recombinant hirudin reduces neointima formation after arterial injury. Nat Med 2:293–298, 1996

80. Dichek DA, Anderson J, Kelly AB, Hanson SR, Harker LA: Enhanced in vivo antithrombotic effects of endothelial cells expressing recombinant plasminogen activators transduced with retroviral vectors. Circulation 93:301–309, 1996

81. Dietrich W, Barankay A, Hahnel C, Richter JA: High-dose aprotinin in cardiac surgery: Three years' experience in 1,784 patients. J Cardiothorac Vasc Anesth 6:324–327, 1992

82. Wachtfogel Y, Kucich U, Hack C, Gluszko P, Niewiarowski S, Colman R, Edmonds LJ: Aprotinin inhibits the contact, neutrophil, and platelet activation systems during simulated extracorporeal perfusion. J Thorac Cardiovasc Surg 106:1–9, 1993

83. Wan S, LeClerc JL, Vincent JL: Inflammatory response to cardiopulmonary bypass: Mechanisms involved and possible therapeutic strategies. Chest 112:676–692, 1997

84. Gott JP, Cooper WA, Schmidt FE Jr, Brown WM III, Wright CE, Merlino JD, Fortenberry JD, Clark WS, Guyton RA: Modifying risk for extracorporeal circulation: Trial of four antiinflammatory strategies. Ann Thorac Surg 66:747–753; discussion 753–744, 1998.

85. Hsu LC: Biocompatibility in cardiopulmonary bypass. J Cardiothorac Vasc Anesth 11:376–382, 1997

86. Redmond JM, Gillinov AM, Stuart RS, Zehr KJ, Winkelstein JA, Herskowitz A, Cameron DE, Baumgartner WA: Heparin-coated bypass circuits reduce pulmonary injury. Ann Thorac Surg 56: 474–478; discussion 479, 1993

87. Bagge L, Thelin S, Hutlman J, Nilsson L, Thorelius J, Hillstrom PA: Heparin-coated CPB-sets increase biocompatibility and reduce endothelial cell damage in pigs. J Cardiothorac Anesth 3:84, 1989.

88. Royston D: The inflammatory response and extracorporeal circulation. J Cardiothorac Vasc Anesth 11:341–354, 1997

89. Rinder C, Fitch J: Amplification of the inflammatory response: Adhesion molecules associated with platelet/white cell responses. J Cardiovasc Pharmacol 27 Suppl 1:S6–S12, 1996

90. Korthius RJ, Anderson DC, Granger DN: Role of neutrophil-endothelial cell adhesion in inflammatory disorders. J Crit Care 9:47–71, 1994

91. Wilson IC, Gardner TJ, DiNatale JM, Gillinov AM, Curtis WE,

Cameron DE: Temporary leukocyte depletion reduces ventricular dysfunction during prolonged postischemic reperfusion. J Thorac Cardiovasc Surg 106:805–810, 1993

92. Litt MR, Jeremy RW, Weisman HF, Winkelstein JA, Becker LC: Neutrophil depletion limited to reperfusion reduces myocardial infarct size after 90 minutes of ischemia: Evidence for neutrophil-mediated reperfusion injury. Circulation 809:1816–1827, 1989

93. Westlin W, Mullane KM: Alleviation of myocardial stunning by leukocyte and platelet depletion. Circulation 80:1828–1836, 1989

94. Breda MA, Drinkwater DC, Laks H, Bhuta S, Corno AF, Davtyan HG, Chang P: Prevention of reperfusion injury in the neonatal heart with leukocyte-depleted blood. J Thorac Cardiovasc Surg 97:654–665, 1989

95. Hachida M, Hanayama N, Okamura T, Akasawa T, Maeda T, Bonkohara Y, Endo M, Hashimoto A, Koyanagi H: The role of leukocyte depletion in reducing injury to myocardium and lung during cardiopulmonary bypass. Asaio J 41:M291–294, 1995

96. Chiba Y, Morioka K, Muraoka R, Ihaya A, Kimura T, Uesaka T, Tsuda T, Matsuyama K: Effects of depletion of leukocytes and platelets on cardiac dysfunction after cardiopulmonary bypass. Ann Thorac Surg 65:107–113; 1998

97. Englander R, Carderelli MG: Efficacy of leukocyte filters in the by-pass circuit for infants undergoing cardiac operations. Ann Thorac Surg 60:S533–S535, 1995

98. Ramamoorthy C, Lynn AM: Con: The use of modified ultrafiltration during pediatric cardiovascular surgery is not a benefit. J Cardiothorac Vasc Anesth 12:483–485, 1998

99. Poston RS, Ennen M, Pollard J, Hoyt EG, Billingham ME, Robbins RC: Ex vivo gene therapy prevents chronic graft vascular disease in cardiac allografts. J Thorac Cardiovasc Surg 116:386–396, 1998

100. Gunn J, Holt CM, Francis SE, Shepherd L, Grohmann M, Newman CM, Crossman DC, Cumberland DC: The effect of oligonucleotides to c-myb on vascular smooth muscle cell proliferation of neointima formation after porcine coronary angioplasty. Circ Res 80:520–531, 1997

101. Isobe M, Suzuki J, Morishita R, Kaneda Y, Sawa Y, Matsuda H, Ogihara T, Horie S, Okubo Y, Amano J: Downregulation of endothelin expression in allograft coronary arteries after gene therapy targeting Cdk2 kinase. Transplant Proc 30:1007–1008, 1998

102. Vassalli G, Dichek DA: Gene therapy for arterial thrombosis. Cardiovasc Res 35:459–469, 1997

103. Fox J, Swain J: Gene Therapy for Cardiovascular Disease. In: Heart Disease: A Textbook of Cardiovascular Medicine. Philadelphia: Saunders, 1996: 663–678

104. Svensson EC, Schwartz LB: Gene therapy for vascular disease. Curr Opin Cardiol 13:369–374, 1998

105. Losordo DW, Vale PR, Symes JF, Dunnington CH, Esakof DD, Maysky M, Ashare AB, Lathi K, Isner JM: Gene therapy for myocardial angiogenesis: Initial clinical results with direct myocardial injection of phVEGF165 as sole therapy for myocardial ischemia. Circulation 98:2800–2804, 1998

106. Baumgartner I, Pieczek A, Manor O, Blair R, Kearney M, Walsh K, Isner JM: Constitutive expression of phVEGF165 after intramuscular gene transfer promotes collateral vessel development in patients with critical limb ischemia. Circulation 97:1114–1123, 1998

107. Isner JM, Baumgartner I, Rauh G, Schainfeld R, Blair R, Manor O, Razvi S, Symes JF: Treatment of thromboangiitis obliterans (Buerger's disease) by intramuscular gene transfer of vascular endothelial growth factor: Preliminary clinical results. J Vasc Surg 28:964–973; 1998

108. Henry T, Annex B, Arzin M, McKendall G, Willerson J, Hendel R, Giordano F, Klein R, Gibson C, Berman D, Luce C, McCluskey E: Double Blind, Placebo Controlled Trial of Recombinant Human Vascular Endothelial Growth Factor. The VIVA Trial American College of Cardiology, New Orleans, 1999

109. Rosengart TK, Lee LY, Patel SR, Sanborn TA, Parikh M, Bergman GW, Hachamovitch R, Szulc M, Kligfield PD, Okin PM, Hahn RT, Devereux RB, Post MR, Hackett NR, Foster T, Grasso TM, Lesser ML, Isom OW, Crystal RG: Angiogenesis gene therapy: Phase I assessment of direct intramyocardial administration of an adenovirus vector expressing VEGF121 cDNA to individuals with clinically significant severe coronary artery disease. Circulation 100: 468–474, 1999

110. Inbal A, Freimark D, Modan B, Chetrit A, Matetzky S, Rosenberg N, Dardik R, Baron Z, Seligsohn U: Synergistic effects of prothrombotic polymorphisms and atherogenic factors on the risk of myocardial infarction in young males. Blood 93:2186–2190, 1999

111. Da Lio AL, Jones NF: New concepts and materials in microvascular grafting: Prosthetic graft endothelial cell seeding and gene therapy. Microsurgery 18:263–266, 1998

112. Seligsohn U, Zivelin A: Thrombophilia as a multigenic disorder. Thromb Haemost 78:297–301, 1997

113. Ernst E: Fibrinogen: An important risk factor for atherothrombotic diseases. Ann Med 26:15–22, 1994

114. Carter AM, Mansfield MW, Stickland MH, Grant PJ: Beta-fibrinogen gene-455 G/A polymorphism and fibrinogen levels: Risk factors for coronary artery disease in subjects with NIDDM. Diabetes Care 19:1265–1268, 1996

115. Colucci M, Scopece S, Gelato AV, Dimonte D, Semeraro N: In vitro clot lysis as a potential indicator of thrombus resistance to fibrinolysis: Study in healthy subjects and correlation with blood fibrinolytic parameters. Thromb Haemost 77:725–729, 1997

116. Green F, Humphries S: Genetic determinants of arterial thrombosis. Baillieres Clin Haematol 7:675–692, 1994

117. Neufeld EJ: Update on genetic risk factors for thrombosis and atherosclerotic vascular disease. Hematol Oncol Clin North Am 12:1193–1209, 1998

118. Redondo M, Watzke HH, Stucki B, Sulzer I, Biasiutti FD, Binder BR, Furlan M, Lammle B, Wuillemin Wa: Coagulation factors II, V, VII, and X, prothrombin gene 20210G—>A transition, and factor V Leiden in coronary artery disease: High factor V clotting activity is an independent risk factor for myocardial infarction. Arterioscler Thromb Vasc Biol 19:1020–1025, 1999

119. Holm J, Hillarp A, Zøller B, Erhardt L, Berntorp E, Dahlback B: Factor V Q506 (resistance to activated protein C) and prognosis after acute coronary syndrome. Thromb Haemost 81:857–860, 1999

120. Meade TW, Ruddock V, Stirling Y, Chakrabarti R, Miller GJ: Fibrinolytic activity, clotting factors, and long-term incidence of ischaemic heart disease in the Northwick Park Heart Study. Lancet 342:1076–1079, 1993

121. Kohler H, Stickland M, Ossei-Gerning N, Carter A, Mikkola H, Grant P: Association of a common polymorphism in the factor XIII gene with myocardial infarction. Thromb Haemost 79:8–13, 1998

122. Iacoviello L, Burzotta F, Di Castelnuovo A, Zito F, Marchioli R, Donati MB: The 4G/5G polymorphism of PAI-1 promoter gene and the risk of myocardial infarction: A meta-analysis. Thromb Haemost 80:1029–1030, 1998

123. Ardissino D, Mannucci PM, Merlini PA, Duca F, Fetiveau R, Tagliabue L, Tubaro M, Galvani M, Ottani F, Ferrario M, Corral J, Margaglione M: Prothrombotic genetic risk factors in young survivors of myocardial infarction. Blood 94:46–51, 1999

124. Eriksson P, Kallin B, van 't Hooft FM, Bavenholm P, Hamsten A: Allele-specific increase in basal transcription of the plasminogen-activator inhibitor 1 gene is associated with myocardial infarction. Proc Natl Acad Sci USA 92:1851–1855, 1995

Index

Activated clotting time, 7
Activated partial thromboplastin
  time, 7, 153
Adenosine, antiinflammatory prop-
  erties of, 46
Adenosine diphosphate (ADP), 47,
  137
  as platelet agonist, 112, 140
Adhesion molecules, 25, 32, 45
  and clinical outcome, 194–195
ADP. *See* Adenosine diphosphate
ADP ribosyltransferase, 39
ADPase, 47, 114
Adventitia, of arterial wall, 31
Aging, effects on endothelial func-
  tion, 43
Alcohol, effects on endothelial func-
  tion, 42
ε-Aminocaproic acid, 158–159
Amoebocyte, 5
Anandamide, 40
Androgens, effects on endothelial
  function, 42
Angiogenesis, 48
Angiogenin, 48
Angiotensin I, 41
Angiotensin II, 33, 40–41
  receptors, 41
Angiotensin-converting enzyme, 41
Angiotensin-converting enzyme in-
  hibitors, 41, 44
  effects on endothelial function, 42
Angiotensinogen, 41
Anticoagulants, endogenous,
  114–115
Antioxidants, effects on endothelial
  function, 42
$α_2$-Antiplasmin ($α_2$-PI), 114, 136–137,
  142, 148f, 151
  activity during cardiopulmonary
    bypass, 157
  deficiency of, 157

plasmin reaction with, 152
Antiplatelet activity, in arterial circulation, 114
Antithrombin, activity in venous circulation, 114–115
Antithrombin III (ATIII), 47, 136–137
  anticoagulant activity of, 131–132
  deficiency, 198, 199t
    acquired, 172, 175
    congenital, 172
  and disseminated intravascular
    coagulation, 94–95
  exogenous, 175–176
    in L-asparaginase therapy, 174
    in cardiopulmonary bypass,
      174–176
    in septic shock, 173–174
  functions of, 171
  in gestational hypertension, 173
  half-life of, 172
  heparin binding to, 170
  inhibition, by plasma elastase, 175
  interaction with heparan, 171
  levels, heparin and, 175–176
  in preeclampsia, 173
  production of, 172
  properties of, 171
Apolipoprotein E, 200
Apoptosis, 49–50
  endothelial, 82, 86–87
  nitric oxide-induced, 50
Apoptosis protein-1, 50
Aprotinin, 13
  therapy with, 156–157, 160–161, 191
Arachidonic acid, 112
  metabolism of, 34
  metabolites, 40
  production of, 33–34
Arginine
  analogues, as competitive antago-
    nists of NOS, 37
  effects on endothelial function, 42

Arginine-glycine-aspartate (RGD), 112, 138
L-Asparaginase therapy, coagulopathy with, 174
Aspirin, 112
  effects on endothelial function, 42
Atherosclerosis, 49
  effects on endothelial function, 43
ATIII. *See* Antithrombin III

Basophils, in inflammatory response, 95–96
Bleeding disorders, 157. *See also* Coagulation; Coagulopathy
Bleeding, post cardiopulmonary bypass, 79
Blood loss, aprotinin and, 161
Bradykinin, 36, 149
  during cardiopulmonary bypass, 154, 154*f*

Calcium
  in coagulation pathways, 137, 140–141
  as cofactor for NOS, 23
  depletion, by heparin administration, 176
Calcium antagonists, effects on endothelial function, 42
Calmodulin, as cofactor for NOS, 23
Calveolin, 36
Cancer chemotherapy, coagulopathy in, 174
Capillaries
  fenestrated (visceral type), 32
  muscle-type, 33
Cardiac failure, peripheral resistance with, 44
Cardiac surgery, adverse outcomes of, variability in, 191–192
Cardiomyopathy, diabetic, 183
Cardiopulmonary bypass
  adverse outcomes of, variability in, 191–192
  antithrombin III repletion in, 174–176
  complement activation in, 18–19
  fibrinolytic response to, 152*f*, 152–156, 154*f*, 161, 176
    clinical correlations with, 157–158
    variation in, 156–157, 175–176
  heparin in, 170

inflammatory response to, 9–10
  initial anticoagulant effect of, 82–83, 161
  procoagulant initiation during, 136, 161
  and systemic inflammatory response syndrome, comparison of, 95
Caspase, 49
Caveolae, 36
CD39, 132
Ceramid, 36
cGMP
  in apoptosis and/or necrosis, 49–50
  physiological functions of, 38–39
  production of, 38
cGMP protein kinase, 45
cGMP-binding phosphodiesterase, 39
cGMP-dependent protein kinases, 38
Chymotrypsin, 9
C1-inhibitor, 136, 151
  deficiency of, 155
Cirrhosis, and tPA clearance, 157–158
Clot retraction, 114
Clotting time, activated, assay, 153
Coagulation, 191
  abnormalities in, perioperative, 79
  activation of, 80–81, 133–135, 134*f*–135*f*
    cardiopulmonary bypass and, 80–81
  and clinical outcomes, 192–193
  contact factor (intrinsic) pathway, 7, 11, 11*f*, 80, 133
    activation of, 134*f*, 135
  cytokines and, 193–194
  evolutionary development of, 7–13
  final common pathway of, 133, 134*f*–135*f*
  pathways of, 7
    cofactors in, 133, 134*f*–135*f*
    interactions of, 133
    modulators of, 136–137
  platelets in, 139–141
  in pregnancy, 172–173
  tissue factor (extrinsic) pathway, 7, 11, 11*f*, 46, 80, 133
    activation of, 133–135, 134*f*
    physiological function of TFPI in regulating, 82

Coagulation proteins (factors),
    24–25, 133–137. *See also spe-
    cific factor*
  evolutionary diversification of, 8
  in inflammatory response, 3
  platelets and, 141–142
  vitamin K-dependent, 9
  vitamin K-nondependent, 9
Coagulin gel formation, 6
Coagulogen, 5–6
  conversion to gel, 6
Coagulopathy
  of cardiopulmonary bypass, 180
  perioperative, 79
Coelomocyte, 5
Collagen
  and platelet adhesion, 110–111, 133
  as platelet agonist, 140
Complement C5b-9, 141, 155m 182.
    See also Membrane attack
    complex (MAC)
Complement factor C1, 12
Complement system
  activation of, 135
    in cardiopulmonary bypass, 18,
    155
  and clinical outcome, 194
  related to membrane attack
    complex, 19
  C4 gene, 194
  during cardiopulmonary bypass,
    18, 154*f*, 155
  heparin-coated bypass circuits
    and, 159–160
  C3/C4/C5 components
    and α₂-macroglobulin, 16, 17*f*
    phylogeny of, 16, 17*f*
  components, 15
    deficiency of, 18
  and cytolytic system, 17–18
  evolutionary development of,
    15–19
  functions of, 15
Connective tissue, of arterial wall, 31
Contact activation, during car-
    diopulmonary bypass, 153
  heparin-coated bypass circuits
    and, 159–160
Contact system, 135–136
Coronary artery occlusion, gene
    therapy for, 211
Coronary vein graft occlusion, gene
    therapy for, 209–211

C-reactive protein, 17, 151
Cyclic guanosine monophosphate.
    See cGMP
Cyclooxygenase, 34, 112
Cytochrome P-450
  evolution of, 21
  membrane association of, 22
  and NOS, relationship between,
    21
  soluble, 22
Cytochrome P-450BM-3, 22
Cytokines, 13
  and clinical outcomes, 193–194
  mast cells and, 97
Cytolysin, 17

DAG. *See* Diacylglycerol
Deep venous thrombosis, 195
Dense granules, 112, 137–138
  contents of, 137
  deficiency, 112
Diabetes mellitus, 183
Diacylglycerol (DAG), metabolism
    of, 34
Disseminated intravascular coagula-
    tion, 93–95, 172–173, 177
  in end-stage hepatic failure, 174
  in septic shock, 173–174

ecNOS. *See* Nitric oxide synthase,
    endothelial
EDHF. *See* Endothelium-derived hy-
    perpolarizing factor
EDRF. *See* Endothelial-derived relax-
    ing factor
Eicosanoids
  as intracellular second messen-
    gers, 34
  in physiological responses, 34
Elastase, 9
  plasma, 175
Endothelial cell(s)
  anticoagulant and antiplatelet fac-
    tors maintained by,
    114–115
  apoptosis, 49, 86–87
  constricting factors released by,
    40–42
  dysregulation of, with cardiopul-
    monary bypass, 79–80
  ecto-ADPase, in inhibition of clot
    formation, 132, 132*f*
  EDRF/NO production by, 35–37

Endothelial cell(s)—*Continued*
  functions of, 131*f*, 131–132
    abnormalities in, 81
  properties of, 131
  prostanoid production by, 33–35
  response to injury, 81
  ultrastructure of, 32–33
Endothelial-derived relaxing factor
    (EDRF), 35
Endothelin-1 (ET-1), 41
  big, 41
Endothelin (ET), 33, 40
  effects on coagulation, 47
  isoforms, 41
Endothelin-converting enzyme, 41
Endothelium
  activation, in response to injury, 82
  and circulatory cells, 44–46
  and coagulation, 46–48
  disruption, in response to injury,
    82
  dysfunction of, 42–44
  functions of, 33, 81, 131*f*, 131–132
  injured, and coagulation distur-
    bances in heart surgery pa-
    tients, 82
  and vascular growth, 48–50
  and vascular integrity, 130–133,
    131*f*
  and vascular permeability, 50–51
Endothelium-dependent hyperpo-
    larization, 39–40
Endothelium-derived hyperpolariz-
    ing factor (EDHF), 33, 40
Endotoxemia, 173–174
Environment, and adverse car-
    diopulmonary outcomes,
    192
Epinephrine, 137, 149
  as platelet agonist, 140
Erythrocytes, and platelet respon-
    siveness, 116
Estrogens, effects
  on endothelial function, 42
  on vascular function, 42
ET. *See* Endothelin
Exercise training, effects on endothe-
    lial function, 42
Extracorporeal oxygenation, 175

Factor I, 136
Factor V, 7, 113–114, 133, 136–137,
    139–141

genetic polymorphisms of, and ar-
    terial thromboembolism,
    200–201, 201*t*
Factor VII, 7, 10–11, 46–47, 80, 113,
    135, 180
  genetic polymorphisms of, and ar-
    terial thromboembolism,
    200–201, 201*t*
Factor VIII, 7, 80, 113–114, 133,
    135–137, 140–141, 151
Factor IX, 11, 80, 113, 135, 137, 141
Factor X, 7, 10–11, 47, 80, 113–114,
    137, 141, 181
  in inflammatory response, 92–93
Factor XI, 10, 25, 135–137, 180
Factor XII, 9–10, 25, 80, 135–137, 153,
    180
  deficiency of, 9–10, 153, 180
Factor XIII, 7, 114–116, 136
  genetic polymorphisms of, and ar-
    terial thromboembolism,
    200–201, 201*t*
Factor V Leiden, 192, 198–200, 199*t*,
    200*f*
Factor V R506Q. *See* Factor V Leiden
Factor C, 25
Factor V Leiden, 156–157
Fibrin, 46, 80, 138, 140
  D-dimers, 142, 152
    aprotinin and, 161
    during cardiopulmonary by-
        pass, 153, 156
  degradation, 142, 152
    aprotinin and, 160
  deposition, 114
  formation, 108
Fibrin clot, formation of, 133
Fibrinogen, 5–6, 111–112, 132,
    137–138, 138*f*, 151
  degradation, 142
  genetic polymorphisms of,
    195–196, 196*f*
    and arterial thromboembolism,
        200–201, 201*t*
  in inflammatory response, 3
Fibrinolysis, 47, 133, 134*f*–135*f*, 135,
    142, 147–152, 148*f*
  aprotinin and, 160–161
  cardiopulmonary bypass and,
    152*f*, 152–156, 154*f*,
    175–176
  and clinical outcomes, 192–193
  genetic variability in, 195–198

regulation, hepatic clearance of tPA and, 151
Fibrinolytic assays, interpretation of, 151
Fibrinopeptide B, 6
Fibroblast growth factor, 48
Fibronectin, 132, 137
Fish oil, effects, on endothelial function, 42
Free fatty acids, regulation, heparin and, 183

Gene therapy
    for angiogenesis, 209, 210*f*
    antiinflammatory, 201, 203–208
    antithrombotic, 201
    clinical uses of, investigatory, 208–212
    inhibitory, 206–208, 207*f*–208*f*
    viral vectors for, 205*t*, 205–206
Genetics, and adverse cardiopulmonary outcomes, 192, 195–198
Glycoprotein Ia, in platelet adhesion, 137
Glycoprotein Ib, in platelet adhesion, 110–111, 132, 134*f*, 137–138, 138*f*, 139
Glycoprotein IIa
    genetic polymorphisms of, 200
    in platelet adhesion, 137
Glycoprotein IIb/IIIa (GpIIb-IIIa), 134*f*–135*f*, 138*f*, 138–141, 178
    conformation change, 111–112
Glycoprotein PF4, immunoglobulin G against, 177–178
Glycosaminoglycans, 47
G-proteins, 34, 137
Growth factors, heparin-binding, 182
Guanylate cyclases, soluble, 38–39

Hageman factor. *See* Factor XII
Hematopoietic cells
    heterotypic interactions of, 108
    homotypic interactions of, 107
Hemocyte, 5
Hemostasis, 5
    arterial, 108–109
    during cardiopulmonary bypass, 155
    cellular and humoral processes in, 130, 130*f*

and immune system, interplay between, 3
    vascular bed specificity of, 4, 47–48
    venous, 108
Heparan
    antithrombin III interaction with, 171
    versus heparin, 171
    properties of, 171
    release, heparin and, 182
Heparan sulfate, 115
Heparin
    adverse effects of, 169–170
    allergy to, 177
    and antithrombin III, 131, 175–176
    binding to antithrombin III, 170
    biochemistry of, 176–177
    calcium depletion by, 176
    in cardiopulmonary bypass, 170
    cellular effects of, 182
    exogenous, immunoglobulin response to, 177–178
    versus heparan, 171
    and heparan release, 182
    immunologically mediated reactions to, 177–178
    and lipoprotein lipase release, 183
    in mast cells, 170
    mechanism of action of, 170
    movement within body, 182–183
    and neointimal proliferation, 49
    and plasma elastase release, 175
    and platelet activation, 178–179
    reversal of, 179–180
    and tissue factor pathway inhibitor release, 180–182
    unfractionated, 170
Heparin cofactor I, 171
Heparin cofactor II, 136–137
Heparin-coated bypass circuits, 159–160
Heparin-induced thrombocytopenic (HIT) syndrome, 177–178
Heparin/protamine complex, adverse effects of, 179–180
Hepatic artery thrombosis, after liver transplantation, 174
Hereditary angioedema, 155
High molecular weight kininogen (HMWK), 7, 10, 133
    during cardiopulmonary bypass, 154, 154*f*
    deficiency of, 153

Histamine, 141
HMWK. *See* High molecular weight kininogen
Horseshoe crab *(Limulus polyphemus)*
  complement-like lytic system, 17
  cytokine-like proteins in, 13–14
  immune/hemostatic system, 2*f*, 2–3, 5
    control of, 6
    initiation of, 6
    localization of, 6
  innate immunity in, 5
Host defense system(s)
  evolution of, 1–2
  primitive, 5–7
Human umbilical vein endothelial cells (HUVEC)
  apoptotic, 86–87
  hypoxia-induced cell death in, 86
HUVEC. *See* Human umbilical vein endothelial cells
Hypercholesterolemia, effects of, on endothelial function, 43
Hyperhomocysteinuria, 198
Hypertension. *See also* Preeclampsia
  effects of, on endothelial function, 43
  endothelial dysfunction in, 44
  gestational, 173
  pulmonary, heparin/protamine complex and, 179–180

I-κ;B, 45–46
IL-1. *See* Interleukin-1
Immunity, 5
Immunoglobulin gene superfamily, 14–15, 25
Inflammatory cells, 92
Inflammatory markers, and clinical outcomes, 192–195
Inflammatory response, 5, 135, 191
  cellular and humoral processes in, 130, 130*f*
  factor Xa in, 92–93
  mast cells in, 95–99
  microvascular, sources of procoagulant activity in, 87*f*, 87–88
  procoagulant initiation during, 136
  reduction
    chemical methods of, 201–202
    genetic methods of, 203–208

    immunologic methods of, 201–202
    physical methods of, 202–203
  thrombin and, 91–92
  vascular bed or organ specificity of, 4
Injury
  complement-dependent lytic pathways in, 25
  innate response to, 24
iNOS. *See* Nitric oxide synthase, inducible
Insulin, effects on endothelial function, 42
Insulin resistance syndrome, 158
Insulin-like growth factor, 48
Integrins, 45, 137
Intercellular adhesion molecules, 14–15, 45
Interferon, 48
Interleukin(s)
  in early animals, 13–14
  evolutionary development of, 13–15
  function of, 25
  IL-1, 13–14
    and coagulation, 193–194
    horseshoe crab, 13–14
  IL-6, and coagulation, 193–194
  IL-10, and coagulation, 193–194
  in inflammation and immunity, 25
Interleukin receptors, in early animals, 14–15
Internal elastic membrane, of arterial wall, 31
Intima, of arterial wall, 31
Ischemia-reperfusion
  bradykinin/nitric oxide-mediated response to, 24
  myocardial, 19
  tissue factor in, 83–84

Kallikrein, 10, 136–137
Kallikrein/kinin system, during cardiopulmonary bypass, 153–154, 154*f*
  heparin-coated bypass circuits and, 159–160
Ketoconazole, 21
Kinin, formation, 135

Large (L) granules, 5–6
Lethal gene, 3

Leukocyte adhesion molecule deficiency syndrome, 4
Leukocyte(s), interactions with endothelial cells, 44–46
Leukocyte-platelet adhesion, 116–118
Leukocyte-platelet conjugates
   during cardiopulmonary bypass, 118–120, 119*f*
   circulating, 118–120
Leukocyte-platelet interactions, receptor-ligand pairs in, 116
Leukotrienes, 34–35
Limulus factor C, 12
Limulus lysate amoebocytic assay, 5
Limulus polyphemus. See Horseshoe crab
Lipoprotein(s), 200
   oxidized, effects on endothelial function, 43
Lipoprotein lipase, release, heparin and, 183
Lipoxygenase, 34
Liver transplantation
   complications of, 174
   and tPA clearance, 157–158
Lysophosphatidylcholine, effects on endothelial function, 43

MAC. *See* Membrane attack complex
α_2-Macroglobulin, 6, 15
Macroglobulin, and complement components C3, C4, and C5, 16
Mast cell mediators, 96–97
Mast cells, 92
   and cytokines, 97
   heparin in, 170
   in inflammatory response, 95–99
Media, of arterial wall, 31
Membrane attack complex (MAC), 15, 17–19, 140
   inhibition of, 19
Membrane attack complex, during cardiopulmonary bypass, 155
Microtubules, platelet, 137–138
Monocyte(s), and platelet adhesion, 122
Monocyte chemotactic peptide-1, 119
Myocardial depression, cytokines and, 19, 193

Myocardial infarct/infarction, 158
   adhesion molecules and, 194–195
   gene therapy for, 211
Myocardial ischemia
   adhesion molecules and, 194–195
   cytokines and, 193

Necrosis, 49–50
   nitric oxide-induced, 50
Neutrophil-activating peptide-2, 116
Nitric oxide (NO), 25, 33, 114
   activity, 19
      mechanisms of, 38–39
      regulation of, 38
   and angiogenesis, 48
   in apoptosis and/or necrosis, 49–50
   and coagulation, 47
   in gene regulation, 39
   in inhibition of clot formation, 132, 132*f*
   metabolism of, 37–38
   and myocardial depression, 19, 193
   and NF-κ;B activity, 46
   and platelet function, 45
   production of, 35
   protein/enzyme interactions of, 39
   and smooth muscle growth, 49
   and vascular permeability, 50
Nitric oxide synthase (NOS), 20, 25–26, 35
   activity, 21
   calcium/calmodulin activation of, 23
   cofactors for, 23
   endothelial (ecNOS), 35
      amino acid sequence of, 36
      characteristics of, 20, 20*t*
      gene, regulation of, 22
      myristoylation, 36
      palmitoylation, 36
      regulation of, 36–37
   evolutionary development of, 20–21
   genes, regulation of, 22–23
   genetic polymorphisms of, 200
   in humans, 22
   inducible (iNOS), 36, 193
      amino acid sequence of, 36
      characteristics of, 20, 20*t*
      gene, regulation, 22

Nitric oxide synthase—*Continued*
  and inflammatory responses, 24
  inhibition of, 37
  isoforms, 20
    genes for, 22
  isoforms of, 35
  neuronal (nNOS), 35
    amino acid sequence of, 36
    characteristics of, 20, 20*t*
    functions, 22–23
    gene, regulation of, 22
  phosphorylation by protein ki-
    nase, 23
  similarity to cytochrome P-450, 21
  synthetic activity, regulation of,
    23–24
S-Nitrosoalbumin, 38
S-Nitrosohemoglobin, 38
nNOS. *See* Nitric oxide synthase,
    neuronal
Norepinephrine, 137
NOS. *See* Nitric oxide synthase
Nuclear factor-&kgr;B, 45–46, 50

Opsonins, 15
Oxidative stress, 49–50. *See also* Re-
    active oxygen species
Oxygen-derived free radicals, 40. *See
    also* Reactive oxygen
    species

PDGF-α, receptors for, 48
Perforin, 17
Peroxynitrite, 37–38
PGI$_2$. *See* Prostacyclin
Phosphatidylserine, 139–141
Phospholamban, 39
Phospholipase A$_2$, calcium-depen-
    dent, 33
Phospholipase C (PLC), 34, 39
Phospholipid, in coagulation path-
    ways, 137
Plasmid DNA, in gene therapy, 204
Plasmin, 9, 134*f*–135*f*, 137, 147–148
  aprotinin and, 160
  during cardiopulmonary bypass,
    153, 176
  formation of, 142, 148
  generation of, 151–152
  reaction with α$_2$-antiplasmin, 152
Plasmin–α$_2$-antiplasmin (PAP) com-
    plex, 152
  aprotinin and, 160–161

during cardiopulmonary bypass,
    153, 155
Plasminogen, 25
  activation of, 147–148, 151–152
  cleavage of, 142
  conversion to plasmin, 142
  growth factors associated with, 10
Plasminogen activator inhibitor 1
    (PAI-1), 47, 148*f*, 149
  active, concentration of, versus
    tPA concentration, 149–151,
    150*f*
  activity
    during cardiopulmonary by-
      pass, 157
    and total tPA antigen, 158
  basal levels of, 149–150
  and clinical outcomes, 192–193
  deficiency of, 151, 157
  elevation of, 158
  genetic polymorphisms, 149, 197*f*,
    197–198
    and arterial thromboembolism,
      200–201, 201*t*
  production, during cardiopul-
    monary bypass, 156
  secretion
    acute-phase increases in,
      149–151
    after cardiopulmonary bypass,
      158
    circadian variation in, 149–150
    in insulin resistance syndrome,
      158
Platelet(s), 137–139
  activation, 80, 110–111, 134*f*, 137,
    138*f*, 139–140
    during cardiopulmonary by-
      pass, 117*f*, 117–118, 155,
      178–179
    effects of, 111
    heparin and, 178–179
    proinflammatory effects, 116
  adhesion, 133, 134*f*, 137–138, 138*f*,
    139
    under high shear, 109–111
  aggregation, 133, 135*f*, 137, 138*f*,
    138–139
  in arterial hemostasis, 108–110
  binding to apoptotic HUVEC,
    86–87
  and coagulation factors, 141–142
  formation of, 137

function, congenital disorders of,
111
glycoprotein receptors, 137–138,
138f. *See also* Glycoprotein
α-granules, 137–139
contents of, 115t, 115–116, 137
heterotypic interactions, 115–121
homotypic interactions, 107–109
interactions with endothelial cells,
44–46
microparticles, 139
microvesicles
production of, 139
shedding of materials from, 139
plasma half-life of, 137
procoagulant activity of, 139–141
P-selectin-positive
circulating, 117–118
effect on PMN and monocytes,
121–122
reactivity, soluble factors of, 116
shape change, 111
surface of, soluble coagulation
cascade on, 112–114
Platelet agonists, 112
released by activation, 112
Platelet count, protamine administration and, 179–180
Platelet endothelial-cell adhesion
molecules, 14–15
Platelet factor, 48
Platelet factor 4, 115–116, 137, 171
Platelet plug, 114
formation of, 111–112, 133,
137–138
Platelet receptor-ligand interactions,
in arterial hemostasis,
108–109, 109f
Platelet-activating factor, 45, 47, 122,
140
PLC. *See* Phospholipase C
Polymorphonuclear (PMN) neutrophils, 92
and platelet adhesion, 118–122
and platelet responsiveness, 116
Potassium channels, calcium-activated, 40
Preeclampsia, 172–173
disseminated intravascular coagulation in, 173
Pregnancy, hypercoagulability in,
172–173
Prekallikrein, 10

deficiency of, 153
Procoagulant initiation, 136
Prostacyclin (PGI$_2$), 33, 114, 132
antiinflammatory properties of, 46
and vascular permeability, 50
Prostaglandins
effects on endothelial function, 43
PGE$_2$, 34
PGF$_{2\alpha}$, 34
PGG$_2$, 34
PGH$_2$, 34, 40
PGI$_2$. *See* Prostacyclin
Protamine
adverse effects of, 179–180
for heparin reversal, 179–180
Protein binding
high-avidity, 16
low-affinity, 16
tight, 16
Protein C, 12, 25, 47, 115, 132,
136–137, 140–141, 157, 171
deficiency, 198–200, 199t, 200f
Protein S, 47, 132, 137, 141, 171
deficiency, 198–200, 199t, 200f
Prothrombin, 46, 141
genetic polymorphisms, and arter-
ial thromboembolism,
200–201, 201t
Prothrombin time, 7
Prothrombinase complex, 11, 46,
113, 141–142
P-selectin, 116–118
immobilized, leukocyte binding
to, 121–122
and platelet adhesion, 118–120
P-selectin glycoprotein ligand-1
(PSGL-1), 118
Pseudopodia, 138
PSGL-1. *See* P-selectin glycoprotein
ligand-1
Pulmonary embolism, 195
Pulmonary hypertension,
heparin/protamine com-
plex and, 179–180
Purines, 33

RANTES, 119
Reactive oxygen species, 33
effects on endothelial function, 43
induction of cell death, 49
Red wine, effects on endothelial
function, 42
Reductive stress, 49

Repair process, evolutionary development of, 13–15

Selectins, 45. *See also* P-selectin
Sepsis syndrome, complement activation in, 18
Septic shock, 173–174
  nitric oxide production in, 19
Serine protease(s), 133, 149
  phylogenetic tree of, 8*f*
Serine protease inhibitors (serpins), 5–6, 136–137
Serotonin, 112, 137
  and clinical outcome, 194
Serpins, 136–137
Shear stress
  in arterial circulation, 110
  in venous circulation, 110
SIRS. *See* Systemic inflammatory response syndrome
Small (S) granules, 5–6
Smooth muscle
  of arterial wall, 31
  cell proliferation, angiotensin II-dependent, 41
  endothelium-dependent hyperpolarization of, 39–40
  relaxation of, 40
  vascular
    cell death, 49
    mitogenesis, 49
    proliferation, 49
Superoxide, 37–38
Superoxide dismutase, 38
Systemic inflammatory response syndrome (SIRS), 3, 12, 14, 23, 95

Tachyplesin, 6
Tenase complex, 141–142
Tetrahydrobiopterin, as cofactor for NOS, 23
TF. *See* Tissue factor
TFPI. *See* Tissue factor pathway inhibitor
TGF. *See* Transforming growth factor
Thioester bond, 16
Thiopentone, 21
Thrombin, 25, 46–47, 80, 140–141, 149
  activity, 12
    during cardiopulmonary bypass, 155
  as anticoagulant, 12
  formation of, 11, 11*f*
  functions of, 136
  generation, 108, 113–114
    after cardiopulmonary bypass, 80
    during cardiopulmonary bypass, 155
      aprotinin and, 160
      heparin-coated bypass circuits and, 159–160
  and inflammatory response, 91–92
  inhibition, 131–132
    during cardiopulmonary bypass, 155
  production of, 180
Thrombin-antithrombin complexes, in preeclampsia, 173
Thrombin/antithrombin (TAT) levels, during cardiopulmonary bypass, 155
Thrombocytopenia. *See* Heparin-induced thrombocytopenic (HIT) syndrome
Thromboembolism
  arterial, genetic factors in, 200–201, 201*t*
  genetic factors in, 198
  venous, genetic factors in, 198–200, 199*t*, 200*f*
Thromboglobulin, 137
Thrombomodulin, 47, 81–82, 115, 132, 136
Thromboplastin. *See* Tissue factor
Thrombosis, 133, 134*f*–135*f*
  genetic variability in, 195, 198–201
  hepatic artery, after liver transplantation, 174
  pathophysiology of, 158
  post cardiopulmonary bypass, 79
Thrombospondin, 48
Thromboxane, 137
Thromboxane A_2, 33, 40, 112
Thromboxane B_2, 112
Thrombus, formation of, 139, 147
Tissue factor (TF), 7, 80, 113, 133, 180–182
  absence of gene for, lethality of, 3
  in coagulation cascade, 10–11
  expression, during cardiopulmonary bypass, 83–85, 85*f*
  synthesis of, 12, 46–47

Tissue factor pathway inhibitor
(TFPI), 47, 82–83
  absence of gene for, lethality of, 3
  clearance of, 181
  functions of, 180
  genetic polymorphisms of, 3, 200
  release, heparin and, 180–182
Tissue plasminogen activator (tPA),
7, 32, 47, 136, 142, 147–148,
148*f*, 171
  active
    in blood, assay, 151
    during cardiopulmonary by-
      pass, 153
  during cardiopulmonary bypass,
      155–156, 176
    aprotinin and, 160
    heparin-coated bypass circuits
      and, 159–160
  and clinical outcomes, 192–193
  genetic variability in, 196–197
  half-life of, 151
  hepatic clearance of, 157–158
    and fibrinolysis, 151
  regulation of, 152
  release
    during cardiopulmonary by-
      pass, 153, 176
    heparin and, 176
  total antigen
    assay, 151
    and PAI-1 activity, 158
TNF. *See* Tumor necrosis factor
tPA. *See* Tissue plasminogen activator
Tranexamic acid, 158–159
Transforming growth factor-α, 48
Transforming growth factor-β, 48,
116
Transforming growth factor (TGF),
effect on smooth muscle
growth, 49
Trypsin, 9
Tumor necrosis factor (TNF), 25
  horseshoe crab, 14
Tumor necrosis factor-α (TNF-α), 43,
48, 119
  and coagulation, 193–194
Tunica adventitia, 32

Tunica intima, 31
Tunica media, 31–32
Type III protamine reaction, 179

Urokinase-type plasminogen activator (uPA), 136, 142, 148
  activation, heparin and, 176
  during cardiopulmonary bypass,
      154*f*, 154–155, 176
  release, heparin and, 176

Vascular cell adhesion molecules, 45
Vascular cells, ex vivo modification
      and reimplantation of, 211
Vascular endothelial growth factor
      (VEGF), 48–49
  gene therapy with, 209, 210*f*
Vascular permeability factor, 48
Vascular smooth muscle cells, gene
      therapy and, 209–211
Vascular wall, anatomy of, 31–32
Vasoconstriction
  angiotensin-dependent, 41
  serotonin-induced, 112
  thromboxane A_2-induced, 112
Vasodilatation, nitric oxide-depen-
      dent, 19
VEGF. *See* Vascular endothelial
      growth factor
Viral vectors, for gene therapy, 205*t*,
      205–206
Vitamin C, effects on endothelial
      function, 42
Vitamin E, effects on endothelial
      function, 42
Vitronectin, 137, 182
von Willebrand factor (vWF), 32,
      47–48, 111–112, 132–133,
      134*f*, 135, 137–138, 138*f*, 139
  in platelet adhesion, 110–111
  polymerization, 139
  subendothelial, platelet attach-
      ment to, 108–109, 109*f*
vWF. *See* von Willebrand factor

Weibel-Palade bodies, 32, 139
White clot syndrome, 177

Zymogens, 133